Neurosecretion and Neuroendocrine Activity (Ed.by BARGMANN et al.)

Contribution: POLENOV, Evolutionary Basis of the General Principle of Neuroendocrine Regulation. Interaction of Peptide and Monoamine Neurohormones in a Dual Control Mechanism

Addendum

Figure legends have had to be included separately, due to postal difficulties with the U.S.S.R. during production.

Fig. 1a-f. Different NSC types (genealogical lines) and their interrelations with the 3rd ventricle or its recesses (*1*) and distribution of the synaptic apparatus of NSC. Note bipolar ependymal (a-c), multipolar neuronal (e, f) type NSC and transitional (d) form of NSC, and ciliary receptor apparatus (*2*) on terminal parts of dendrites making contact with CSF and on surface of NSC perikarya (p. 16)

Fig. 2. Structure of brain of *Amphioxus* larva (according to BOEKE, 1908). *1* eye, *2* infundibular organ, *3* ventricle of brain, *4* medullary canal, *5* neuropore (p. 16)

Fig. 3a-f. Various interrelations between axonal terminals and dendrites of peptidergic (*dark*) and monoaminergic (*stippled*) NSC and capillaries, glandular cells and 3rd ventricle. (a) In median eminence neurosecretory axonal contacts (*1*) with capillaries (*2*) that continue into portal vein (*3*) from which capillaries of AP originate (*4*); (b) axo-adenar indirect simple (*1*) and direct synaptoid (*2*) contacts in proadenohypophysis and mesoadenohypophysis of Teleostei; (c) simple axo-adenar contacts with connective tissue layer (*1*) and basement membrane (*2*) and synaptoid contacts (*3*) in IL; (d) in PP axo-vasal contact (*1*) with capillary (*2*) of general circulation (*3*) entered also by capillaries from adrenal medulla (*4*); (e) dendro-ventricular contacts (*1*); (f) axo-ventricular contacts (*1*). Arrows indicate pathways of neurohormones: *black*: peptide, *stippled*: monoamine, *double*: both neurohormones (p. 17)

Fig. 4. Two tentative stages of evolution of hypothalamo-hypophysial neurosecretory complex (b, c), NSC and their synaptic apparatus, and *Amphioxus* infundibular organ (a). Note peptidergic "Gomori-positive" (*1*), "Gomori-negative" (*2*), monoaminergic (*3*), ependymal type NSC and peptidergic "Gomori-positive" (*4*), "Gomori-negative" (*5*), and monoaminergic neuronal type NSC, axo-vasal contact terminals of NSC with capillaries of ventral meninx (*7*), with surface of primitive median eminence (*8*) and inside of it (*9*), with capillaries localized on the border of IL and PP (*10*) and inside of the latter (*11*); simple indirect axo-adenar contacts with cells of IL separated by connective tissue septum (*12*) and one basement membrane (*13*), direct axo-adenar synaptoid contacts (*14*); dendro-ventricular (*15*) and axo-ventricular (*16*) contacts with cavity of 3rd ventricle and its recesses; capillaries draining neurosecretory centers (*17*); residual cavity of hypophysis (*18*), AP (*19*); double arrows (*20*) show means of communication (dual control) by peptide and monoamine neurohormones on AP via portal blood flow (p. 18)

Fig. 5. General principle of dual neuroendocrine control of visceral organ functions and possible ways of neuroconductive regulation of functions of neurosecretory and chromaffin cells (neuro-endocrine reflex arc). *(1)* peptidergic "Gomori-

Springer-Verlag Berlin Heidelberg New York 1978

positive" NSC, *(2)* peptidergic "Gomori-negative" NSC, *(3)* monoaminergic NSC, *(4)* median eminence with fiber terminals of "Gomori-positive" and "Gomori-negative" peptidergic and monoaminergic NSC; *(5)* PP with terminals of peptidergic "Gomori-positive" fiber, *(6)* terminals of peptidergic and adrenergic fibers in IL and *(7)* in tuberal part of AP, *(8)* main part of AP, *(9)* double arrow showing influence of peptide adenohypophysiotropic neurohormones and monoamines on AP via portal bloodstream. *(10)* optic chiasm, *(11)* exteroceptor (retina), *(12)* afferent pathway from retina, *(13)* interneuron of optic pathway in corpora quadrigemina, *(14)* pathway from optic center to monoaminergic centers of brain stem, *(15)* monoaminergic neurons of brain stem, *(16)* adrenergic pathways to hypothalamic NSC of various types, *(17)* monoaminergic pathways to interneurons of hypothalamus, *(18)* neurons of medial hypothalamus (for example, dorsomedial nucleus), *(19)* neuron of anterior hypothalamus (for instance, suprachiasmatic nucleus), *(20)* pathways to various types of NSC and hypothalamic neurons from suprahypothalamic areas of brain (for instance from limbic system). *(21)* neuron of brain stem projecting to vegetative centers of spinal cord, *(22)* vegetative preganglionic neuron of spinal cord, *(23)* vegetative postganglionic neuron that innervates adrenal medulla, *(24)* chromaffin cell, *(25)* interoceptor, *(26)* afferent neuron of spinal ganglion, *(27)* interneuron of afferent pathway from spinal cord, *(28)* pathway of viscerotropic neurohormones from PP via general circulation - paraadenohypophysial pathway of peptide neurohormones (black arrow), *(29)* influence of tropic hormones of AP (light arrow) on: *(30)* thyroid gland (TH), *(31)* adrenal cortex (ACTH), *(32)* Langerhans islets (STH), *(33)* ovary (FSH, LH, LTH), *(34)* entry of catecholamines of suprarenal gland into general circulation (stippled arrow); *(35)* main vessel of general circulation, *(36)* influence of viscerotropic peptide and catecholamine neurohormones on visceral organs (double arrow), *(37)* blood vessel, *(38)* kidney (for example, effect of ADH), *(39)* uterus, and *(40)* different peripheral endocrine glands: *solid lines* indicate well known interneuronal pathways, *cross hatched*: hypothetical pathways, small arrows show direction of nerve impulse (p. 21)

Fig. 6. Evolution of neuroendocrine reflex and general principle of neuroendocrine regulation (modified diagram of E. and B.SCHARRER, 1963). Receptor-secretory cell *(1)*, receptor cell *(2)*, NSC *(3)*, neurohaemal organ *(4)*, neurons of analyzing centers *(5)*. *Solid dots*: phylogenetically ancient direct pathways of neurohormonal influence on target-organs *(6)*, *light circles*: indirect pathways of neurohormonal influence via peripheral endocrine glands *(7)* and *encircled small dots*: indirect pathways of neurohormonal influence via central endocrine glands *(8)* (p. 23)

Errata

Page	Line	Instead of	Should read
17	1	(Fig. 3a)	(Fig. 3e)
18	13	(Figs. 3d,4b)	(Figs. 3c,4b)
19	16	(Figs. 1c,f,4c)	(Figs. 1e,f,4c)
22	37	(Konstantinova, 1977;	(Konstantinova, 1978;
22	46	of the EP	of the AP
23	27	(Fig. 6)	(Fig. 5)
24	6	3d,f,4b,c	3e,f,4b,c
24	8 and 32	Konstantinova, 1977).	Konstantinova, 1978).
24	47	"every day life", at such ...	"every day life", and at such ...
26	21	Konstantinova, 1977).	Konstantinova, 1978).
27	18	neuroendocrine relations	neuro-endocrine relations

Neurosecretion and Neuroendocrine Activity

Evolution, Structure and Function

Proceedings of the
VIIth International Symposium on Neurosecretion
Leningrad, August 15-21, 1976

Edited by
W. Bargmann, Kiel; A. Oksche, Giessen;
A. Polenov, Leningrad; B. Scharrer, New York

With 168 Figures

Springer-Verlag Berlin Heidelberg New York 1978

Professor Dr. W. BARGMANN
Anatomisches Institut der Universität
2300 Kiel/FRG

Professor Dr. A. OKSCHE
Zentrum für Anatomie und Cytobiologie
der Justus Liebig-Universität
6300 Giessen/FRG

Professor Dr. A. L. POLENOV
Laboratory of Neuroendocrinology
Sechenov Institute of Evolutionary Physiology
and Biochemistry, Academy of Sciences of the USSR
Leningrad/USSR

Professor Dr. B. SCHARRER
Department of Anatomy
Albert Einstein College of Medicine
Bronx, New York 10461/USA

ISBN-13: 978-3-642-66887-6 e-ISBN-13: 978-3-642-66885-2
DOI: 10.1007/978-3-642-66885-2

Library of Congress Cataloging in Publication Data. International Symposium on Neurosecretion, 7th, Leningrad, 1976. Neurosecretion and neuroendocrine activity. Includes bibliographies and index. 1. Neuroendocrinology-Congresses. 2. Neurosecretion-Congresses. 3. Nervous system-Evolution-Congresses. I. Bargmann, Wolfgang, 1906-. II. Title. QP356.4.I59.1976a. 591.1'88. 78-5861.

Softcover reprint of the hardcover 1st edition 1978

Offsetprinting and bookbinding: Brühlsche Universitätsdruckerei, Lahn-Giessen.
2127/3130-543210

The VIIth International Symposium on Neurosecretion took place in the Conference Hall of the Academy of Sciences in Leningrad, August 1976, under the direction of Prof. Andrey Polenov (Leningrad). The meeting was held under the auspices of

Scientific Council in the Combined Problems of Physiology of Man and Animals
Sechenov Institute of Evolutionary Physiology and Biochemistry
Pavlov Institute of Physiology
Pavlov First Leningrad Medical Institute
Zhdanov State University of Leningrad
All-Union Scientific Society of Anatomists, Histologists and Embryologists

This volume contains the abstracts and speeches given at the meeting, but these are not printed in the sequence they were actually given. Acknowledgment is made to Dr. Morris (Oxford), Prof. J. Priedkalns (Adelaide), and Dr. R. Snipes (Giessen) for editorial review of the texts. Dr. B. Krisch (Kiel) was responsible for compiling the index. The editors are grateful to Springer-Verlag (Berlin Heidelberg New York) for their careful consideration in the publishing of this volume.

Contents

Ontogenesis of Neurosecretory Systems

Structure and Function of Neurosecretory Systems in the Brain of Vertebrates

Caudal Neurosecretory System of Fishes

Structure and Function of Neurosecretory Systems in Invertebrates

Concluding Remarks

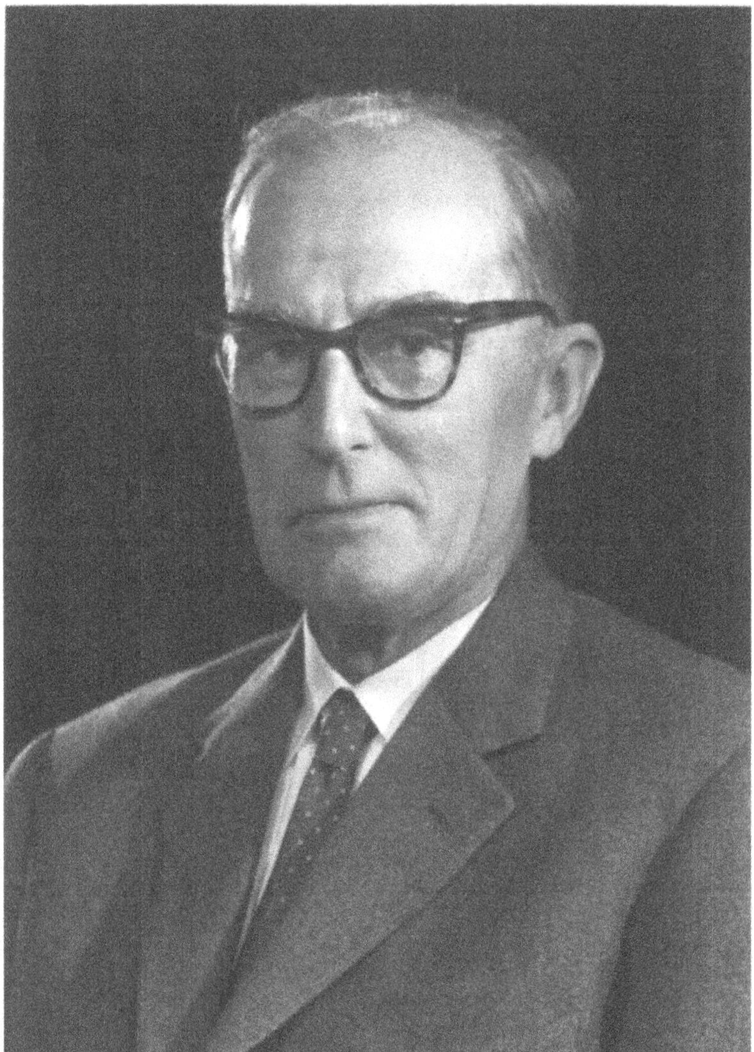

Mathias Thomsen 1896–1976. In memoriam

This volume is dedicated to the memory of Dr. Mathias THOMSEN, one of the pioneers in the study of neurosecretion, who was born in Copenhagen on October 9, 1896 and died there on July 3, 1976. His long and fruitful scientific career was spent in the Danish capital, where from 1927-1967 he was professor of zoology at the Veterinary and Agricultural University. Following his retirement, until his terminal illness, he continued with his research work as a distinguished guest investigator at the Institute of General Zoology of the University of Copenhagen.

A true scholar with a broad knowledge in biology, Mathias THOMSEN amassed a distinguished academic record which was given recognition by his election to a number of prestigious organizations, among them the Royal Danish Academy of Sciences and Letters and the Academy of Zoology of India. In collaboration with his wife Ellen, he made important contributions to the elucidation of neurosecretory and hormonal phenomena in insects. Those of us privileged to know him from the earlier Symposia on Neurosecretion remember him not only for his meticulously prepared presentations, but for his fine human qualities, his high integrity, sensitivity, and keen judgement.

Wolfgang BARGMANN (Kiel)
Andreas OKSCHE (Giessen)
Andrey POLENOV (Leningrad)
Berta SCHARRER (New York)

Opening Remarks

A. L. POLENOV
Laboratory of Neuroendocrinology, Sechenov Institute of Evolutionary Physiology and Biochemistry, Academy of Sciences of the USSR, Leningrad, USSR

Dear Colleagues! Dear Friends! Ladies and Gentlemen!

On behalf of the National Organizing Committee and myself, I am glad to welcome you, in this historic building of the Academy of Sciences on the banks of the Neva, to our heroic Leningrad, a city of intellectual and cultural progress and of revolutionary traditions.

Peter the Great founded our wonderful city, which became an outlet to Europe, "a window to the West." It is through this "window" that a renovating, reviving ray of light penetrated into the secluded, patriarchal, boyard Russia and gave rise to rapid progress in all fields of life in Russia, including the field of science that is of particular importance for us. The original development of a number of sciences now serving the prosperity of our Motherland is connected with the name of Peter I.

It is significant that we have gathered on "Vasilyevsky, glorious Island," as it is praised in an old Russian song, on its Strelka (Point) near the famous Rostral Columns. It is the place where, as Peter I said in the poem "The Bronze Horseman" by A.S. PUSHKIN, "Ships flying flags of different countries will come to visit us." It has come true. You, our dear guests, have come to Leningrad from many countries just as vessels carrying flags of different nations came to Saint Petersburg at the time of Peter I.

Our city is named after Lenin, a brilliant thinker, an outstanding statesman, and the founder of a new type of state. Here in Petrograd, in Smolny, Lenin formed the first socialist government, which in its first decrees assigned an important role to science in the development of a young socialist state. Later the scope of scientific research and the development of different sciences reached a level never seen before. Large scientific centers sprang up in formerly backward outlying districts that have now become Soviet National Republics. The result of these changes can be seen at this symposium where neuroendocrinologists have come from different parts of our expansive country, from the shores of the Pacific to the Baltic, from the Arctic to the Caspian and Black Seas. There are scientists present from Novosibirsk, Rostov-on-Don, Tashkent, Ufa, and other large scientific centers that were once remote provincial towns of old Russia.

Our city is famous for its scientific traditions. Outstanding scientists known all over the world have worked in Petersburg-Leningrad and at its Academy of Sciences. They are the neurologists B.M. BEKHTEREV, I.P. PAVLOV, and L.A. ORBELI (the founder of the Sechenov Institute of Evolutionary Physiology and Biochemistry of the Academy of Sciences of the USSR), the histologists and cytologists A.S. DOGIEL, A.A. MAKSIMOV, A.A. ZAVARZIN, D.N. NASONOV, the zoologists K. BARR, L.S. BERG, and Ye.N. PAVLOVSKY.

We are proud of the fact that neuroendocrinologists of Leningrad were invited by the International Committee on Neurosecretion Symposia to organize the Seventh International Symposium. This proposal was supported by leading Soviet neuroendocrinologists, and by our joint efforts we have managed to organize this important meeting of neuroendocrinologists.

I believe that Leningrad's neuroendocrinologists are justified in holding this symposium on neurosecretions in their native city. In 1945 when I was a student at the Leningrad University, my dear teacher, the late Prof. N.L. GERBILSKY, suggested the subject of my investigation, the role of hypothalamic neurosecretion in the regulation of the gonadotropic function of the hypophysis of Teleostei. The results of this student work were published in 1949-1950. At about this time at Moscow University, Prof. L.B. LEVINSON and a group of his students independently undertook research on neurosecretion of bees and amphibians, in particular its cytomorphological and cytochemical aspects. Their findings were published in 1947-1949.

Since the 1950s Leningrad has become a pioneering center in the USSR in the development of the study of neurosecretion. The First All-Union Symposium on Neurosecretion (1962) and the First All-Union Conference on Neuroendocrinology (1974) were held in Leningrad. Major research teams working in the field of neuroendocrinology and neurosecretion are concentrated in Leningrad. These are the groups of Prof. V.G. BARANOV and Prof. M.I. MITYUSHEF (Pavlov Institute of Physiology), Prof. I.I. GRACHEV and Dr. I.A. BARANNIKOVA (The Leningrad University), and Prof. T.B. ZHURAVLEVA (First Pavlov Leningrad Medical Institute). Additional studies on neurosecretion are carried out in other institutions of Leningrad.

In the late 1950s investigations on neurosecretion were already undertaken on a wide scale in our country. Large schools for the study of neurosecretion were established, headed by Prof. B.V. ALESHIN (Kharkov), Prof. A.A. VOITKEVICH (Obninsk), Prof. B.G. NOVIKOV (Kiev), Prof. M.S. MITSKEVICH (Moscow), and Prof. A.A. GALOYAN (Erevan).

On behalf of the Organizing Committee and all Soviet endocrinologists, I am especially glad to welcome our guests whose names are connected with the initiation and development of the study of neurosecretion, our great friends, members of National Academies, Prof. Berta SCHARRER (USA), Prof. W. BARGMANN (FRG), and Prof. M. GERSCH (GDR).

Many leading scientists who have devoted their lives to the development of the study of neurosecretion are present at this meeting. We are also indebted to them for large contributions to the development of original branches in neuroendocrinology. I refer to Prof. F. STUTINSKY, Prof. R. ACHER, Prof. R. MILIN, Prof. J. FLAMENT-DURAND, Prof. G. STERBA, and others. Among the participants we also see many talented scientists of the younger generation.

Some participants have come to the symposium with their families. I am glad to welcome them and to wish them a good time in Leningrad.

Regrettably, Prof. K. AKERT, Prof. I. ASSENMACHER, Prof. J. BARRY, Prof. H. BERN, Prof. H.-G. GOSLAR, Prof. H. KOBAYASHI, Prof. A. OKSCHE, Prof. Th. SCHIEBLER, and some others could not attend our symposium.

I consider it my duty to express deep sorrow on this occasion about the untimely deaths of Prof. Sir Francis KNOWLES, Prof. H. HELLER, and Prof. A.A. VOITKEVICH. I invite all of you to rise for a minute's silence in their memory.

Since the First International Symposium on Neurosecretion held in Naples in 1955, the study of neurosecretion has developed into a new branch of neurobiology - neuroendocrinology. During the past years it has been established that neurosecretory function includes not only the classic peptidergic "Gomori-positive" neurosecretory cells, but monoaminergic cells as well. Immunocytochemical and electron-microscopic investigations have revealed peptidergic "Gomori-negative" neurosecretory cells and new neurohemal organs, insights of particular importance. These findings have greatly extended the area of research concerning the problem of neurosecretion. While in Naples some 50 participants attended the symposium, at the symposia in Kiel (1969) and in London (1973) there were over 100, and this meeting is attended by about 250 participants. Symposia on neurosecretion have now reached the level of a conference.

The main topic of this symposium - evolutionary aspects of neuroendocrinology - was suggested by the National Organizing Committee and approved by the International Committee on Neurosecretion Symposia. Evolutionary aspects have been selected intentionally, and not by chance. Everyone here is well aware that the origin and initial development of the problem of neurosecretion were based on an evolutionary approach by the founders of this school - Professors E. and Berta SCHARRER, Prof. B. HANSTRÖM, and Prof. W. BARGMANN. Later this approach became traditional. The same orientation holds for our national approach to biology by K. BARR, I.I. MECHNIKOV, A.O. KOVALEVSKY, O.A. ORBELI, I.M. SECHENOV, A.N. SEVERTSEV, and I.I. SCHMALHAUSEN. The evolutionary perspective in the field of neuroendocrinology is widely practiced by the schools of Prof. N.L. GERBILSKY, Prof. A.A. VOITKEVICH, Prof. B.G. NOVIKOV, and Prof. M.S. MITKEVICH.

The Organizing Committee has selected papers for presentation bearing in mind the main topic of the symposium. These are communications dealing with three major approaches in elucidating the general evolutionary events responsible for the structure and function of neurosecretory elements: (1) phylogenetic development of neurosecretory elements and their function, (2) ontogenetic development of neurosecretory elements and their function, and (3) the role of neuroendocrine mechanisms in realizing species adaptation, i.e., mechanisms causing the evolutionary process. The latter approach is, according to Prof. N.L. GERBILSKY, the subject of ecologic histophysiology.

Half of the reports and demonstrations deal with evolutionary aspects. The majority of them are concerned with the role of different types of neurosecretory cells in the regulation of homeostasis and of the function of endocrine glands, primarily that of the adenohypophysis. The latter problem is still regarded as most controversial and attracts much attention by neuroendocrinologists.

The other half are concerned with various aspects of neurosecretion, featuring two main problems: (1) investigation of neural and hormonal mechanisms regulating the function of neurosecretory cells and neurosecretory centers as a whole, and (2) investigation of the role of neurosecretory systems in the regulation of adaptive reactions of the organism.

The latter problem has received much attention all over the world in connection with the great urgency for studies on the influence of environmental phenomena on human beings and animals. This work has given rise to extensive research aimed at exploring outer space, the oceans of the world, and at developing measures for the protection of nature from increasing air pollution.

Today we are opening the Seventh International Symposium on Neurosecretion. We hope that it can be regarded not only as an important meeting where we shall discuss many interesting problems and results of our research work, but also as a good learning ground for young investigators.

This symposium is an important event for Soviet neuroendocrinologists because foreign scientists can see for themselves the scope and diversity of research being carried out in our country.

The Organizing Committee is well aware that the program of the symposium is overloaded. We shall attempt to alternate our work with rest and recreation as much as possible. I hope our dear guests will have a very enjoyable time in Leningrad and be able to see the sights of our beautiful city, to visit its wonderful museums and suburbs and make friends with the people of Leningrad.

I wish you every success.

Evolutionary Aspects of Neuroendocrinology

Current Concepts on the Evolution of the Neurosecretory Neuron*

B. SCHARRER
Department of Anatomy, Albert Einstein College of Medicine, Bronx, New York 10461, USA

Neurosecretory neurons can be defined as nerve cells that engage in secretory activity to a degree which greatly surpasses that of conventional neurons, and which is comparable to that of gland cells. The capacity of these specialized neuronal elements for controlling effector cells by means of neurohormonal signalling and the absence, at least in classic neurosecretory neurons, of contacts with postsynaptic cells represent significant deviations from the norm as formulated by the neuron doctrine. What is the rationale for the phenomenon of neurosecretion, and what is its place within the spectrum of neurochemical mediation?

The most satisfactory approach to this problem seems to be provided by the *evolutionary history* of neuronal elements, the command cells of metazoans. In essence, the conceptual model of the ancestral neuron is based on its phylogenetic derivation from a less differentiated, pluripotential epithelial element. Therefore, the primitive nerve cell can be viewed as a functionally versatile structure, endowed with the capacity to dispatch both long-distance and localized chemical signals. This concept is supported by a comparative analysis of neuroregulatory mechanisms encompassing all multicellular organisms, and based on the premise that the most elementary integrative systems existing today may resemble those of our remote ancestors (PAVANS DE CECCATTY, 1974).

Cytologic signs of neurosecretory activity as well as experimental evidence for the operation of neurohormones are found throughout the entire metazoan series. Some of the neurons of the lowest eumetazoans, the coelenterates, display neurosecretory granules comparable to those in higher animals with regard to their staining properties and electron microscopic appearance (LENTZ, 1968; DAVIS, 1974). Moreover, in sponges, cell types that do not even satisfy all of the criteria of primitive neurons contain cytoplasmic inclusions of a similar kind (PAVANS DE CECCATTY, 1966, 1974). Neurosecretory granules are abundant in the nervous system of planarians. In the ganglia of annelids, over one half of all neurons are of the neurosecretory type.

Even more relevant is the fact that distinctive hormonal functions and other "nonconventional" neuroregulatory roles can be ascribed to the neurosecretory neurons of these primitive forms.

---

*Part of the studies referred to in this article have been supported by research grants NB-05219, NB-00840, and 5 PO-1-NS-07512 from the U.S.P.H.S. and by N.S.F. grant BMS 74-12456.

Tests with isolated neurosecretory granules of the coelenterate *Hydra* reveal that their content regulates growth and differentiation, especially during regeneration (LENTZ, 1968). This neuromediator also seems to participate in the induction of gametogenesis and sexual differentiation (BURNETT and DIEHL, 1964). Similarly, neurosecretory control from a distance, of growth during development and regeneration and of certain reproductive events has been demonstrated in planarians (LENTZ, 1968; GRASSO and BENAZZI, 1973) and in annelids (HAUENSCHILD, 1974).

The salient point is that none of these primitive invertebrates seems to possess "regular" glands of internal secretion. Therefore, at this level, the nervous system is the only agency available for carrying out all of the required endocrine functions. Neurohormones are thus the phylogenetically oldest bloodborne chemical messengers, and the endocrine type of coordination accounts for a relatively large sector of neuronal activities in lower invertebrates. In other words, far from being a latecomer, the neurosecretory neuron dates back to the very beginning of the development of neural structures. Furthermore, its versatility indicates that it has remained closer to the nerve cell precursor than has the more specialized "conventional" neuron.

Evidently, an important factor in the increasing *diversification of neuronal types* and activities at consecutive levels of the evolutionary scale is the degree and manner in which the neurons' inherited capacity for the manufacture of secretory products is used.

A decisive step in this process of specialization was the acquisition, by arthropods and vertebrates, of an endocrine apparatus proper, since it relieved neurons from doing double duty. On the one hand, the gradual evolution of higher integrative centers gave rise to vast numbers of neurons equipped for rapid, precisely localized, "synaptic" transmission. These neurons make only restricted use of chemical mediators in the form of neurotransmitters. On the other hand, cells producing neurohormonal mediators took over a novel and highly significant role, that of *mediation between the two systems of integration* (see MARTINI and GANONG, 1976). In this capacity, the neurosecretory neuron represents the final common pathway transmitting neural directives to the first way station of the endocrine apparatus, a role for which this cell, having retained its dual capacity, seems to be made to order (see SCHARRER, 1970, 1972, 1974, 1976).

In view of this shift in functional significance, it is perhaps surprising that first order neurohormonal mechanisms, obligatory in lower invertebrates, still occur in mammals, including man. In the latter, one-step mechanisms such as the neurosecretory control over "terminal" effector cells in the kidney or mammary gland would seem to be unnecessary. Yet, their existence makes sense in an evolutionary perspective, i.e., when interpreted as carry-overs from systems operating by necessity in phylogenetically less advanced forms.

An unexpected and challenging result of the detailed ultrastructural analysis of the neuroendocrine axis was the realization that not all of the neurosecretory neurons dispatch their messenger substances via the general or the special portal circulation. Synaptoid release sites of neurosecretory neurons were found to occur in close vicinity to, or even in contiguity with, their apparent cells of destination. The latter are not restricted to endocrine elements, but include a variety of somatic structures, among them various exocrine gland cells and muscle fibers. Furthermore, some neurosecretory neurons establish synapselike relationships with other neurons (see SCHARRER, 1976). These observations suggest localized, i.e., *neurotransmitterlike actions* on the part of neurosecretory mediators. The existence of nonhormonal modes of information transfer by peptidergic neurons eliminates the sharp dividing line originally thought to separate conventional from classic neurosecretory neurons. Now the latter actually blend into a continuum of diverse neurochemical activities.

What makes the discovery of synaptoid structures between neurons fascinating is that they go hand in hand with increasing physiologic evidence in support of the concept that nonconventional (peptidergic) neuroregulators may modulate certain forms of synaptic interneuronal communication. This kind of neurophysiologic activity represents a novel form of information transfer which may indeed turn out to be quite important (see, for example, CONSTANTINIDIS et al., 1974; STERBÁ, 1974; BROWN and VALE, 1975; McCANN and MOSS, 1975; PLOTNIKOFF et al., 1975; PRANGE et al., 1975; VINCENT and ARNAULD, 1975; BROWNSTEIN et al., 1976; GUILLEMIN et al., 1976; DE WIED et al., 1976).

Thus far, the evolutionary interpretation of the phenomenon of neurosecretion presented here has been based on morphologic and physiologic evidence. Can it be further substantiated by tracing the *biochemical history* of neurosecretory mediators? Even though the picture is imcomplete, particularly with respect to the situation in lower forms, a few general trends are beginning to emerge.

In contradistinction to those used in much smaller amounts by conventional nerve cells, the chemical messengers operating in classic neurosecretory neurons of vertebrates and invertebrates are proteinaceous in nature. Furthermore, the biologically active polypeptides of many, though not all, neurosecretory neurons are bound to special proteins, called neurophysins (see WALTER, 1975; WATKINS, 1975), which are responsible for the selective stainability of neurosecretory material throughout the animal kingdom. Aside from serving as carrier molecules, these proteins may play an active role of their own (PILGRIM, 1974).

The rather detailed biochemical information on neurohypophyseal hormones reveals an impressive structural similarity throughout the entire vertebrate series that speaks for a common evolutionary origin (ACHER, 1974; HELLER, 1974; CARRAWAY and LEEMAN, 1975; WALLIS, 1975). The same holds for the neurophysins, another old and strikingly homologous class of neuronal products (CAPRA and WALTER, 1975). Their phylogenetic history within the vertebrate series is illustrated by the fact that neurophysins can be identified as far down as the cyclostomes by their cross-reaction with antihuman antisera (see ZIMMERMAN, 1976).

The existence of analogous proteinaceous compounds in invertebrates can be deduced from certain histochemical and biochemical data, sporadic though they still are. For example, a chromatophorotropin chemically identified in a crustacean shows a close resemblance to some of the small hypophysiotropic peptides of mammals (FERNLUND and JOSEFSSON, 1972). Moreover, pigment concentration in two types of integumentary cells of this arthropod can be elicited by a chemically synthesized octapeptide (JOSEFSSON, 1975). In this context, another item of interest is the demonstration of immunoreactive thyrotropin-releasing factor in the ganglia of some gastropods (GRIMM-JØRGENSEN et al., 1975), where its function obviously must differ from that of a vertebrate hypophysiotropin.

In sum, none of the data cited speaks against the concept that the characteristic products of presently existing neurosecretory neurons have a common ancestry. In the course of a long evolutionary history, a proteinaceous precursor molecule may have gradually given rise to several subclasses of closely related compounds that took over a variety of special activities. Conversely, there are indications of the principle of hormone economy in that some of these chemical entities perform more than one physiologic function (see BARKER and GAINER, 1974; HORST and SPIRT, 1974; WITTER, 1975).

In *conclusion*, peptidergic neurons represent a highly specialized minority, capable of long distance (neurohormonal) as well as close range (neurohumoral) and intermediate forms of information transfer to various effector cells. The versatility of these neurons seems to be the result of a long evolutionary history that, in higher organisms, has culminated in their central role as mediators between the nervous and the endocrine integrative systems.

References

ACHER, R.: Chemistry of the neurohypophysial hormones: an example of molecular evolution. Handbook of Physiology. Sect. 7. Endocrinology. GREEP, R.O., ASTWOOD, E.B. (eds.). 1974, Vol. IV, part 1, pp. 119-130

BARKER, J.L., GAINER, H.: Peptide regulation of bursting pacemaker activity in a molluscan neurosecretory cell. Science 184, 1371-1373 (1974)

BROWN, M., VALE, W.: Central nervous system effects of hypothalamic peptides. Endocrinology 96, 1333-1336 (1975)

BROWNSTEIN, M.J., PALKOVITS, M., SAAVEDRA, J.M., KIZER, J.S.: Distribution of hypothalamic hormones and neurotransmitters within the diencephalon. In: Frontiers in Neuroendocrinology. MARTINI, L., GANONG, W.F. (eds.). New York: Raven Press 1976, Vol. IV, pp. 1-23

BURNETT, A.L., DIEHL, N.A.: The nervous system of *Hydra*. III. The initiation of sexuality with special reference to the nervous system. J. Exp. Zool. 157, 237-249 (1964)

CAPRA, J.D., WALTER, R.: Primary structure and evolution of neurophysins. Ann. N.Y. Acad. Sci. 248, 397-407 (1975)
CARRAWAY, R., LEEMAN, S.E.: The amino acid sequence of a hypothalamic peptide, neurotensin. J. Biol. Chem. 250, 1907-1911 (1975)
CONSTANTINIDIS, J., GREISSBÜHLER, F., GAILLARD, J.M., HOVAGUIMIAN, T., TISSOT, R.: Enhancement of cerebral noradrenaline turnover by thyrotropin-releasing hormone: evidence by fluorescence histochemistry. Experientia 30, 1182-1183 (1974)
DAVIS, L.E.: Ultrastructural studies of the development of nerves in *Hydra*. Am. Zool. 14, 551-573 (1974)
FERNLUND, P., JOSEFSSON, L.: Crustacean color-change hormone: amino acid sequence and chemical synthesis. Science 177, 173-175 (1972)
GRASSO, M., BENAZZI, M.: Genetic and physiologic control of fissioning and sexuality in planarians. J. Embryol. Exp. Morphol. 30, 317-328 (1973)
GRIMM-JØRGENSEN, Y., McKELVY, J.F., JACKSON, I.M.D.: Immunoreactive thyrotrophin releasing factor in gastropod circumoesophageal ganglia. Nature 254, 420 (1975)
GUILLEMIN, R., LING, N., BURGUS, R.: Endorphines, peptides, d'origine hypothalamique et neurohypophysaire à activité morphinomimêtique. Isolement et structure molêculaire de l'α-endorphine. C.R. Acad. Sci., D (Paris) 282, 783-785 (1976)
HAUENSCHILD, C.: Endokrine Beeinflussung der geschlechtlichen Entwicklung einiger Polychaeten. Fortschr. Zool. 22, 75-92 (1974)
HELLER, H.: Molecular aspects in comparative endocrinology. Gen. Comp. Endocrinol. 22, 315-332 (1974)
HORST, W.D., SPIRT, N.: A possible mechanism for the anti-depressant activity of thyrotropin releasing hormone. Life Sci. 15, 1073-1082 (1974)
JOSEFSSON, L.: Structure and function of crustacean chromatophorotropins. Gen. Comp. Endocrinol. 25, 199-202 (1975)
LENTZ, T.L.: Primitive nervous systems. New Haven-London: Yale University Press 1968
McCANN, S.M., MOSS, R.L.: Putative neurotransmitters involved in discharging gonadotropin-releasing neurohormones and the action of LH-releasing hormone on the CNS. Life Sci. 16, 833-852 (1975)
MARTINI, L., GANONG, W.F. (eds.): Frontiers in Neuroendocrinology. New York: Raven Press 1976, Vol. IV
PAVANS DE CECCATTY, M.: Ultrastructures et rapports des cellules mésenchymateuses de type nerveux de l'Eponge *Tethya lyncurium* Lmk. Ann. Sci. Nat. Zool. (12) 8, 577-614 (1966)
PAVANS DE CECCATTY, M.: The origin of the integrative systems: a change in view derived from research on coelenterates and sponges. Perspect. Biol. Med. 17, 379-390 (1974)
PILGRIM, C.: Histochemical differentiation of hypothalamic areas. Prog. Brain Res. 41, 97-110 (1974)
PLOTNIKOFF, N.P., WHITE, W.F., KASTIN, A.J., SCHALLY, A.V.: Gonadotropin releasing hormone (GnRH): neuropharmacological studies. Life Sci. 17, 1685-1692 (1975)
PRANGE, A.J., WILSON, I.C., BREESE, G.R., LIPTON, M.A.: Behavioral effects of hypothalamic releasing hormones in animals and men. Prog. Brain Res. 42, 1-9 (1975)
SCHARRER, B.: General principles of neuroendocrine communication. In: The Neurosciences: Second Study Program. SCHMITT, F.O. (ed.) New York: The Rockefeller Univ. Pr. 1970, pp. 519-529
SCHARRER, B.: Neuroendocrine communication (neurohormonal, neurohumoral, and intermediate). Prog. Brain Res. 38, 7-18 (1972)

SCHARRER, B.: The spectrum of neuroendocrine communication. In: Recent Studies of Hypothalamic Function. Int. Symp. Calgary, 1973. Basle: Karger 1974, pp. 8-16

SCHARRER, B.: Neurosecretion - comparative and evolutionary aspects. In: Prog. Brain Res. 45, 125-137 (1976)

STERBA, G.: Ascending neurosecretory pathways of the peptidergic type. In: Neurosecretion - the Final Neuroendocrine Pathway. KNOWLES, F., VOLLRATH, L. (eds.). VI. Int. Symp. on Neurosecretion, London, 1973. Berlin-Heidelberg-New York: Springer-Verlag 1974, pp. 38-47

VINCENT, J.D., ARNAULD, E.: Vasopressin as a neurotransmitter in the central nervous system: some evidence from the supraoptic neurosecretory system. Prog. Brain Res. 42, 57-66 (1975)

WALLIS, M.: The molecular evolution of pituitary hormones. Biol. Rev. 50, 35-98 (1975)

WALTER, R. (ed.): Neurophysins: carriers of peptide hormones. Ann. N.Y. Acad. Sci. 248 (1975)

WATKINS, W.B.: Immunohistochemical demonstration of neurophysin in the hypothalamoneurohypophysial system. Int. Rev. Cytol. 41, 241-284 (1975)

WIED, D. de, WIMERSMA GREIDANUS, T.B. van, BOHUS, B., URBAN, I., GISPEN, W.H.: Vasopressin and memory consolidation. Prog. Brain Res. 45, 181-194 (1976)

WITTER, A.: The in vivo fate of brain oligopeptides. Biochem. Pharmacol. 24, 2025-2030 (1975)

ZIMMERMAN, E.A.: Localization of hypothalamic hormones by immunocytochemical techniques. In: Frontiers in Neuroendocrinology. MARTINI, G., GANONG, W.F. (eds.). New York: Raven Press 1976, Vol. IV, pp. 25-62

Evolutionary Basis of the General Principle of Neuroendocrine Regulation. Interaction of Peptide and Monoamine Neurohormones in a Dual Control Mechanism

A. L. POLENOV
Laboratory of Neuroendocrinology, Sechenov Institute of Evolutionary Physiology and Biochemistry, Academy of Sciences of the USSR, Leningrad, USSR

A. Introduction

Almost half a century has passed since the investigation of neurosecretory function began. Numerous data concerning the structure and function of the classic "Gomori-positive" hypothalamohypophyseal neurosecretory system have accumulated. During roughly the last fifteen years new findings on the neurosecretory function of the "Gomori-negative" tuberohypophyseal neurosecretory system consisting of both peptidergic and monoaminergic elements have been obtained. A flow of new, frequently rather contradictory, data has changed previous concepts of the mechanisms involved in the neurosecretory control of endocrine glands, in particular of the adenohypophysis.

In the present report we shall summarize our views on the evolution of the hypothalamic neurosecretory cells and then formulate our concept of a universal dual neuroendocrine control of visceral organs, including endocrine glands, by peptide and monoamine neurohormones. Our concept is based on a morphofunctional study on the formation of the hypothalamohypophyseal complex in the ontogeny and phylogeny of vertebrates as well as comparative histophysiologic data on the role of the hypothalamus-posterior pituitary neurosecretory system in the development of stress reactions. We shall dwell only upon views of a general character; more detailed findings will be reported and demonstrated by my co-workers and students at the present symposium.

B. General Principles Regarding the Evolution of the Hypothalamic Peptidergic and Monoaminergic Neurosecretory Cells

At present peptidergic (Gomori-positive and Gomori-negative), adrenergic, and serotoninergic (monoaminergic) neurosecretory (neuroendocrine) cells (NSC) are recognized in the hypothalamus. These four types of NSC seem to develop during phylogeny and ontogeny from a general cellular source and to form four parallel genealogic lines (Fig. 1). We asume that genealogic lines are characteristic of all elements of the nervous tissue.

It is well known that the neuroectodermal cells lining the neural tube are the primordial form of the neurosecretory cells as well as all other elements of the nervous tissue. These cells seem to

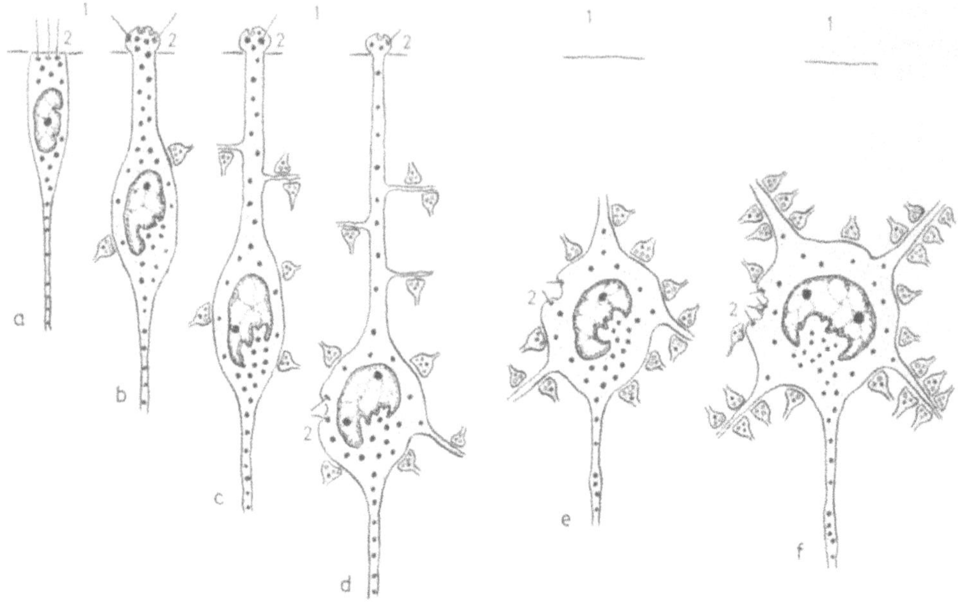

Fig. 1

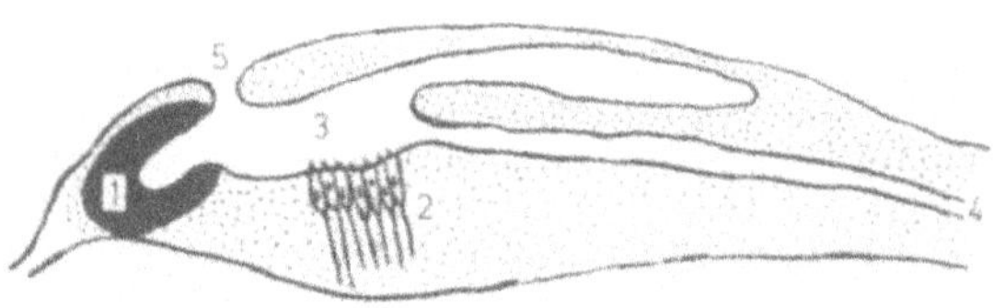

Fig. 2

be capable of reception of stimuli (they possess cilia) as well as exocrine secretion. After the neuropores are closed, as in the case of Amphioxus larvae (Fig. 2), these cells seem to transform into cells of internal secretion, because the hormones they produce enter the cerebrospinal fluid (CSF). Due to this well known fact endocrine secretion is to a certain degree characteristic of many definitive elements of the nervous tissue. During evolution some of these elements intensified their endocrine function. Later this led to the formation of neuroendocrine cells in different regions of the definite nervous system. During phylogeny, and to a lesser degree ontogeny, peptidergic and monoaminergic hypothalamic NSC of vertebrates go through two putative main stages.

At the first stage unipolar and bipolar, so-called ependymal type NSC predominate in the hypothalamus (Figs. 1a-c, 3e, 4a,b). The perikarya of these NSC lie either in the ependymal lining or are subependymal. These NSC seem to have a receptor function since their apical ends and/or intraventricular bulbs of their dendrites making contact with the CSF have cilia (see VIGH-TEICHMANN and VIGH, 1974). At the same time in the region of

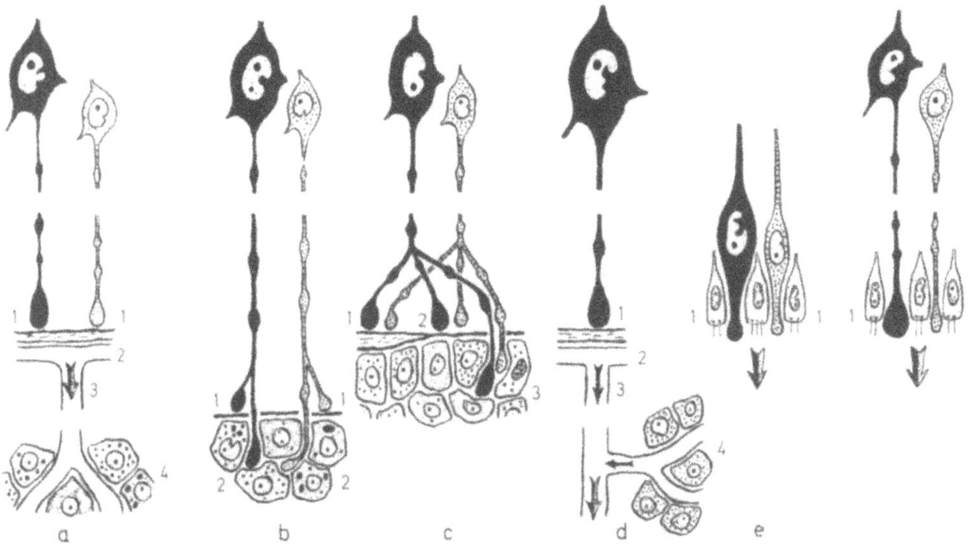

Fig. 3

these dendroventricular contacts (Fig. 3a) the secretory substance is discharged, possibly by a microapocrine or macroapocrine process (MÜLLER et al., 1971; VAN OORDT et al., 1974; McCANN and ROSENBLUTH, 1974; EFIMOVA, 1976). A considerable amount of the neurosecretory material (NSM), however, is transported by axons and accumulated in their terminal parts. The ependymal type of NSC is devoid of or poor in synapses predominantly of axosomatic type of synapses (see VIGH-TEICHMANN and VIGH, 1974).

The infundibular organ of Amphioxus and the paraventricular organ of Submammalia are the result of accumulation of the perikarya of ependymal type NSC. The peptidergic and monoaminergic ependymal type NSC either prevail in adult animals, or they are numerous among the NSC of the preoptic, periventricular and infundibular nuclei, as is the case in the phylogenetically more ancient species among Anamnia, for instance Cyclostomata, Acipenseridae and Urodela. A small number of bipolar NSC have been found in the periventricular and infundibular nuclei of reptiles. In Anamnia, however, numerous very well developed multipolar neuronal type NSC are observed in the above-mentioned nuclei. It should be noted that these NSC are more numerous in phylogenetically younger than in phylogenetically old groups (POLENOV, 1968; VIGH-TEICHMANN and VIGH, 1974; KONSTANTINOVA, 1978, in this volume). In early ontogeny some NSC in birds pass the "ependymal" stage (DENISIEVSKY, 1967). Neurosecretory formations at this stage of development have a poor blood supply (Fig. 4a,b); only peptidergic neurosecretory centers of Teleostei are richly vascularized.

Most axons of both types of the NSC run to the neurohemal regions, where they form predominantly primitive axovasal neurosecretory contacts with pial plexus separating the brain from

Fig. 4

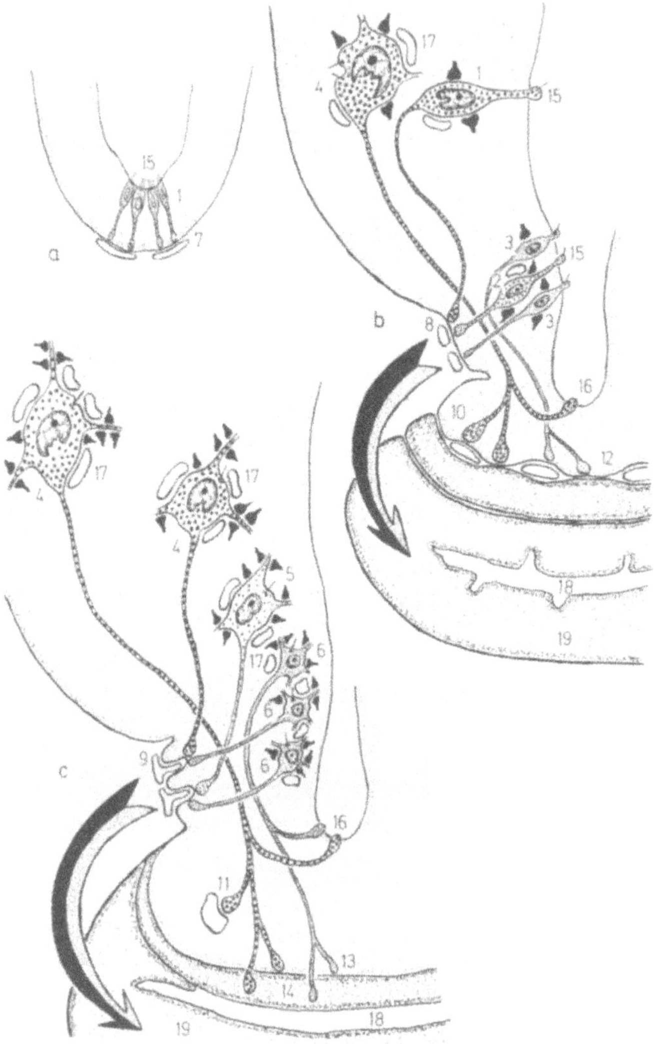

the adenohypophysis (Fig. 4a,b). It is noteworthy that under conditions of traumatic regeneration, caused by deafferentation of the hypothalamus as in experiments by HALASZ, peptidergic Gomori-positive neurosecretory fibers grow into the brain sheath and form primitive axovasal contacts similar to those of the phylogenetically ancient type (DANILOVA and POLENOV, 1977). These data confirm once more one of the main principles of evolutionary morphology and physiology (ORBELI, 1959), according to which phylegenetically older morphofunctional characteristics come forth under pathologic conditions. The ependymal type of NSC may also form indirect axoadenar neurosecretory contacts with the connective tissue septa at the border of the glandular cells and the hypophyseal intermediate lobe (IL) (Figs. 3d, 4b). Less frequently, axon terminals penetrate into the CSF of the infundibular and hypophyseal recesses, where they form axoventricular contacts. Thus, released by axon terminals, peptide and monoamine neurohormones may enter the blood circulation, connective tissue septa, and the intercellular clefts, as well as the CSF. Such primitive organization of neurohemal regions is characteristic of Cyclostomata, adult fish (except Elasmobranchii, Teleostei), phylogenetically ancient groups of amphibians, reptiles, and birds, as well as all vertebrates at the early stages of their ontogeny (BARGMANN, 1966; POLENOV, 1968; POLENOV and GARLOV, 1971; POLENOV et al., 1972, 1974, 1976; POLENOV and BELENKY, 1973; BELENKY et al., 1973; VIGH-TEICHMANN and VIGH, 1974; TSUNEKI and GORBMAN, 1975).

At the second stage of the evolution of vertebrates, the multipolar peptidergic and monoaminergic neuronal types of the NSC predominate. They are practically no longer connected by dendrites with the lumen of ventricle III (Figs. 1c,f, 4c). These NSC sank rather far into the brain tissue. In evolution the NSC tend to move even further from the ventricle (POLENOV, 1968; VIGH-TEICHMANN and VIGH, 1974). At this stage of development, neurosecretory centers, especially "magnocellular" elements, have a very rich vascularization. During the ontogeny of vertebrates the number of processes of the NSC increases. The neuronal type of the NSC seem to retain their receptor function because their perikarya have short cilia penetrating the intercellular clefts (SENCHIK and PISUGIN, 1974). Sometimes accumulations of these cilia together with synaptic boutons form complicated receptor apparatuses that seem to be capable of hemoreception (PLUZHNIKOV et al., 1978, in this volume). The number of synapses on the neuronal type of NSC increases in the course of evolution. Axosomatic synapses on NSC prevail at the earlier stages of ontogeny and phylogeny. In addition to these, numerous axodendritic synapses appear in phylogenetically younger species (see VIGH-TEICHMANN and VIGH, 1974).

Perfect axovasal neurosecretory contacts with the basal lamina of the pericapillary spaces and their derivatives, intervascular channels, are predominantly present in the neuronal type of the NSC. Intervascular channels are characteristic of neurohemal organs of highly organized, phylogenetically young groups of Anamnia (Teleostei, Anura). These vertebrates, especially highly organized groups within the various classes (Elasmobranchii, Teleostei, Anura, Crocodilia, Mammalia), have also perfect direct axoadenar synaptoid neurosecretory contacts (Figs. 3b,c, 4c) localized among glandular cells of different lobes of the adenohypophysis, but chiefly in the IL (BARGMANN, 1966; POLENOV, 1968; ZAMBRANO et al., 1972; POLENOV and BELENKY, 1973; KAUL and VOLLRATH, 1974; BAGE et al., 1975). However, in addition primitive indirect axoadenar contacts with a connective tissue layer and with one basal membrane are also frequent. In some classes of vertebrates axoventricular contacts (Figs. 3f, 4c) at the site of infundibular recesses are very well developed (POLENOV, 1968; WITTKOWSKI, 1973; VIGH-TEICHMANN and VIGH, 1974). Appearance of synapses formed by axon terminals of the neuronal type peptidergic NSC (extrahypothalamic pathways) on the perikarya of neurons in different parts of the CNS (see STERBA, 1974) and of conventional monoaminergic neurons represents the highest degree of evolution of NSC. In this case peptides and monoamines act as neurotransmitters.

C. Main Evolutionary Steps in the Establishment of Relationships Between Peptidergic and Monoaminergic Axon Terminals and Tissue Elements in the Adenohypophysis and Neurohypophysis

I. Adenohypophysis

Data on the dual neurosecretory "innervation" of the IL in different vertebrate species are beyond doubt (see KNOWLES, 1967; BAUMGARTEN et al., 1972; POLENOV et al., 1974). In all vertebrates, terminals of peptidergic A_1- and A_2-type axons (d of granules = 1500-3000 Å and 1000-1500 Å respectively) and monoaminergic B-type axons (d = 600-1100 Å) form different types of axoadenar contacts (Figs. 3c, 4b,c) with the glandular cells of the IL. In Teleostei all three types of axoadenar contacts (Fig. 3b) have been described in the proadenohypophysis and mesoadenohypophysis which are homologues of the anterior pituitary (AP) (see KAUL and VOLLRATH, 1974; EKENGREN, 1975). This might be explained by the fact that the AP of Teleostei has no portal vascular system. It is known that highly organized idioadaptive features occur in Teleostei. Similar interrelations between the two types of fibers seem to exist also in the tuberal lobe of reptiles, birds, and mammals (VIGH-TEICHMANN and VIGH, 1974). Thus, the function of the glandular cells of the IL (Figs. 3, 4, 5), and partly of the AP, is controlled by peptide as well as monoamine (more precisely, catecholamine) neurohormones.

II. Median Eminence (Proximal Neurosecretory Contact Region - PNCR - in Cyclostomata and Primitive Fish)

In this neurohemal organ three main types of terminals - peptidergic A_1, A_2, and monoaminergic B - make contact with capillaries of the portal circulation (Figs. 3a, 4b,c, 5). During phylogeny in vertebrates and ontogeny in the frog, the relative number of A-terminals (especially A_1) decreases and that of B-terminals increases greatly. In the external zone of the median eminence of mammals generally only A_2- and a great many B-terminals persist (see POLENOV and BELENKY, 1973; POLENOV et al., 1976). These changes parallel those of axovasal contacts, which vary from primitive contacts via a wide connective tissue layer to very narrow pericapillary spaces. It should be underlined that we have never seen any monoaminergic axoaxonal synapses on peptidergic fibers and their terminals in the external zone of the median eminence in any of the specimens studied. These morphologic data allow us to conclude that peptide adenohypophysiotropic neurohormones as well as monoamines enter the portal circulation. Many authors assume that catecholamines enter the portal blood (BARGMANN, 1966; KNOWLES, 1967; LEONARDELLI and BARRY, 1967; WURTMAN, 1970; DIERICKX, 1974; OKSCHE et al., 1974).

Fig. 5

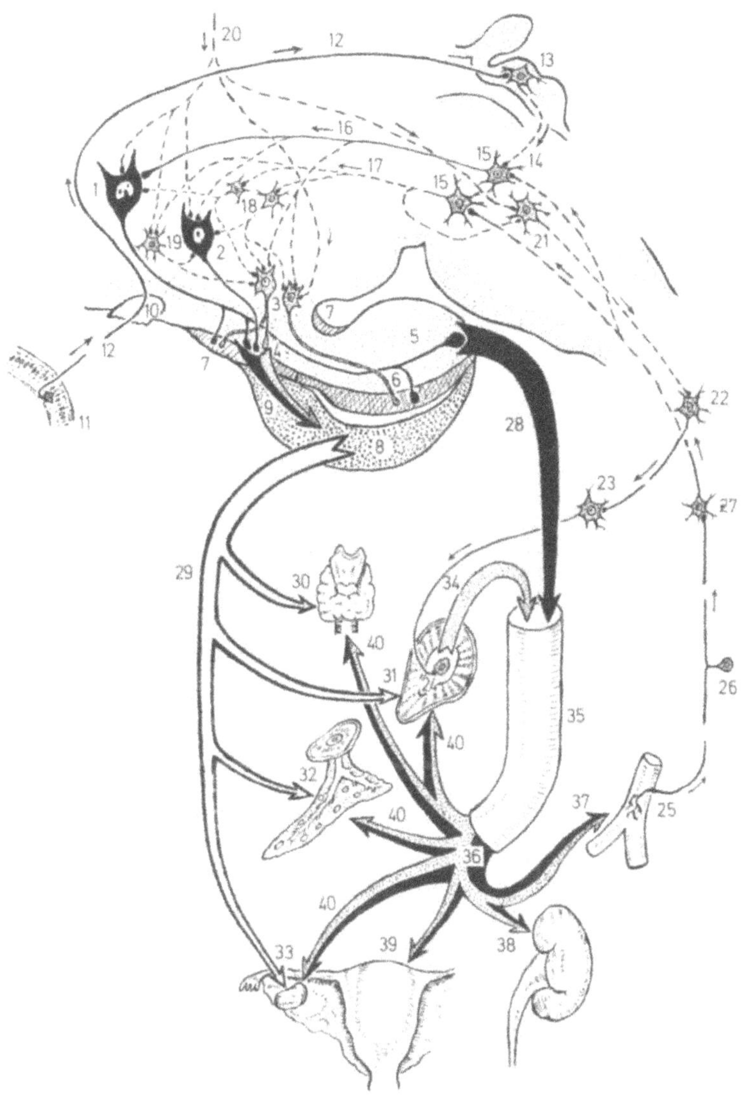

A synchronous reaction of peptidergic and monoaminergic terminals has been found in some experiments (adrenalectomy in mice and rats) and during metamorphosis in amphibians at the light (PAF method) and electron microscopic levels and in Falck preparations (KONSTANTINOVA and DANILOVA, 1975; BELENKY et al., 1973). Thus, the increased number of PAF-positive fibers in the external zone parallels accumulation of electron-dense granules in A- and B-terminals as well as intensity of fluorescence. On the contrary, presence of a large number of synaptic vesicles and a small number of granules is in accordance with the availability of scarce PAF-positive material and lower intensity of fluorescence. These data show that peptide and monoamine terminals act together, and that the combination of these two types of neurohormones entering the portal blood circulation seems to be necessary to control the function of the glandular cells of the AP.

Results of experiments performed by McCANN and his co-workers, who cultivated an isolated AP together with a fragment of a basal hypothalamus in vitro, support our assumption. Release of LH is observed in these experiments. Increased secretion of LH and FSH occurs if dopamine is added to the medium in which these tissues are included. This effect is not observed, if noradrenaline, dopamine, or serotonin are added to the medium in which only the AP is incubated. No stimulation of the AP in vivo is seen if the same monoamines are injected into the portal circulation (see KAMBERI and McCANN, 1969; SCHNEIDER and McCANN, 1970). Presence of APUD cells which assimilate and decarboxylate precursors of monoamines in the AP is indirect evidence that monoamines enter the AP (TAKOR et al., 1973).

Thus, the function of the glandular cells of the AP as well as the IL is controlled both by peptide and monoamine neurohormones. Peptide neurohormones are contained both in the Gomori-positive (possibly in CRH) and in Gomori-negative (possibly in GnRH) neurosecretory substances. The mechanism of this dual control is not yet clear. We suppose that monoamines (catecholamines) play a less specialized role than adenohypophysiotropic neurohormones in this process. It is quite possible that monoamines intensify or diminish the influence of peptide neurohormones or even change the nature of their influence.

III. Posterior Pituitary (PP)

In contrast to the median eminence, in the PP, reduction of monoaminergic and progressive increase of peptidergic A_1-terminals making contact with the capillaries of the general circulation is observed in the course of evolution (POLENOV and BELENKY, 1973). Thus, only A_1-terminals make contact with the capillaries in the PP of mammals (Figs. 3d, 4c, 5). B-type terminals are very scarce in the PP. They occur predominantly at the border of the IL or inside it (Figs. 3c, 4c). Only in Cyclostomata and fish (except Teleostei), B-terminals form axovasal contacts where catecholamines as neurohormones enter the general circulation (Fig. 4b). It is well known that a small number of adrenergic sympathetic fibers in the mammal PP innervate muscle cells of vessels (KONSTANTINOVA, 1977; BJÖRKLUND et al., 1973). Absence of monoaminergic axovasal contacts in the mammal PP shows that peptide (viscerotropic according to our terminology) neurohormones (vasopressin, oxytocin) are released into the capillaries under "every day life" conditions without any participation of monoamines.

D. PP and Chromaffin Tissue

Both peptide and monoamine neurohormones, predominantly catecholamines, are necessary to regulate the function of the glandular cells of the EP and the IL. It is well known that only viscerotropic peptide neurohormones are discharged from the PP into the general circulation in large amounts under stressful situations. The question arises as to how peptide neurohormones alone exert their influence upon practically all visceral organs (POLENOV, 1968; PRONIN and SULAKVALIDZE, 1969). It is also well known, however, that under stressful conditions great amounts of noradrenaline and adrenaline are released from the peripheral neuroendocrine apparatus, adrenal, and extra-adrenal chromaffin tissue (Figs. 3d, 5), into the general circulation (see CLEGG and CLEGG, 1969; SMITTEN, 1972).

So we assume that interaction of peptide hypothalamic neurohormones and catecholamines from the chromaffin tissue at the level of the visceral organ cells, peripheral endocrine glands included, is possible (Fig. 5). Influence of peptide viscerotropic neurohormones upon these glands under stressful situations is realized via a para-adenohypophyseal pathway (POLENOV, 1968). This influence may possibly be both stimulatory (small doses) and inhibitory (large doses). It has been shown that adrenaline and noradrenaline as well as vasopressin and oxytocin affect the function of the same organs. Examples are epithelial cells of kidney tubules and digestive tract glands or smooth muscle of vessels and digestive tract (GENETSINSKY, 1964; CLEGG and CLEGG, 1969; BOGACH, 1974). Both groups of neurohormones may have very similar or very different influences upon these organs.

Thus we have reason to assume that neuroendocrine regulation of the function of the visceral organs, peripheral endocrine glands included, is realized by peptide and catecholamine neurohormones (Fig. 6).

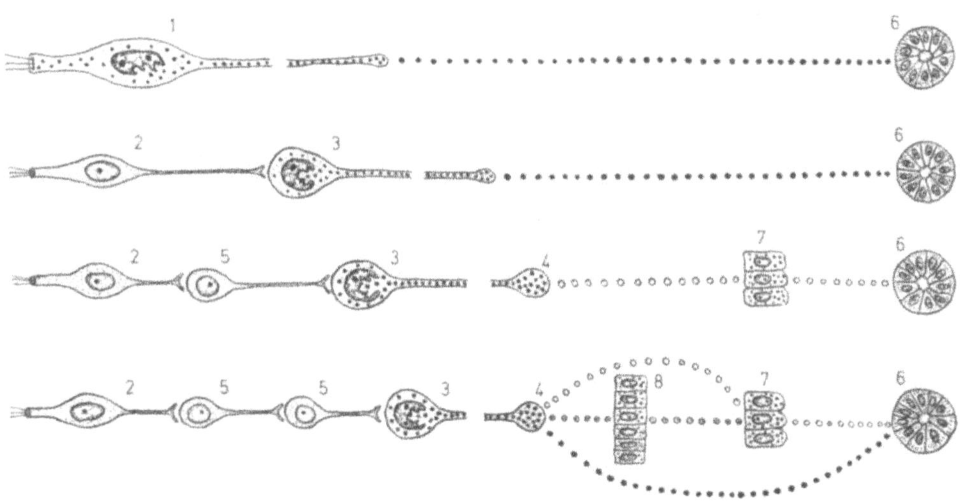

Fig. 6

E. Dual Neurotropic Effects of Neurohormones

It should perhaps be emphasized that both peptide and monoamine (predominantly noradrenaline and serotonin) hypothalamic neurohormones, especially in low vertebrates, seem to be discharged also at dendroventricular and axoventricular contacts (Figs. 3d,f, 4b,c) into the CSF of the third ventricle and its recesses (SCHARRER and SCHARRER, 1963; BARGMANN, 1966; STERBA, 1966, 1974; POLENOV, 1968; POLENOV and GARLOV, 1971; KONSTANTINOVA, 1977). A close topographic arrangement of both kinds of elements forming the hypothalamoventricular neuroendocrine system has been found. This speaks once more for a *dual* long range influence of these neurohormones, this time via the CSF. They seem to exert their influence upon some circumventricular and vascular (vascular plexus and vascular sac in fish) organs, and in general upon the CSF. In this way the neurohormones exert their neurotropic effect. The presence of some adenohypophysiotropic neurohormones, vasopressin, oxytocin, and monoamines in the CSF is well established (see SCOTT et al., 1974; VIGH-TEICHMANN and VIGH, 1974; SETALO et al., 1975).

F. Interrelations Between the Hypothalamo-AP and Hypothalamo-PP Systems

At present, three systems are generally recognized in the hypothalamohypophyseal neurosecretory complex: hypothalamus-AP, hypothalamus-IL, and hypothalamus-PP. The first system consists of peptidergic Gomori-positive neurosecretory neurons of the "magnocellular" nuclei. The hypothalamus-IL system is formed by peptidergic Gomori-positive neurosecretory cells and adrenergic neurosecretory cells of the arcuate nucleus and its homologues, which "innervate" the IL. The hypothalamus-AP system is composed of both Gomori-positive, Gomori-negative peptidergic NSC, and monoaminergic NSC. The latter occur in the infundibular (arcuate) and periventricular nuclei (see KONSTANTINOVA, 1977). Gomori-positive NSC are present not only in the well known nuclei, but are also diffusely distributed in numerous small "additional" NSC groups (nuclei) Gomori-negative peptidergic NSC are larger than monoaminergic NSC and, as immunofluorescence histochemical and electron microscopic studies show, are diffusely distributed in the hypothalamus. They are also found in some "parvicellular" nuclei (infundibular, periventricular and ventromedial nuclei) (see LEONARDELLI and BARRY, 1967; OKSCHE et al., 1974; VIGH-TEICHMANN and VIGH, 1974; NAIK, 1975; SETALO et al., 1975).

Numerous investigations show that the functional role of the hypothalamus-PP system and the hypothalamus-IL system comes into play under stressful conditions, and especially in relatively long (up to some days) stressful situations as well as under pathologic conditions. The hypothalamo-AP system functions mainly in "every day life," at such stages of the life cycle of animals as metamorphosis, pregnancy, lactation, and also stress situations, especially under short term conditions (POLENOV, 1968, 1975).

Ontogenetic and phylogenetic studies of the hypothalamohypophyseal complex show that the hypothalamus-PP system and the hypothalamus-IL system appear and begin to function earlier than the hypothalamus (median eminence)-AP system (BELENKY et al., 1973; POLENOV and BELENKY, 1973; ALESHIN, 1974; PEARSON and LICHT, 1974). It is reasonable to assume that the para-adenohypophyseal way of influence, using viscerotropic peptide neurohormones, is phylogenetically older than the transadenohypophyseal way of influence using adenohypophysiotropic peptide neurohormones (Fig. 5). This assumption is supported by evidence indicating that the peripheral endocrine glands appear and begin to function at earlier ontogenetic stages in the vertebrates than the adenohypophysis (see LEVINA, 1973; MITSKEVICH, 1974). This phenomenon is especially prominent in lower vertebrates (YAKOVLEVA, 1949; BARANNIKOVA, 1974). It is also well known (see SCHARRER and SCHARRER, 1963) that in the course of evolution of almost every type of Protostomia and Deuterostomia, NSC and the systems which regulate visceral functions and reproduction appear first (Fig. 6). Later, in phylogenetically young groups peripheral endocrine glands are formed, and in the last stage "central" endocrine glands appear (y-organ in crustaceans, corpora allata in insects, subneural gland in Tunicata and adenohypophysis in Craniata).

It is well known that all humorally functioning defensive mechanisms of the organism are mobilized under stressful situations. The humoral way of regulation is phylogenetically very ancient. Moreover, we regard stress as an almost pathologic state. According to Orbeli's conception (1959), phylogenetically more ancient mechanisms come forth under pathologic situations. Hence it becomes clear why the para-adenohypophyseal neuroendocrine mechanism of hypothalamic regulation, which is phylogenetically old, goes into action under stressful and pathologic conditions. Thus, it might be supposed that the phylogenetically younger hypothalamus-AP system "insures" itself by the readiness of the more ancient hypothalamus-PP system under critical accidental situations.

During the evolution of vertebrates, the role of the hypothalamic monoaminergic neurosecretory apparatus becomes more and more important in the regulation of the phylogenetically younger hypothalamus-AP system. This is manifested by an increase of the number of monoaminergic neurosecretory centers during evolution, and in the median eminence by an increase of the number of axovasal contacts formed by axons of monoaminergic NSC (POLENOV and BELENKY, 1973).

G. Neuronal Regulation of the Neuroendocrine Centers

At the very outset of the evolution of Deuterestomia, a primitive ependymal type of NSC able to receive stimuli from the CSF appear to have been devoid of a synaptic apparatus. Later, single axosomatic synapses arise on the ependymal type of the NSC, and some reduction of receptor function takes place in lower vertebrates (Figs. 1, 4). In very well developed species of vertebrates (Teleostei, mammals) in which the neuronal type of NSC possesses a highly developed synaptic apparatus, cilia (most prominent in Teleostei) are also sometimes retained. The cilia seem to be responsible for the perception of substances dissolved in the tissue fluid surrounding the perikarya as well as for physicochemical properties of the fluid (see SENCHIK et al., 1976; PLUZHNIKOV et al., 1977). The availability of receptors at the site of the magnocellular neurosecretory centers has been reported (see VIGH-TEICHMANN and VIGH, 1974). The main regulatory input to NSC, however, is realized by the synaptic apparatus.

It is well established that adrenergic synapses prevail on the hypothalamic peptidergic and monoaminergic NSC (OKSCHE et al., 1974; SENCHIK et al., 1976; KONSTANTINOVA, 1977). The perikarya of the respective adrenergic neurons are located in the hypothalamus as well as the medulla oblongata and the pons Varolii (BJÖRKLUND et al., 1975). Some evidence speaks for a direct influence of serotoninergic and cholinergic neurons situated in the brain stem as well as in the forebrain (for instance, limbic system) upon the function of NSC. It is supposed that the main centers which receive information from interceptors and exteroceptors destined for NSC are localized in the reticular formation of the brain stem. From these centers impulses are transmitted to the hypothalamic NSC and possibly also to the chromaffin cells of the peripheral neuroendocrine system (Fig. 5). It is quite possible that the synchronous reaction of the peptidergic and monoaminergic NSC of the hypothalamus are provided for by conventional neurons of the CNS.

Thus, two main types of neurosecretory (neuroendocrine) cells are contained in the hypothalamus: (1) large peptidergic Gomori-positive and Gomori-negative cells and (2) small monoaminergic cells. These elements are components of two central neurosecretory (neuroendocrine) apparatuses. Their activity is controlled and integrated by neurons of the CNS, in particular by those of adrenergic nature. The role of the monoaminergic neuroendocrine apparatus and especially that of the neuronal controlling and integrative centers of the CNS, becomes more and more important in the evolution of vertebrates.

The result of the interaction of both hypothalamic neurosecretory apparatuses is that peptide and monoamine neurohormones produced by NSC together exert dual control over the function of the glandular cells of the AP and the IL and possibly also over the activity of some circumventricular, vascular organs, and of the CNS as a whole.

The hypothalamic-AP system, consisting of peptidergic and monoaminergic NSC accomplishes neurohormonal regulation of functions, predominantly of the peripheral endocrine glands via the median eminence and the AP, i.e., via the transadenohypophyseal way. This type of neuroendocrine regulation is phylogenetically young.

The hypothalamo-PP, predominantly peptidergic, system via the PP, i.e., via the para-adenohypophyseal way, interacts with the peripheral adrenergic neuroendocrine apparatus (chromaffin tissue). This is especially pronounced under prolonged stressful pathologic situations. In this case, dual control over the visceral organ functions, including those of peripheral endocrine glands, is realized. This mechanism of neuroendocrine regulation is phylogenetically ancient.

We do not consider this report to be complete. It is merely an attempt to systematize a large accumulation of factual material in the field of neuroendocrinology and to present diagramatically very complicated neuroendocrine relations that constitute the basis for the regulation and integration of adaptive trophic and reproductive functions of the organism.

References

ALESHIN, B.V.: Mechanisms of hypothalamic regulation of adenohypophysial functions. Prog. Physiol. Sci. (Moscow) 5, 48-81 (1974)

BAGE, G., EKENGREN, Bo., FERNHOLM, Bo., FRIDBERG, G.: The pituitary gland of the roach, *Leuciscus rutilus*. III. The pars intermedia and its innervation. Acta Zoologica 56, 43-60 (1975)

BARANNIKOVA, I.A.: Some peculiarities of the formation of neurosecretory systems and development of endocrine functions in the ontogenesis of fishes. In: Hormonal Factors of Individual Development. ASTAUROV, B.L. (ed.). Moscow: Nauka 1974, pp. 61-71

BARGMANN, W.: Neurosecretion. Int. Rev. Cytol. 19, 183-201 (1966).

BAUMGARTEN, H.G., BJÖRKLUND, A., HOLSTEIN, A.F., NOBIN, A.: Organization and ultrastructural identification of the catecholamine nerve terminals in the neural lobe and pars intermedia of the rat pituitary. Z. Zellforsch. Mikrosk. Anat. 126, 483-517 (1972)

BELENKY, M.A., CHETVERUKHIN, V.K., POLENOV, A.L.: The hypothalamo-hypophysial system of the frog, *Rana temporaria*. II. Functional morphology of the external zone of the median eminence during metamorphosis. Gen. Comp. Endocrinol. 21, 250-261 (1973)

BJÖRKLUND, A., LINDVALL, O., NOBIN, A.: Evidence of an incertohypothalamic dopamine neurone system in the rat. Brain Res. 89, 29-43 (1973)

BJÖRKLUND, A., MOORE, R.Y., NOBIN, A., STEMOVI, U.: The organization of tubero-hypophyseal and reticulo-infundibular catecholamine neuron systems in the rat brain. Brain Res. 51, 171-191 (1975)

BOGACH, P.G.: Peristaltic activity of the small intestine. In: Handbook of Physiology - Physiology of Digestion. SOLOVIEV, A.V. (ed.). Leningrad: Nauka 1974, pp. 447-521

CLEGG, P.C., CLEGG, A.G.: Hormones, Cells and Organisms (The Role of Hormones in Mammals). Stanford: Stanford University Press 1969

DANILOVA, O.A., POLENOV, A.L.: "Gomori-positive" neurosecretion in the rat after deafferentation of the median basal hypothalamus. Cell Tissue Res. 176, 121-130 (1977)

DENISIEVSKY, A.W.: Histogenesis der neurosekretorischen Zellen des Vogelhypothalamus. In: Problems of the Hypothalamic Neurosecretion. I. Problems of the Hypothalamic Physiology. NOVIKOV, B.G. (ed.). Kiev: Kiev Univ. Press 1967, pp. 96-107

DIERICKX, K.: Identification of adenohypophysiotropic neurohormone producing neurosecretory cells in *Rana temporaria*. In: Neurosecretion - the Final Neuroendocrine Pathway. KNOWLES, F., VOLLRATH, L. (eds.). VI Internat. Symposium on Neurosecretion. Berlin-Heidelberg-New York: Springer-Verlag 1974, pp. 170-181

EFIMOVA, N.A.: Liquor-Contacting Neurosecretory Cells in the Preoptic Nucleus of Juvenile Acipenseridae. Evolutionary Aspects of Neuroendocrinology. Proc. VII Internat. Symposium on Neurosecretion. POLENOV, A.L., BELENKY, M.A. (eds.). Leningrad 1976, p. 48

EKENGREN, Bo.: The aminergic innervation of the pituitary gland in the roach, *Leuciscus rutilus*. Cell Tissue Res. 158, 169-175 (1975)

GINTSINKSKY, A.G.: Physiological Mechanisms of Water Metabolic Equilibrium. Moscow-Leningrad: Nauka 1974

KAMBERI, I.A., McCANN, S.M.: Effect of biogenic amines, FSH-releasing factor (FRF) and other substances on the release of FRH by pituitaries incubated in vitro. Endocrinology 85, 815-824 (1969)

KAUL, S., VOLLRATH, L.: The goldfish pituitary. II. Innervation. Cell Tissue Res. 154, 231-249 (1974)

KNOWLES, F.: Neuronal properties of neurosecretory cells. In: Neurosecretion. IV Internat. Symposium on Neurosecretion. STUTINSKY, F. (ed.). Berlin-Heidelberg-New York: Springer-Verlag 1967, pp. 8-19

KOBAYASHI, H., MATSUI, T., ISHII, S.: Functional electron microscopy of the hypothalamic median eminence. Int. Rev. Cytol. 29, 281-381 (1970)

KONSTANTINOVA, M.S.: Monoaminergic structures within the hypothalamo-hypophyseal complex in the phylogenesis of vertebrates. In: Neurosecretion and Neuroendocrine Activity, BARGMANN, W., OKSCHE, A., POLENOV, A., SCHARRER, B. (eds,).VIIth Internat.Symposium on Neurosecretion. Berlin-Heidelberg-New York: Springer-Verlag 1978, pp.52-55

KONSTANTINOVA, M.S., DANILOVA, O.A.: Distribution of catecholamines in the median eminence of the adrenalectomized rats. Bull. Exp. Biol. Med. (Moscow) 80, 100-102 (1975)

LEONARDELLI, J., BARRY, J.: Etude des modifications de l'activité monoamine oxydasique au niveau de l'appareil hypothalamo-hypophysaire chez le cobaye mâle après castration bilatérale. C. R. Soc. Biol. (Paris) 161, 1314-1317 (1967)

LEVINA, S.E.: Formation of Reproductive System of Some Sections of Endocrine Regulations in Embryonic Development of Man. Thesis 1973

McCANN, O.C., ROSENBLUTH, J.: Sensory and secretory catecholamine-containing cells bordering the third ventricle of the toad brain. In: Neurosecretion - the Final Neuroendocrine Pathway. VI Internat. Symposium on Neurosecretion. KNOWLES, F., VOLLRATH, L. (eds.). Berlin-Heidelberg-New York: Springer-Verlag 1974

MITSKEVICH, M.S.: Some aspects of the problem of hormonal control mechanisms in prenatal life. Ontogenes (Moscow) 5, 557-566 (1974)

MÜLLER, H., STERBA, G., WEISS, J.: Beiträge zur Hydrencephalokrinie. III. Elektronenmikroskopische Untersuchungen über die Ausleitung von Neurosekret in den Liquor. Z. Wiss. Zool. (Leipzig) 183, 156-180 (1971)

NAIK, D.V.: Immuno-electron microscopic localization of luteinizing hormonoreleasing hormone in the arcuate nuclei and median eminence of the rat. Cell Tissue Res. 157, 437-455 (1975)

OKSCHE, A., OEHMKE, H.Y., HARTWIG, H.G.: A Concept of Neuroendocrine Cell Complexes. Neurosecretion - the Final Neuroendocrine Pathway. VI Internat. Symposium on Neurosecretion. KNOWLES, F., VOLLRATH, L. (eds.). Berlin-Heidelberg-New York: Springer-Verlag 1974, pp. 154-164

OORDT, P.C.W.J., van, GOOS, H.J.Th., PEUTE, J., TERLOU, M.: Structural and Functional Aspects of Two Types of Gomori-negative Neurosecretory Centers in the Caudal Hypothalamus of Amphibia. Neurosecretion - the Final Neuroendocrine Pathway. VI Internat. Symposium on Neurosecretion. KNOWLES, F., VOLLRATH, L. (eds.). Berlin-Heidelberg-New York: Springer-Verlag 1974, pp. 182-192

ORBELI, L.A.: Basic problems and methods of evolutionary physiology. In: Evolution of Nervous System Functions. Leningrad: Medgiz 1959, pp. 3-15

PEARSON, A.K., LICHT, P.: Embryology and cytodifferentiation of the pituitary gland in the lizard, *Anolis carolinensis*. J. Morphol. 144, 85-118 (1974)

PLUZHNIKOV, L.T., SENCHIK, Yu.I., POLENOV, A.L.: Functional Morphology of the Synaptic Apparatus of the Nucleus Praeopticus Peptidergic Neurosecretory Cells in the Carp, *Cyprinus carpio* L. VII Internat. Symposium on Neurosecretion. Berlin-Heidelberg-New York: Springer-Verlag 1978, this volume

POLENOV, A.L.: Hypothalamic Neurosecretion. Leningrad: Nauka 1968

POLENOV, A.L.: Morpho-Functional Foundations of Neurosecretory (Peptidergic) and Adrenergic Regulating Mechanisms of the Hypothalamus. Proc. XI All-Union Congress of I.P. Pavlov Physiological Society. CHENIGOVSKY, V.N. (ed.). Leningrad: Nauka 1970, Vol. I, pp. 311-315

POLENOV, A.L.: Hypothalamic control of reproduction in fish. In: Hormonal Regulation of the Sexual Cycle of Fishes. Part I. BARANNIKOVA, I.A. (ed.). Moscow: Pyzhchevaya Promyshlennost 1975, pp. 54-69

POLENOV, A.L., BELENKY, M.A.: Some regularities of the development of neurohemal parts of the hypothalamo-hypophysial neurosecretory system in ontogenesis and phylogenesis of vertebrates. J. Evol. Biochem. Physiol. (Leningrad) 11, 355-363 (1973)

POLENOV, A.L., BELENKY, M.A., KONSTANTINOVA, M.S.: The hypothalamo-hypophysial system in the lamprey, *Lampetra fluviatilis* L. I. The neurohypophysis. Cell Tissue Res. 150, 505-519 (1974)

POLENOV, A.L., GARLOV, P.E.: The hypothalamo-hypophysial system in Acipenseridae. I. Ultrastructural organization of large neurosecretory terminals (Herring bodies) and axo-ventricular contacts. Z. Zellforsch. Mikrosk. Anat. 116, 349-374 (1971)

POLENOV, A.L., GARLOV, P.E., KONSTANTINOVA, M.S., BELENKY, M.A.: The hypothalamo-hypophysial system in Acipenseridae. II. Adrenergic structures of the hypophysial neurointermediate complex. Z. Zellforsch. Mikrosk. Anat. 128, 470-481 (1972)

PRONINA, N.N., SULAKVELIDZE, T.S.: Hormones and Regulation of Water Metabolism. Antidiuretic Hormone. Leningrad: Nauka 1969

SCHARRER, E., SCHARRER, B.: Neuroendocrinology. New York-London: Columbia University Press 1963

SCHNEIDER, H.P.G., McCANN, S.M.: Mono- and indolamines and control of LH-secretion. Endocrinology 86, 1127-1133 (1970)

SCOTT, D.E., KOZLOWSKI, G.P., SHERIDAN, M.N.: Scanning electron microscopy in the ultrastructural analysis of the mammalian cerebral ventricular system. Int. Rev. Cytol. 37, 349-386 (1974)

SENCHIK, Yu.I., PLUZHNIKOV, L.T., POLENOV, A.L.: Peculiarities of the ultrastructure and distribution of synapses on neurosecretory cells of different size of the Nucleus preopticus in *Cyprinus carpio* L. Tsitologiia (Leningrad) 18, 275-283 (1976)

SÉTÁLÓ, G., VIGH, S., SCHALLY, A.V., ARIMURA, A., FLERKÓ, B.: LH-RH-containing neural elements in the hypothalamus. Endocrinology 96, 135-142 (1975)
SMITTEN, N.A.: Sympato-Adrenal System in Phylo- and Ontogenesis of Vertebrates. Moscow: Nauka 1972
STERBA, G.: Zur cerebrospinalen Neurokrinie der Wirbeltiere. Verh. Dtsch. Zool. Ges. in Jena. Zool. Anz. Suppl. 29, 393-440 (1966)
STERBA, G.: Das oxytocinerge neurosekretorische System der Wirbeltiere. Beitrag zu einem erweiterten Konzept. Zool. Jb. Physiol. 78, 409-423 (1974)
TAKOR TAKOR, T., PEARSE, A.G.E.: Cytochemical identification of human and marine pituitary corticotrophs and somatotrophs as APUD cells. Histochemie 37, 207-214 (1973)
TSUNEKI, K., GORBMAN, A.: Ultrastructure of the anterior neurohypophysis and the pars distalis of the lamprey, *Lampetra tridentata*. Gen. Comp. Endocrinol. 25, 487-508 (1975)
VIGH-TEICHMANN, I., VIGH, B.: The infundibular cerebrospinal fluid-containing neurons. Ergeb. Anat. Entwicklungsgesch. 50, 1-91 (1974)
WITTKOWSKI, W.: Elektronenmikroskopische Untersuchungen zur funktionellen Morphologie des tubero-hypophysären Systems der Ratte. Z. Zellforsch. Mikrosk. Anat. 130, 101-148 (1973)
WURTMANN, R.J.: Brain catecholamines and control of secretion from the anterior pituitary gland. In: Hypothalamic Hormones of the Hypothalamus: Assay and Chemistry. MEITES, J. (ed.). Baltimore: Williams and Wilkins 1970, pp. 184-194
YAKOVLEVA, I.V.: Independence of the thyroid gland activity of hypophysial thyropropic function in postembryonic development of Acipenseridae. Dokl. Akad. Nauk SSSR 69, 281-284 (1949)
ZAMBRANO, D., NISHIOKA, R.S., BERN, H.A.: The Innervation of the Pituitary Gland of Teleost Fishes. Brain-Endocrine Interaction, Median Eminence: Structure and Function. Internat. Symposium. KNIGGE, K.M., SCOTT, D.E., WEINDL, A. (eds.). Basle: Karger 1972

Molecular Evolution of Neurohypophyseal Hormones and Neurophysins

R. ACHER
Laboratory of Biologic Chemistry, University of Paris VI, 96, Boulevard Raspail, 75006 Paris, France

Following the discovery of the pressor, oxytocic, and antidiuretic activities in posterior pituitary powders, about seventy years ago, two opposing views were held about the number of molecules responsible for these activities. According to the unitary conception, defended by ABEL, MAC ARTHUR, and later by VAN DYKE, a single protein displayed all these biologic properties; this so-called "mother-molecule" would be extracted from the gland under mild conditions and isolated by fractionated salt precipitation. In contrast, the multimolecule conception led DUDLEY, KAMM, and later DU VIGNEAUD, FROMAGEOT, and their co-workers to purify and characterize two active peptides from mammalian glands, the one, oxytocin, possessing oxytocic and milk-ejecting activities, the other vasopressin, possessing the pressor and antidiuretic activities. The question arose whether the actual hormone was the protein, the peptides being only cleavage products, or whether oxytocin and vasopressin were natural hormones.

In 1955, we showed that the multiactive protein of the ox was not a pure molecule but a complex comprising two active peptides, oxytocin and vasopressin, and an inactive protein, a kind of carrier for which we have suggested the name "neurophysin" (ACHER et al., 1955; ACHER et al., 1956). Later we isolated the complex from five mammalian species and carried out the dissociation in the same way so that neurophysin was recognized as a general neurohypophyseal hormone-binding protein (J. CHAUVET et al., 1960; M.T. CHAUVET et al., 1976).

The molecular ratio oxytocin/vasopressin/neurophysin was first calculated to be 1:1:1 because a molecular weight of 20,000 was adopted for neurophysin on the basis of ultracentrifugation data. However, further characterization of neurophysin has shown that, on the one hand, two isoproteins very similar in size and amino-acid sequence, were often present in the complex, and on the other hand, that the molecular weight of each, determined by SDS electrophoresis and amino-acid analysis, was about 10,000. So a stoichiometric ratio between one mole of active peptide and one mole of inactive protein seems to exist in the complex. Because of that, an attractive hypothesis is that one neurophysin is specific for oxytocin and the other for vasopressin. In fact DEAN and HOPE (1968) have shown that neurosecretory granules can be separated into two types, one containing oxytocin and the so-called neurophysin-I, and the other vasopressin and the so-called neurophysin-II. The association can be explained either by a common biosynthetic precursor or by the need for a hormone carrier for transport from the hypothalamus to the posterior pituitary gland. Up to now, the biologic significance of the association remains ambiguous.

I shall examine first the evolution of neurohypophyseal hormones (for a recent review see ACHER, 1974), I shall then report recent results on mammalian neurophysins (for reviews see HOPE and PICKUP, 1974; BRESLOW, 1974; ACHER, 1976), and finally I shall discuss briefly the biologic relationships between neurohypophyseal hormones and neurophysins (ACHER, 1976).

A. Neurohypophyseal Hormones

I. Purification

Whatever the biologic significance of the association between neurophysins and neurohypophyseal hormones might be, the use of the complex as a procedure for the purification of active peptides turned out to be very successful (ACHER et al., 1958). The procedure is fast and gives high yields. For the first step, one precipitates the complex from posterior pituitary extracts by use of sodium chloride; for the second step, one dissociates the complex by means of trichloroacetic acid, which precipitates only neurophysins but leaves neurohypophyseal hormones in the supernatant solution; for the third step, one separates the two hormones usually present by chromatography of a single ion-exchange. The complex can be reconstituted (J. CHAUVET et al., 1960); so, in species in which intrinsic neurophysins do not give high yields for any reason, it is convenient to add beef or horse neurophysin and to operate under the usual conditions. Because the procedure needs only a few hundred mg of posterior pituitary powder, it could be applied not only to mammals but also to small but abundant species such as chicken or frog (1 g represents 1500 and 10,000 glands respectively).

During the last 5 years it was often necessary to perform isolation of neurohypophyseal hormones with only a few dozens or one hundred glands from small and rare species such as egg-laying mammals or lungfishes, and a more sensitive method was elaborated. In this procedure all the proteins of the posterior pituitary extract are directly precipitated with trichloroacetic acid. Then the peptides, which are in the supernatant solution, are separated by chromatoelectrophoresis on paper. With this microtechnique, 25-50 mg of posterior pituitary powder (10 Echidna for 25 mg), approx. 0.03-0.10 mg of neurohypophyseal hormone can be obtained. Approximately 0.01 mg (10 nmol) are necessary for determining the amino-acid composition and approximately 0.05-0.2 mg (50-200 nmol) for establishing the amino-acid sequence.

By using these procedures successively, we were able to isolate and characterize, over a period of 15 years, the neurohypophyseal hormones of about 40 species belonging to seven out of eight classes of vertebrates. Six new neurohypophyseal hormones have been chemically characterized in the course of this exploration.

II. Structure

From these studies, the conclusion can be drawn that on the one hand, each species usually has two neurohypophyseal peptides, on the other, that the neurohypophyseal hormones are evolutionarily very stable because the same hormones are generally found in species belonging to the same class.

Four main groups can clearly be distinguished in vertebrates. These groups are:

1. The mammals, including primitive prototherian mammals such as Echidna, in which oxytocin and arginine or lysine vasopressin have been found.

2. The nonmammalian tetrapods, namely birds, reptiles, amphibians, and lungfishes, in which two different peptides, mesotocin (Ile^8-oxytocin) and arginine vasotocin have been characterized.

3. The bony fishes, including primitive bony fishes such as Polypterus, in which isotocin (Ser^4-Ile^8-oxytocin) and arginine vasotocin have been identified.

4. Finally the cartilaginous fishes, which show a rather great hormone heterogeneity in contrast to the other classes. Two particular features have to be noted: cartilaginous fishes, namely rays, sharks, and chimaeras have arginine vasotocin like all the other nonmammalian vertebrates, but the amount is very small; the second hormone differs in each subgroup. In four species of rays, glumitocin (Ser^4-Gln^8-oxytocin) has been characterized.

More recently, purification of the hormones of a small shark, the spiny dogfish *Squalus acanthias*, has been undertaken. Two oxytocin-like peptides in addition to arginine vasotocin were disclosed. The amounts were approximately equal; chemical and pharmacologic characterizations of these two hormones have been carried out. They are valitocin (Val^8-oxytocin) and aspargtocin (Asn^4-oxytocin). For the first time two oxytocin-like peptides are clearly identified in a vertebrate species, and it remains to be determined whether both peptides are produced by a single gland or not.

In the chimaeras, the ratfish *Hydrolagus colliei* has been examined by PICKERING and HELLER (1969), and a peptide having the amino-acid composition of oxytocin has been isolated. The presence of oxytocin in a fish is rather puzzling.

III. Phylogeny

Figure 1 summarizes the characteristics of the six oxytocin-like and the three vasopressin-like hormones known to date. All these peptides have nine amino-acid residues, six of which are invariant. In the oxytocin-like family, substitutions occur only in

	1 2 3 4 5 6 7 8 9	1 2 3 4 5 6 7 8 9
Mammals (except pig)	Cys-Tyr-Ile-*Gln*-Asn-Cys-Pro-*Leu*-Gly-NH_2 oxytocin	Cys-Tyr-*Phe*-Gln-Asn-Cys-Pro-*Arg*-Gly-NH_2 arginine vasopressin
Pig	Cys-Tyr-Ile-*Gln*-Asn-Cys-Pro-*Leu*-Gly-NH_2 oxytocin	Cys-Tyr-*Phe*-Gln-Asn-Cys-Pro-*Lys*-Gly-NH_2 lysine vasopressin
Birds, reptiles, amphibians, lungfishes	Cys-Tyr-Ile-*Gln*-Asn-Cys-Pro-*Ile*-Gly-NH_2 mesotocin	Cys-Tyr-*Ile*-Gln-Asn-Cys-Pro-*Arg*-Gly-NH_2 vasotocin
Bony fishes (paleopterygians and neopterygians)	Cys-Tyr-Ile-*Ser*-Asn-Cys-Pro-*Ile*-Gly-NH_2 isotocin	Cys-Tyr-*Ile*-Gln-Asn-Cys-Pro-*Arg*-Gly-NH_2 vasotocin
Cartilaginous fishes (rays)	Cys-Tyr-Ile-*Ser*-Asn-Cys-Pro-*Gln*-Gly-NH_2 glumitocin	vasotocin (?)
Cartilaginous fishes (sharks)	Cys-Tyr-Ile-*Gln*-Asn-Cys-Pro-*Val*-Gly-NH_2 valitocin	vasotocin (?)
	Cys-Tyr-Ile-*Asn*-Asn-Cys-Pro-*Leu*-Gly-NH_2 aspargtocin	vasotocin (?)

Fig. 1. Structures of neurohypophyseal hormones found in vertebrates. (In cartilaginous fishes, arginine vasotocin was identified by chromatographic and pharmacologic procedures)

positions 4 and/or 8. In position 4, a polar residue, namely glutamine, serine, or asparagine is always present. In position 8, a nonpolar residue such as leucine, isoleucine, or valine is almost always present, with the exception of glutamine in glumitocin. It is of interest to note that this latter hormone, in contrast to the five other oxytocin-like peptides, displays a very poor rat oxytocic activity. A hydrophobic residue in position 8 is probably crucial for the specific binding to the rat-uterus receptor.

In the vasopressin-like family the only vasopressin-like peptide found up to now in nonmammalian vertebrates is arginine vasotocin. The change of arginine vasotocin into arginine vasopressin usually present in mammals is due to the replacement in position 3 of isoleucine by phenylalanine; this substitution of an aliphatic residue for an aromatic one, a single interchange between two hydrophobic residues, produces an increase of the rat antidiuretic activity and a loss of the secondary oxytocic activity displayed by vasotocin.

Figure 2 shows the successive amino-acid substitutions in the two evolutionary lines. It is of interest to note that there is a clear-cut division between nonmammalian tetrapods and mammals. Both neurohypophyseal hormones are changed, and this double change may be explained by a specialization for new functions: lactation on the one hand and antidiuresis on the other.

Figure 3 combines chemical and paleontologic data to trace a hypothetic evolution of the neurohypophyseal hormones. If there is a great complexity in cartilaginous fishes, in contrast from bony fishes to mammals, two evolutionary lines could be distinguished: the oxytocin line with three steps (isotocin, mesotocin, oxytocin) and the vasopressin line with only two steps (arginine vasotocin and vasopressin).

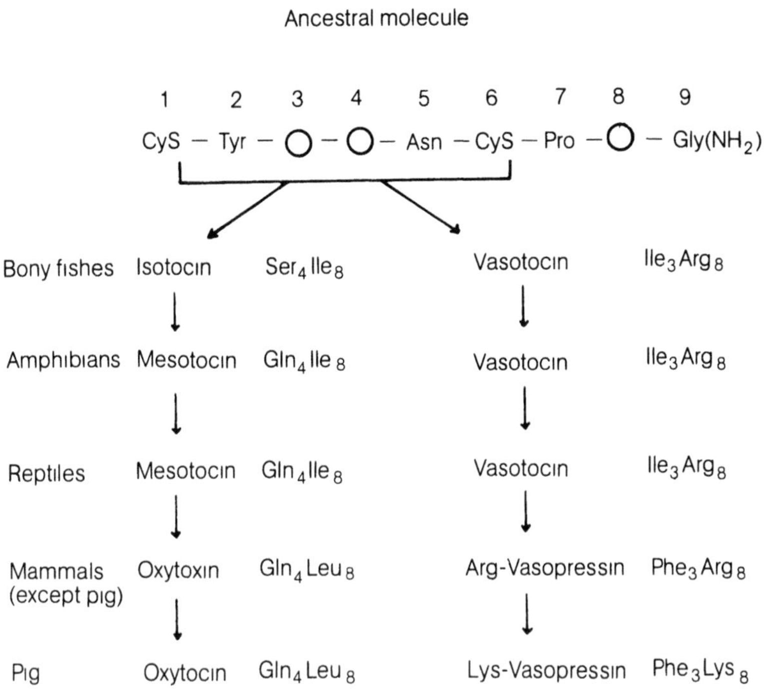

Fig. 2. Hypothetical scheme of evolution of neurohypophyseal hormones. One-gene duplication and series of subsequent single substitutions in positions *3*, *4*, or *8* produce two molecular lines. Substituted amino acids and their positions in hormone are listed to *right* of each hormone

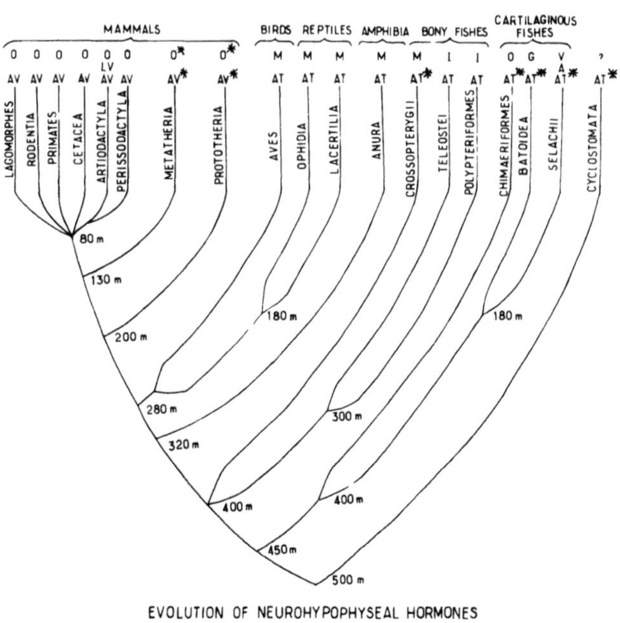

Fig. 3. Neurohypophyseal hormones and species evolution according to paleontologic data. Letters indicate hormones identified in modern representatives of groups (asterisk means that identification is not chemical but pharmacologic): *O* - oxytocin, *AV* - arginine vasopressin, *LV* - lysine vasopressin, *M* - mesotocin, *I* - isotocin, *A* - aspargtocin, *V* - valitocin, *G* - glumitocin, *AT* - arginine vasotocin. Numbers give time in millions of years since divergence

B. Neurophysins

Neurophysins are characterized by the following properties:

1. The ability to give a stoichiometric and reversible complex with the neurohypophysial hormones.

2. A peculiar amino-acid composition, a high content of glutamic acid (10-14 residues out of 100), and, especially, a high content of proline (8-9 residues), which is unusual in animal proteins.

3. A very high number of disulfide bridges in the molecule - seven bridges for a polypeptide chain of approximately 100 residues. So the conformation is probably different from those of the known proteins.

I. The Number of Neurophysins

The first problem is to determine the number of different neurophysins found in the gland, and this problem has not yet been fully resolved. As a matter of fact, the number of components detected by electrophoresis on polyacrylamide gel seems to depend upon the species and, in a given species, upon the time elapsed between death and removal of the gland, and also upon the pH of the extraction; in particular, cleavages or deletions at the ends of the single polypeptide chain have been observed, and two or three components can be derived from the same molecule. Because of that, it is difficult to estimate the real number of molecular species. Neurophysins are usually called neurophysin-I, -II, or -III, according to their relative electrophoretic migrations to the anode, but this nomenclature introduces some confusion when a comparison is made from one species to the other. We have proposed another nomenclature that I shall indicate later.

According to HOPE and PICKUP (1974), in the ox and the pig, two major components neurophysin-I and neurophysin-II and a minor component neurophysin-III or -C are present in approximate proportions 3:3:1 when the extraction is carried out in a strong acidic medium 0.1 *N* HCl. However we (CHAUVE et al., 1975a, 1976) and others (WUU and CRUMM, 1976a) have observed that in the pig, neurophysin-I is a truncated form of neurophysin-III, so the number of neurophysins in this species does not appear greater than two. On the other hand, WATKINS (1973) found in sheep a major component and two minor components in the approximate proportions 5:1:1. We have purified the major neurophysin from sheep pituitary, which represents about 70% of the total amount of neurophysins (CHAUVET et al., 1975a). The other components are more difficult to isolate, and it is not clear whether these are degradation products or other molecular species.

II. Characterization

So far, a few mammalian neurophysins have been isolated, and complete characterization has been made only for ox, sheep, and pig neurophysins. On the basis of the structural data from several laboratories including ours, we have proposed to distinguish provisionally two phylogenetic lines of neurophysins that we called MSEL-neurophysins and VLDV-neurophysins according to the amino-acid residues in positions 2, 3, 6, and 7. One-letter symbols are used for indicating the amino acids: M - methionine, S - serine, E - glutamic acid, L - leucine, etc. (Fig. 4).

In our structural nomenclature, the so-called neurophysin-I of the pig, neurophysin-II of the ox, and neurophysin-III of the sheep evidently belong to the same family, differences in electrophoretic migrations due to secondary factors having introduced the confusion.

Ovine, bovine, and porcine MSEL-neurophysins have been isolated by a three-step procedure. The first step is the isolation of the neurohypophyseal hormone-neurophysin complex by salt precipitation, as mentioned before. The second is the dissociation of the complex by molecular sieving on Sephadex G-25 in 0.2 *M* acetic acid, which gives "crude" neurophysin. The third step is ion-exchange chromatography of this material onto Diethylaminoethyl-Sephadex A-50 at pH 5.9, by using an ionic strength gradient. The first peak (A) contains MSEL-neurophysin, and the second peak (B) usually contains VLDV-neurophysin as well as degraded forms (Fig. 5).

Purified MSEL-neurophysins of ox, sheep, and pig have been split by trypsin after oxydation of the disulfide bridges. The eight tryptic fragments have been sequenced and isolated by peptide mapping.

On the other hand, proteins were cleaved by chymotrypsin, pepsin, and thermolysin, and the resulting peptides were purified and characterized in the same way. These overlapping peptides

Comparison between N-terminal sequences of mammalian neurophysins

Neurophysins	Sequence
MSEL-neurophysins	1 5 10 15 20 25 27
Bovine	Ala-Met-Ser-Asp-Leu-Glu-Leu-Arg-Gln-Cys-Leu-Pro-Cys-Gly-Pro-Gly-Gly-Lys-Gly-Arg-Cys-Phe-Gly-Pro-Ser-Ile-Cys
Porcine	— —
Ovine	— —
VLDV-neurophysins	1 27
Bovine	— Val-Leu — — Asp-Val — Thr — — — — — — — — — — — — — — — — — — —
Porcine	— Val-Leu — — Asp-Val — Lys — — — — — — — — — — — — — — — — — — —
Human	— Ala-Pro — — Asp-Val — Lys — — — — — — — — — — — — — — — — Asn — —

The dashes represent residues identical with those of bovine MSEL-neurophysin

Fig. 4. Two types of mammalian neurophysins. MSEL-neurophysins and VLDV-neurophysins (details in the text)

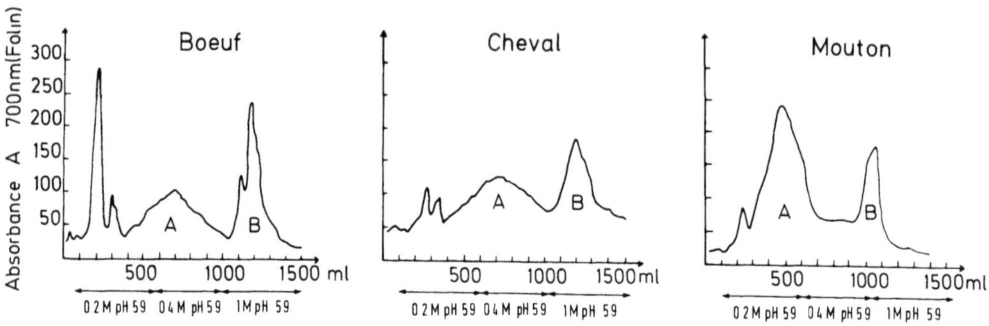

Fig. 5. Purification of MSEL-neurophysins *(Peak A)* by ion-exchange chromatography on Diethylaminoethyl-Sephadex-A-50 (cf. Fig. 4)

MSEL- NEUROPHYSINS

Ovine: [1] Ala-Met-Ser-Asp-[5] Leu-Glu-Leu-Arg-Gln-[10] Cys-Leu-Pro-Cys-Gly-[15] Pro-Gly-Gly-Lys-Gly-[20] Arg-Cys-Phe-Gly-Pro-[25] Ser
Bovine: ———
Porcine: ———

Ovine: [26] Ile-Cys-Cys-Gly-[30] Asp-Glu-Leu-Gly-Cys-[35] Phe-Val-Gly-Thr-Ala-[40] Glu-Ala-Leu-Arg-Cys-[45] Gln-Glu-Glu-[48] Ile-Tyr-[50] Leu
Bovine: ——— -Asn- ———
Porcine: ——— -Asn- ———

Ovine: [51] Pro-Ser-Pro-Cys-[55] Gln-Ser-Gly-Gln-Lys-[60] Pro-Cys-Gly-Ser-Gly-[65] Gly-Arg-Cys-Ala-Ala-[70] Ala-Gly-Ile-Cys-Cys-[75] Asn
Bovine: ———
Porcine: ———

Ovine: [76] Asp-Glu-Ser-Cys-[80] Val-Thr-Glu-Pro-Glu-[85] Cys-Arg-Glu-Gly-[89] Ile-[90] Gly-Phe-[92] Pro Arg-Arg-[95] Val
Bovine: ——— -Ile- / -Val- ———
Porcine: ——— -Ala-Ser- — -Leu- ——— -Ala

Fig. 6. Amino-acid sequences of ovine, bovine, and porcine MSEL-neurophysins

allow us to order the tryptic fragments so that a single amino-acid sequence has been determined for the three molecules (CHAUVET et al., 1975a, 1976) (Fig. 6).

Our amino-acid sequence of bovine MSEL-neurophysin, although considerably different from the one published previously under the name neurophysin-II (WALTER et al., 1971), has recently been completely confirmed (WUU and CRUMM, 1976b). Our sequence of porcine MSEL-neurophysin is in agreement with that proposed by WUU et al. (1971, also, WUU and CRUMM, 1976a), so that these structures can now be regarded as well established.

The general pattern of MSEL-neurophysin is that of a 95-residue polypeptide chain. In the three species, the 14 cysteine residues are in the same positions, so it can be assumed that the seven disulfide bridges are identical. In fact there are very few differences: a single substitution between sheep and ox in position 48, and five substitutions between sheep and pig in positions 48, 89, 92, and 95. Apparently variations occur mainly in the C-terminal part of the molecule. It may be recalled that the three species belong to the same mammalian order, Artiodactyla, and that sheep and ox belong to the suborder Ruminantia, while pig belongs to the suborder Suiformes.

The structural studies on the second family, VLDV-neurophysins, have progressed much more slowly because the amount seems lower and the molecule is less stable. So far, only N-terminal sequences have been published. From the results presented by WUU and CRUMM (1973), the VLDV-neurophysin of the pig could differ by 17 residues from MSEL-neurophysin of the same species, so the two molecules clearly belong to two distinct phylogenetic lines.

C. Biologic Relationships Between Neurohypophyseal Hormones and Neurophysins

A considerable amount of work has been carried out on the relationships between neurohypophyseal hormones and neurophysins. They deal with the possible existence of a common precursor and with the carrier hypothesis. I shall briefly examine these two aspects.

I. The Possible Biosynthetic Common Precursor

Recent studies on peptide hormones have shown that most of them are manufactured as larger prohormones, that means as a polypeptide chain that is cleaved before secretion into an active shorter peptide and an inactive fragment. For instance, proinsulin, proparathormone, and progastrin have been isolated. It seems reasonable to assume that oxytocin and vasopressin are primarily synthesized as larger molecules. Are neurophysins fragments of these larger molecules? The evidence for this conception is up to now only indirect and consists in cytologic and biochemical data.

It has long been known that the so-called neurosecretory material found in granules of paraventricular or supraoptic neurons gave specific staining reactions such as Bargman-Gomori's chrome-hematoxylin or Sloper's performic acid alcian blue, and could be identified with cystine-rich proteins and possibly with neurophysins. More recent studies, particularly with immunofluorescence (HOPE and PICKUP, 1974) or immunoperoxidase (SOKOL et al., 1976) techniques have shown the presence of neurophysin-like material in cell bodies of magnocellular neurons in paraventricular and supraoptic nuclei. According to HOPE and PICKUP (1974), the immunofluorescent material follows a path from the hypothalamus to the posterior pituitary gland, which is identical to the path followed by the peptide hormones.

According to SOKOL et al. (1976), in Brattleboro rats, which suffer "diabetes insipidus" because they lack arginine vasopressin, about half of the magnocellular neurons in the supraoptic and paraventricular nuclei were devoid both of immunoperoxidase-reactive neurophysin and vasopressin. On the other hand, PICKERING et al. (1975) have observed that in homozygote Brattleboro rats, one of the three neurophysin components detected in normal rats by polyacrylamide-gel electrophoresis is absent and have deduced that this neurophysin (neurophysin A) is biosynthetically related to vasopressin. Because the dual disappearance of vasopressin and a neurophysin seems to correspond to a single gene mutation and occurs in homozygotes, this finding gives support from a genetic standpoint to the common precursor thesis.

SACHS and TAKABATAKE (1964) have tried to prove that vasopressin is biosynthesized as a large molecule, possibly a protein, by using a pulse-chase technique with infusion of ^{35}S-cysteine into the third ventricle of dogs. After 1.5 h, a labeled protein was observed in the hypothalamic median eminence but no labeled vasopressin; puromycin was added to stop the protein synthesis. After an additional 4.5 h labeled vasopressin was present, probably arising through cleavage of the labeled protein. Chemical (molecular weight, electrophoretic migration) and immunologic properties of the labeled protein seem similar to those of neurophysins. Because neurohypophyseal hormones and neurophysins were identified in the neurosecretory granules of the ox posterior pituitary gland (DEAN and HOPE, 1968; HOPE and PICKUP, 1974), it appears very likely that the biosyntheses of both substances are closely related. So far, however, the possible common precursors have not been isolated and characterized.

II. The Possible Role of Carrier for Neurophysins

It may be observed that each type of neurophysin isolated from ox or pig displays virtually the same binding affinity for oxytocin or vasopressin ($K_D = 1 \times 10^{-4}$ *M* at pH 7.4) and is also able to bind neurohypophyseal hormones from lower vertebrates (BRESLOW, 1974; ACHER, 1976). Therefore, there is apparently no specificity in the binding *within* the neurohypophyseal hormone family. This fact does not eliminate a possible role of carrier, but merely indicates that this function is not highly specialized. The role of neurophysins might be to prevent the diffusion of the small hormones outside the granules during the transport and before secretion through exocytosis.

BRESLOW and co-workers (1974) have shown that the first three amino-acid residues of the peptide hormone are involved in the binding, and have used synthetic tripeptides for determining the number of binding sites on neurophysins. From NMR and CD studies, they have concluded that each mole of neurophysin can bind one mole of peptide hormone, and that the single tyrosine of the protein is moving during the association. However, the hormone-bindung site of neurophysins has not yet been located and we must await X-ray studies on the complex to determine the three-dimensional structure of the association.

III. Ontogeny of Neurohypophyseal Hormones and of Neurophysins

A last point that one should consider in a report on evolution of neurohypophyseal peptides and proteins is the ontogeny of the molecules. "Haeckel's Law," based on morphologic data, claims that ontogenesis recapitulates phylogenesis. If this law is true at the molecular level, fetal proteins of mammals should be more similar to homologous proteins from lower vertebrates than the adult ones.

A study both of neurohypophyseal hormones and neurophysins may shed some light on their biologic relationships. We have looked for arginine vasotocin, a nonmammalian hormone, in bovine fetus either at the age of 7-9 months or at the age of 4-5 months, and we have not found this primitive hormone. However, VIZSOLYI and PERKS (1969) have isolated and characterized arginine vasotocin from the posterior pituitary gland of the sheep and the seal at midgestation. On the other hand, PAVEL and collaborators (MILCU et al., 1963) have presented data suggesting that arginine vasotocin is present in the pineal gland of adult mammals. Therefore, it seems that the biosynthesis of this hormone remains active in adults in some nerve tissues other than the hypothalamus. PAVEL (1971) has suggested that pineal arginine vasotocin may be elaborated by secretory ependymal cells, regarded as the most primitive secretory cells of the brain.

We have also recently investigated fetal-bovine neurophysins (CHAUVET et al., 1975b). Bovine MSEL-neurophysin of fetuses at the age of 7-9 months has been purified. Apparently at this stage of development, MSEL-neurophysin is largely dominant, as is arginine vasopressin when compared with oxytocin. We have characterized fetal MSEL-neurophysin and found that the amino-acid sequence is identical with that of adult MSEL-neurophysin. This finding might be taken as an indirect argument for the common precursor, since the variation of the amount of arginine vasopressin seems always parallel with that of the same MSEL-neurophysin.

Further data, especially on neurophysins from lower vertebrates, are necessary to show the parallel evolution of neurohypophyseal hormones and neurophysins, and perhaps to discover the evolution of their precursors.

References

ACHER, R.: Chemistry of the neurohypophysial hormones: an example of molecular evolution. Handbook of Physiology. Sect. 7. Endocrinology. Washington, D.C.: American Physiol. Soc. 1974, part 1, pp. 119-130

ACHER, R.: Les neurophysines. Aspects moléculaires et cellulaires. Biochimie 58, 895-911 (1976)

ACHER, R., CHAUVET, J., OLIVRY, G.: Sur l'existence éventuelle d'une hormone unique neurohypophysaire. I. Relations entre l'ocytocine, la vasopressine et la protéine de Van Dyke extraites de la neurohypophyse du boeuf. Biochim. Biophys. Acta 22, 421-427 (1956)

ACHER, R., LIGHT, A., VIGNEAUD, V. du: Purification of oxytocin and vasopressin by way of a protein complex. J. Biol. Chem. 233, 116-120 (1958)

ACHER, R., MANOUSSOS, G., OLIVRY, G.: Sur les relations entre l'ocytocine et la vasopressine d'une part et la protêine de Van Dyke d'autre part. Biochim. Biophys. Acta 16, 155-156 (1955)

BRESLOW, E.: The neurophysins. Adv. Enzymol. 40, 271-333 (1974)

CHAUVET, M.T., CHAUVET, J., ACHER, R.: The complete amino acid sequence of the major ovine neurophysin (MSEL-neurophysin); comparison with a reinvestigated bovine MSEL-neurophysin. FEBS Lett. 58, 234-237 (1975a)

CHAUVET, M.T., CHAUVET, J., ACHER, R.: Foetal bovine MSEL-neurophysin: comparison with adult homologous neurophysin. FEBS Lett. 62, 89-92 (1975b)

CHAUVET, M.T., CHAUVET, J., ACHER, R.: The neurohypophysial hormone-binding proteins: complete amino-acid sequence of ovine and bovine MSEL-neurophysins. Eur. J. Biochem. 69, 475-485 (1976a)

CHAUVET, M.T., COFFE, G., CHAUVET, J., ACHER, R.: On the biological significance of neurophysins: presence of a major neurophysin in the sheep. FEBS Lett. 53, 331-333 (1975)

CHAUVET, M.T., COFFE, G., CHAUVET, J., ACHER, R.: Les neurophysines des Mammifêres: êvolution et signification biologique. C. R. Soc. Biol. 170, 257-268 (1976)

CHAUVET, J., LENCI, M.T., ACHER, R.: L'ocytocine et la vasopressine du mouton: reconstitution d'un complexe hormonal actif. Biochim. Biophys. Acta 38, 266-272 (1960)

DEAN, C.R., HOPE, D.B.: The isolation of neurophysin-I and -II from bovine pituitary neurosecretory granules separated on a large scale from other subcellular organelles. Biochem. J. 106, 565-573 (1968)

HOPE, D.B., PICKUP, J.C.: Neurophysins. Handbook of Physiology, Sect. 7. Endocrinology. Washington, D.C.: American Physiol. Soc. 1974, Vol. IV, part 1, pp. 173-189

MILCU, S.M., PAVEL, S., NEACSU, C.: Biological and chromatographic characterization of a polypeptide with pressor and oxytocic activities isolated from bovine pineal gland. Endocrinology 72, 563-566 (1963)

PAVEL, S.: Evidence for the ependymal origin of arginine vasotocin in the bovine pineal gland. Endocrinology 89, 613-614 (1971)

PICKERING, B.T., HELLER, H.: Oxytocin as a neurohypophysial hormone in the holocephalian elasmobranch fish, *Hydrolagus collei*. J. Endocrinol. 45, 597-606 (1969)

PICKERING, B.T., JONES, C.W., BURFORD, G.D., McPHERSON, M., SWANN, R.W., HEAP, P.F., MORRIS, J.F.: The role of neurophysin proteins: suggestions from the study of their transport and turnover. Ann. N.Y. Acad. Sci. 248, 15-35 (1975)

SACHS, H., TAKABATAKE, Y.: Evidence for a precursor in vasopressin biosynthesis. Endocrinology 75, 943-948 (1964)

SOKOL, H.W., ZIMMERMAN, E.A., SAWYER, W.H., ROBINSON, A.G.: The hypothalamic-neurohypophysial system of the rat: localization and quantitation of neurophysin by light microscopic immunocytochemistry in normal rats and in Brattleboro rats deficient in vasopressin and a neurophysin. Endocrinology 98, 1176-1188 (1976)

VIZSOLYI, E., PERKS, A.M.: New neurohypophysial principle in foetal mammals. Nature 223, 1169-1171 (1969)

WALTER, R., SCHLESINGER, D.H., SCHWARTZ, I.L., CAPRA, J.D.: Complete amino acid sequence of bovine neurophysin-II. Biochem. Biophys. Res. Commun. 44, 293-298 (1971)

WATKINS, W.B.: The isolation and biochemical characterization of three neurophysins of the sheep. J. Endocrinol. 59, 17-29 (1973)

WUU, T.C., CRUMM, S.E.: Amino acid sequence of porcine neurophysin-II. 9th Int. Congr. Biochem., Stockholm, 1973, Abstract Db 9

WUU, T.C., CRUMM, S.E.: Characterization of porcine neurophysin-III. Its resemblance and possible relationship to porcine neurophysin-I. J. Biol. Chem. 251, 2735-2739 (1976a)

WUU, T.C., CRUMM, S.E.: Amino acid sequence of bovine neurophysin-II: a reinvestigation. Biochem. Biophys. Res. Commun. 68, 634-639 (1976b)

WUU, T.C., CRUMM, S.E., SAFFRAN, M.: Amino acid sequence of porcine neurophysin-I. J. Biol. Chem. 246, 6043-6063 (1971)

Morphofunctional Evolution of the Neurohemal Regions of the Hypothalamo-Hypophyseal System

M. A. BELENKY

Laboratory of Neuroendocrinology, Sechenov Institute of Evolutionary Physiology and Biochemistry, Academy of Sciences of the USSR, Leningrad, USSR

The aim of the present report is to anylyze the structural and functional evolution of the median eminence (ME) and the neural lobe (NL), with special reference to lower vertebrates since it is evident that the development of neuroendocrine control mechanisms can be more easily studied in these species. Though numerous papers deal with the structure and ultrastructure of both neurohemal zones, few of them are primarily concerned with the comparative morphologic analysis of these organs (WINGSTRAND, 1966; POLENOV, 1968a,b; KOBAYASHI et al., 1970; RODRÍGUEZ, 1971; RODRÍGUEZ and GIMENEZ, 1972; POLENOV and BELENKY, 1973). For more complete references see POLENOV and BELENKY (1973).

In Cyclostomata (*Lampetra fluviatilis* L.) the ME is rather small and occupies the rostral region of the floor of the third ventricle. Three zones can be recognized: an ependymal (tanycyte) zone, an internal zone, containing the fibers of the hypothalamo-hypophyseal tract, and an external zone (EZ). The latter usually contains a small amount of paraldehyde-fuchsin positive (PAF+) material. A weak monoamine fluorescence has been seen in the EZ with the use of Falck's technique (TSUNEKI et al., 1975).

Three types of nerve fibers and their terminals are present in the ME (Fig. 1). Peptidergic A_1 and A_2 types have granules 120-180 nm and 100-160 nm in diameter, respectively. Monoaminergic fibers have granules up to 100 nm in diameter. A_2 fibers predominate in the EZ of the lamprey ME. There are few B-type fibers (Fig. 2). Different types of nerve terminals and tanycyte vascular "endfeet" make contact with a dense connective-tissue layer located between the brain surface and the hypophyseal pars distalis (PD). The lamprey ME lacks a primary portal plexus (TSUNEKI and GORBMAN, 1975, and our personal observations). The capillaries supplying the PD are seen just under the connective-tissue layer. They also surround the cords of glandular cells. It is suggested that both peptide and monoamine neurohormones may diffuse through the connective-tissue layer and affect the function of the PD. It seems likely that the secondary capillary plexus supplying the PD arises earlier in evolution than the primary portal capillaries abutting the brain surface. The stroma of the lamprey ME is probably formed exclusively by tanycytes.

In Elasmobranchii and Chondrosteoidei the extent of the axo-vascular contact region in the ME increases, mainly due to the greater size of this organ. Deep invaginations of the contact surface are seen only in the Elasmobranchii ME (POLENOV, 1968b; KNOWLES et al., 1975). These two groups of fishes, as well as Polypteridae and Holostei, have a distinct portal circulation

(WINGSTRAND, 1966), although their portal system is primitive. It lacks capillary loops, the so-called "intervascular channels" (KNOWLES, 1965) etc.

In Chondrosteoidei (*Acipenser güldenstädti* Brandt and *A. ruthenus* L.) the percentage of B-type terminals increases and that of A_1 terminals decreases, compared to the lamprey ME (Fig. 2). Few pituicytes are seen in the ME of these species.

The teleostean (*Cyprinus carpio* L.) neurohypophysis-PD complex shows signs of great secondary specialization. There is no typical vascular-portal system that connects the hypothalamus to the PD. Numerous A_1-, A_2-, and B-type terminals are separated from the glandular cells of the PD by relatively thin connective-tissue septa connected with the pericapillary spaces of vessels supplying this complex. Some terminals, mainly of A_1 and A_2 types, make contact with these capillaries. Direct synaptoid axoadenohypophyseal cell contacts are few. The percentage of B-type terminals is rather high, especially in the rostral PD (proadenohypophysis), while monoaminergic fibers appear to be relatively few in the PD, using Falck's technique (see KONSTANTINOVA, 1976). It seems likely that in Teleostei the neurohypophyseal roots penetrating the PD are a functional equivalent of the ME of other vertebrate species.

Beginning with Amphibia, particularly the anuran species (*Rana temporaria* L.), the extended zone of the axovascular contacts is mainly due to numerous capillary loops and intervascular channels deeply penetrating the EZ of the ME. The percentage of B-type terminals in the EZ of the frog ME increases, compared to that of homologous organs in fishes. These changes are more distinct in mammals. Although the percentage of monoaminergic terminals has not been established in these species, at least 35-40% of all terminals in the EZ of the albino rat and mouse belong to type B, i.e., they are probably of a monoaminergic nature (AJIKA and HÖKFELT, 1973, and personal observations). The number of pituicytes in mammals is much larger, especially in the region of the hypothalamohypophyseal tract.

The NL-intermediate lobe (IL) complex originates earlier in evolution or at least outstrips the ME in its development. In lampreys the NL occupies the main part of the floor of the recessus infundibuli. Three zones similar to those in the ME can be recognized in the NL (Fig. 1). Two types of peptidergic fibers (types A_1 and A_2) and monoaminergic B-type fibers have been revealed in the NL. The granules in the peptidergic terminals of the NL are somewhat larger than those in the ME of the same species. A_2 terminals are the most frequent in the lamprey NL. B-type and especially A_1-type fibers are few. All nerve terminals and tanycyte-vascular endfeet are in contact with the connective-tissue septa separating the NL and the IL. Numerous capillaries of the regular circulation are located there. It seems likely that both peptide and monoamine neurohormones may be discharged from the nerve terminals into these blood vessels. Some of the neurohormones probably diffuse through the connective tissue septa that regulate the function of the IL glandular cells. Mostly tanycytes are seen in the lamprey NL; pituicytes are extremely rare.

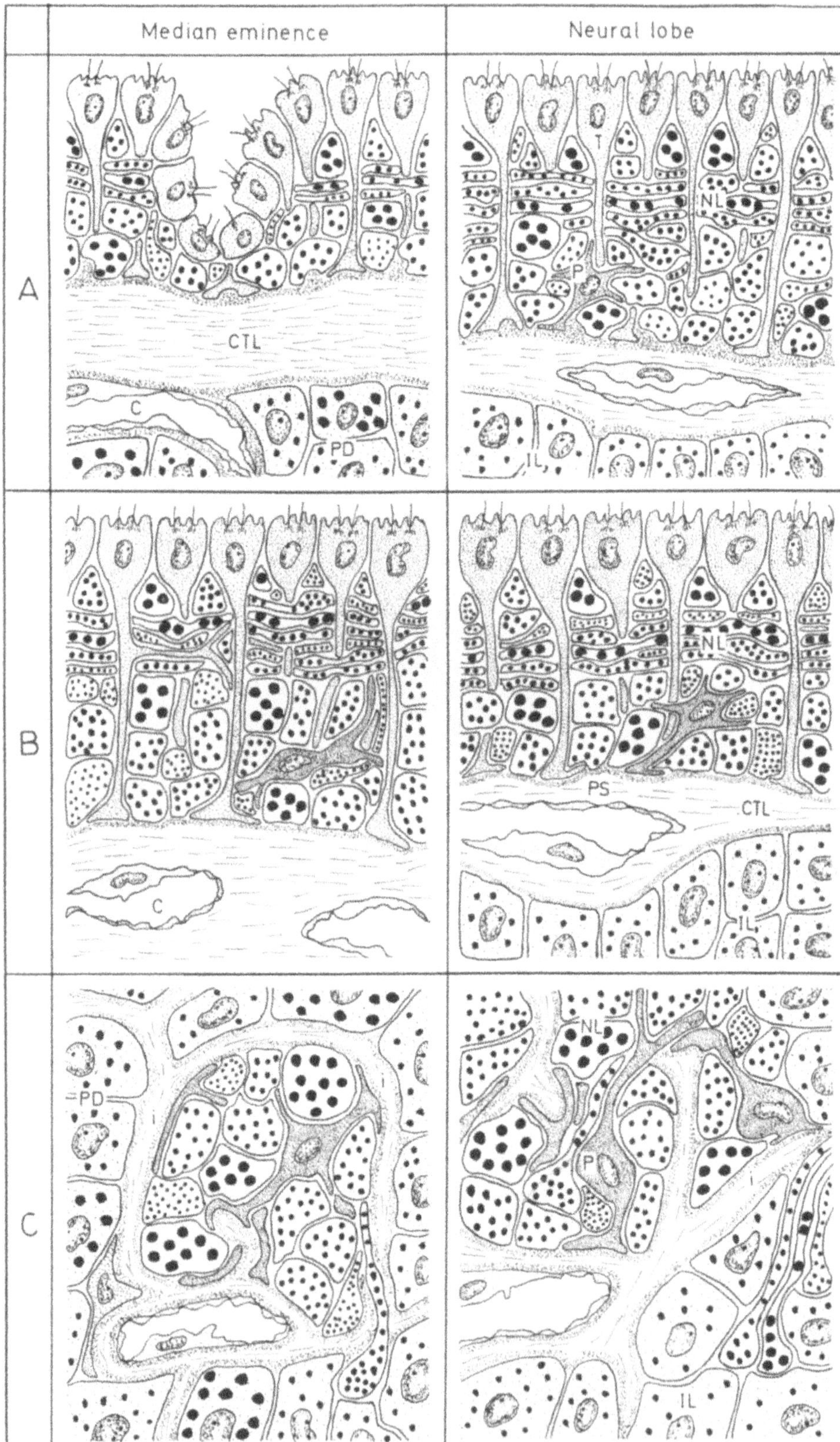
Median eminence
Neural lobe
A
B
C
CTL
C
PD
T
NL
P
IL
PS
i

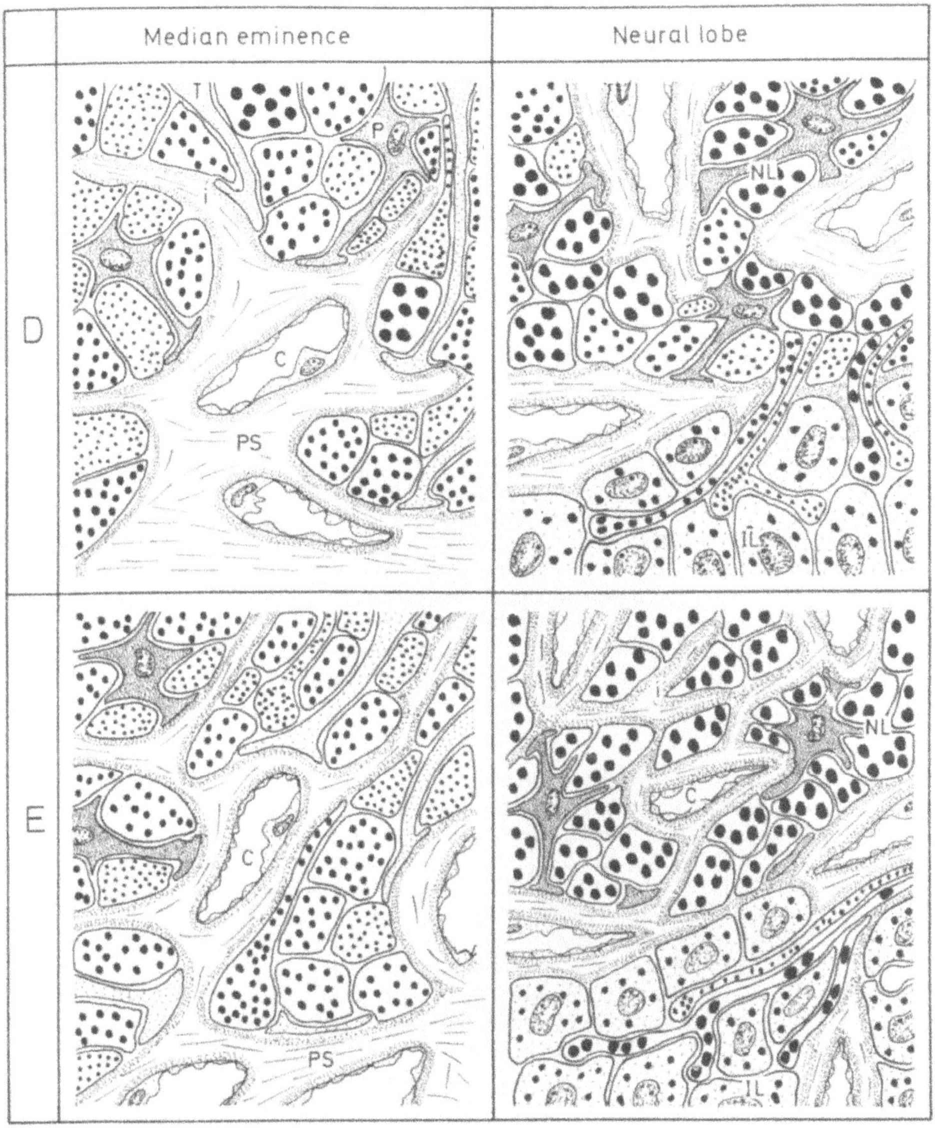

▲
◀ Fig. 1A-E. Diagram of phylogenetic transformations of ME and NL - intermediate lobe complex in Cyclostomata (A), Chondrosteoidei (Acipenseridae) (B), Teleostei (C), Amphibia (D), and Mammalia (E). Modified from POLENOV and BELENKY (1973). ● A_1 fibers, • A_2 fibers, • B fibers, *C* - capillary, *CTL* - connective tissue layer, *i* - intervascular channel, *IL* - intermediate lobe, *NL* - neural lobe, *P* - pituicyte, *PD* - pars distalis, *PS* - pericapillary space, *T* - tanycyte

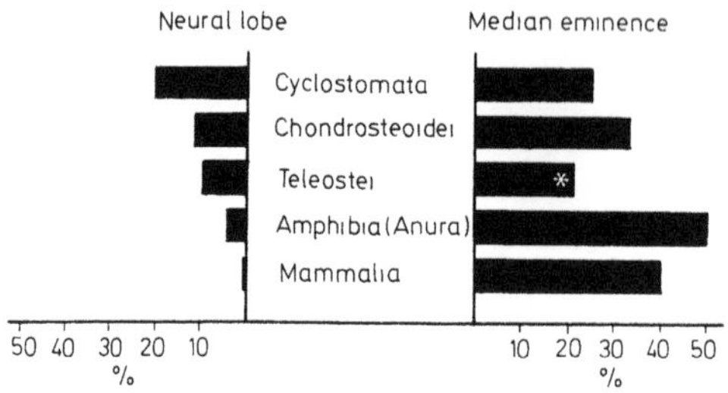

Fig. 2. Percentage of monoaminergic B-type terminals in EZ of ME and NL of different species. * - data from complex neurohypophysis-proximal pars distalis of *C. carpio*

In Elasmobranchii numerous peptidergic and monoaminergic fibers grow into the IL and make direct synaptoid contact with the glandular cells. This is probably due to high idioadaptive-type secondary specialization. Some neurosecretory terminals are in contact with the blood capillaries (POLENOV, 1968a,b). Although Acipenseridae (Chondrosteoidei) occupy a higher evolutionary position than Elasmobranchii, they probably have a close relation to the main trunk of the vertebrate phylogenetic tree. Their NL-IL complex retains the same general mode of structural organization as that of Cyclostomata. The extent of the axovascular contact zone increases in these fish, due exclusively to numerous tubular roots deeply penetrating the IL. In the NL of Acipenseridae the percentage of A_1 terminals is distinctly higher, and B-type terminals are less frequent than in the lamprey NL. Pituicytes are rather frequent, their cytoplasm contains many fibrils.

The roots of the neurohypophysis penetrate the IL (meta-adenohypophysis) of teleostean fishes. Numerous A_1 and A_2 terminals and only a few B-type terminals make contact with the blood capillaries of the regular circulation, whereas all types of terminals form direct synaptoid axoadenohypophyseal contacts with the glandular cells of the IL. Some nerve terminals are separated from the glandular cells by connective-tissue septa, basement membrane and/or pituicyte processes. The blood capillaries usually accompany the roots of the NL and strongly developed intervascular channels penetrate deeply into both NL and IL parenchyma. Numerous pituicytes contain many fibrils. Distinct desmosomes are frequently seen between the pituicyte processes (KORNIENKO and BELENKY, 1976).

In amphibians, anuran species in particular, the NL represents a solid structure penetrated by a network of wide capillaries and intervascular channels. Axovascular contacts are formed mainly by A_1-type peptidergic terminals. Monoaminergic fibers are more frequent near the IL. Some peptidergic and monoaminergic fibers pass into the IL and reach the glandular cells.

In mammals the extent of axovascular contacts increases due to a three-dimensional capillary network and numerous intervascular channels penetrating the NL. Peptidergic elements in the NL of the mouse and rat belong to type A_1. The NL of these species contain only few B-type terminals. These terminals are mainly seen on the border with the IL, and together with A_1 fibers in the latter.

From the present data it is evident that in the course of evolution the percentage of monoaminergic terminals increases in the EZ of the ME and decreases in the NL (Fig. 2). Monoaminergic terminals are concentrated in two main regions: in the EZ of the ME and on the border between the NL and IL and/or in the latter. It seems likely that this position of monoaminergic elements is due to their role in the dual peptidergic and monoaminergic regulation of functions of the hypophyseal PD and IL (POLENOV, 1970; POLENOV and BELENKY, 1973; POLENOV, 1977, in this volume). On the other hand, the percentage of A_2 terminals increases in the ME. An opposite correlation has been revealed in the NL. Thus, only one morphologic type of peptidergic terminal is seen in both the EZ of the ME (type A_1) and the NL (type A_2) of mammals.

Both peptidergic and monoaminergic fibers, even in Cyclostomata, have the main ultrastructural signs characteristic of higher vertebrates. The mode of discharge of peptide and monoamine neurohormones is probably similar in different species.

The concentration of synaptic vesicles near the "active" zones in the sites of contact between the nerve terminals and both pituicytes and tanycytes in the ME and NL has been described by many authors. It seems likely that these pictures mainly reflect the release of neurohormones. These active contacts are especially prominent in species such as Cyclostomata, Acipenseridae, etc., with a limited extent of the zone of direct axovascular contacts (without neuroglial cuffs). The quantity of peptide and monoamine neurohormones being discharged directly into the pericapillary space increases in the course of evolution. The possibility cannot be excluded, however, that the active zones at the sites of neuroglial junctions represent the signs of innervation of these auxiliary elements.

Distinct pictures of recapitulation of the ancestral features have been revealed in the early ontogenesis of different species, *R. temporaria* in particular. One can mention, for example, the low percentage of monoaminergic fibers in the EZ of the ME, superficial position of the primary portal vessels, lack of capillary loops and intervascular channels, etc. As in phylogeny, so also during early ontogeny the NL develops faster than the ME. The NL is relatively quickly separated from the floor of the third ventricle and reaches its definitive structural organization. On the other hand, the ME develops rapidly only during frog metamorphosis (BELENKY et al., 1973). In the course of evolution the NL is gradually segregated from the floor of the third ventricle, and in many species the NL lacks a direct connection with the brain ventricle. The NL resembles typical endocrine organs with respect to its structural organization and arrangement of the blood vessels and auxiliary neuroglial elements. On the other hand, the ME retains the simple (primitive) three-layered structure characteristic of the primary neurohemal contact region in the floor of the third ventricle.

Thus, the progressive divergence and development leading to the specialization of functions of both neurohemal regions have been revealed in phylogenesis and ontogenesis. The evolutionary transformations in the NL and the ME are primarily concerned with the changes in the percentages of different nerve terminals, the complication of the blood-supply system, the increased extent of the neurovascular contact region, and the differentiation of the auxiliary neuroglial elements.

References

AJIKA, K., HÖKFELT, T.: Ultrastructural identification of catecholamine neurones in the hypothalamic periventricular-arcuate nucleus-median eminence complex with special reference to quantitative aspects. Brain Res. 57, 97-117 (1973)

BELENKY, M.A., CHETVERUKHIN, V.K., POLENOV, A.L.: The hypothalamo-hypophysial system of the frog *Rana temporaria*. II. Functional morphology of the external zone of the median eminence during metamorphosis. Gen. Comp. Endocrinol. 21, 250-261 (1973)

KNOWLES, F.: Neuroendocrine correlations at the level of ultrastructure. Arch. Anat. Microsc. Morphol. Exp. 54, 343-358 (1965)

KNOWLES, F., VOLLRATH, L., MEURLING, P.: Cytology and neuroendocrine relations of the pituitary of the dogfish, *Scyliorhinus canicula*. Proc. R. Soc. Med. 191, 507-525 (1975)

KOBAYASHI, H., MATSUI, T., ISHII, S.: Functional electron microscopy of the hypothalamic median eminence. Int. Rev. Cytol. 29, 281-381 (1970)

KONSTANTINOVA, M.S.: Distribution of monoamines in the hypothalamus and hypophysis of the carp *Cyprinus carpio*. J. Evol. Biochem. Physiol. (Leningrad) 12, 192-193 (1976)

KORNIENKO, G.G., BELENKY, M.A.: The ultrastructure of the neurohypophysis-metaadenohypophysis complex in sazan females before spawning. (In Russian). Tsitologiia 18, 1205-1212 (1976)

POLENOV, A.L.: Hypothalamic Neurosecretion. (In Russian). Leningrad: Nauka 1968a

POLENOV, A.L.: On the evolution of the median eminence - the proximal neurosecretory contact region in some fishes (Elasmobranchii, Chondrosteoidei). Arch. Anat. Histol. Embryol. Norm. Exp. 51, 553-561 (1968b)

POLENOV, A.L.: Morpho-functional foundations of neurosecretory (peptidergic) and adrenergic regulating mechanisms of the hypothalamus. In: Proceedings of the XIth All-Union Congress of I.P. Pavlov Physiological Society (in Russian). CHERNIGOVSKY, V.N. (ed.). Leningrad: Nauka 1970, Vol. I, pp. 311-315

POLENOV, A.L.: Evolutionary basis of a general principle of neuroendocrine regulation - interaction of peptide and monoamine neurohormones (a dual control). This volume, pp. 15-30

POLENOV, A.L., BELENKY, M.A.: Some regularities of the development of neurohemal parts of the hypothalamo-hypophysial neurosecretory system in onto- and phylogenesis of vertebrates. J. Evol. Biochem. Physiol. (Leningrad) 9, 355-363 (1973)

RODRÍGUEZ, E.M.: The comparative morphology of neural lobes of species with different neurohypophysial hormones. In: Subcellular Organization and Function in Endocrine Tissues. HELLER, H., LEDERIS, K. (eds.). Cambridge: University Press 1971, pp. 263-291

RODRÍGUEZ, E.M., GIMENEZ, A.: Comparative aspects of nervous control of pars intermedia. Gen. Comp. Endocrinol. 3, 97-107 (1972)
TSUNEKI, K., GORBMAN, A.: Ultrastructure of the anterior neurohypophysis and the pars distalis of the lamprey, *Lampetra tridentata*. Gen. Comp. Endocrinol. 25, 487-508 (1975)
TSUNEKI, K., KOBAYASHI, H., YANAGISAWA, M., BANDO, T.: Histochemical distribution of monoamines in the hypothalamo-hypophysial region of the lamprey, *Lampetra japonica*. Cell Tissue Res. 161, 25-32 (1975)
WINGSTRAND, K.G.: Comparative anatomy and evolution of the hypophysis. In: The Pituitary Gland. HARRIS, G.W., DONOVAN, B.T. (eds.). London: Butterworths 1966, pp. 58-126

Monoaminergic Structures Within the Hypothalamo-Hypophyseal Complex in the Phylogenesis of Vertebrates

M. S. KONSTANTINOVA

Laboratory of Neuroendocrinology, Sechenov Institute of Evolutionary Physiology and Biochemistry, Academy of Sciences of the USSR, Leningrad, USSR

The morphology and the functional significance of monoaminergic (MA) structures within the hypothalamohypophyseal complex of vertebrates have recently been extensively studied by the Falck-Hillarp technique.

An accumulation of MA bipolar nerve cells making direct contact with the cerebrospinal fluid (CSF) via their dendrites and containing dopamine (DA), noradrenaline (NA), and serotonin (5-HT) occurs in the hypothalamic ventricular wall in all nonmammalian types (VIGH, 1971; KONSTANTINOVA, 1973, 1975). The most developed system of these MA CSF-contacting nerve cells has been found in cyclostomes and fish (BAUMGARTEN, 1972; KONSTANTINOVA, 1973). This system is reduced in amphibians, reptiles, and birds, and is absent in mammals (BAUMGARTEN, 1972). Both sensory and secretory functions of MA CSF-contacting nerve cells have been suggested (VIGH, 1971; BAUMGARTEN, 1972). The release of monoamines into the CSF via dendrites and via axons in the region of their terminals could be supposed. In the hypothalamus of mammals four groups of MA nerve cells, having no direct contact with the CSF, are located in the periventricular region (1) in rostral and middle hypothalamus, (2) in the arcuate nucleus, (3) in dorsal, and (4) in caudal hypothalamic areas (BJÖRKLUND and NOBIN, 1973). MA nerve cells the axons of which terminate in neurohemal organs (SCHARRER, 1969), making typical axovascular contacts with capillaries of the portal system and common circulation, and axoglandular contacts with endocrine cells of intermediate lobe (IL) (BARGMANN et al., 1976; POLENOV, 1970), should be called neurosecretory cells, which produce their effect via neurohormones (the arcuate nucleus, the system of MA CSF-contacting nerve cells).

In the hypothalamus DA, NA, and 5-HT terminals have been discovered near the capillaries in the median eminence (ME) in mammals (BJÖRKLUND et al., 1973) and in the structures homologous to the ME in lower vertebrates (POLENOV et al., 1976). Monoamines as well as peptide neurohormones are probably released from the ME into the blood of the portal vessels and may regulate the function of the anterior hypophysis (POLENOV, 1970). Axovascular contacts of MA terminals in the neural lobe (NL) are especially developed in cyclostomes and ancient fish. The release of MA from the MA terminals into the capillaries connected with the common circulation has been postulated (POLENOV et al., 1972, 1976).

Indirect axoglandular contacts of MA terminals with endocrine cells in IL of cyclostomes and chondrostei, and axoglandular synaptoid contacts in IL of elasmobranchs, teleosts, and tetra-

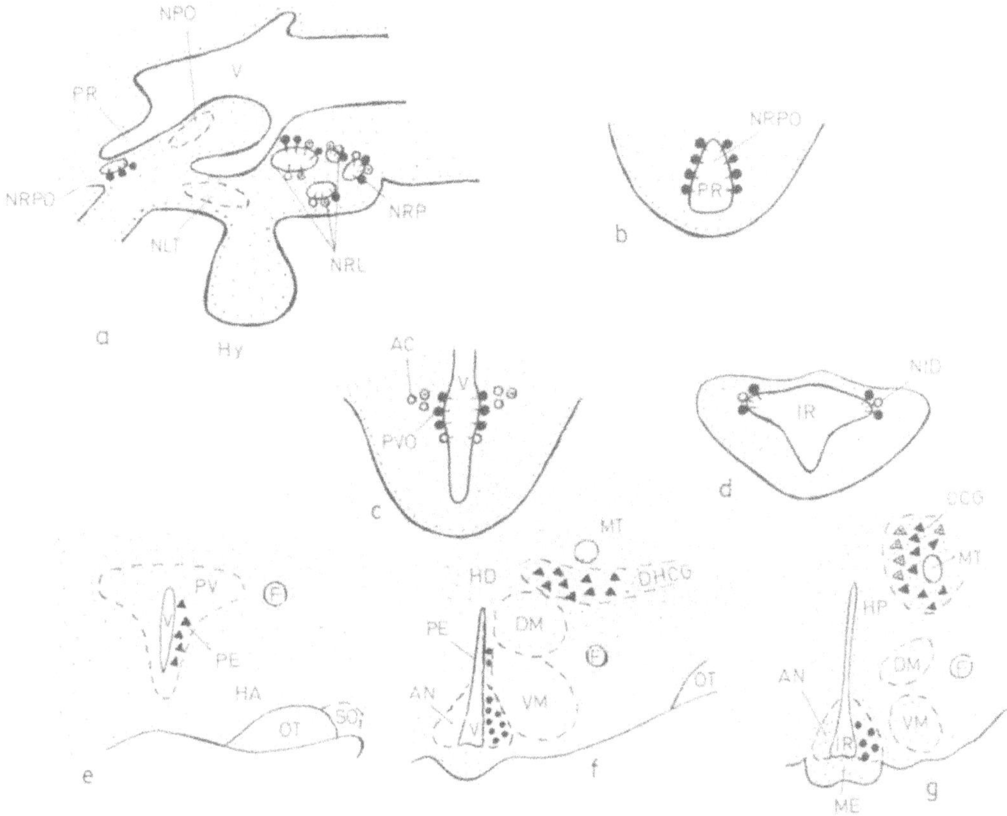

Fig. 1a-g. Schematic drawing of distribution of hypothalamic monoamine cell bodies in vertebrates. a) in teleosts, modified from EKENGREN (1975); b-d) in amphibians, modified from VAN OORDT et al. (1974); e-g) in mammals, modified from BJÖRKLUND and NOBIN (1973). Terms: *NRPO* - nucleus recessus preopticus, *NPO* - nucleus preopticus, *NLT* - nucleus lateralis tuberis, *Hy* - hypophysis, *NRL* - nucleus recessus lateralis, *NRP* - nucleus recessus posterioris, *PR* - preoptic recess, *PVO* - paraventricular organ, *AC-PVO* - accompanying cells, *V* - third ventricle, *IR* - infundibular recess, *NID* - nucleus infundibularis dorsalis, *PE* - periventricular nucleus, *PV* - paraventricular nucleus, *F* - fornix, *HA* - anterior hypothalamic area, *OT* - optic tract, *SO* - supraoptic nucleus, *AN* - arcuate nucleus, *ME* - median eminence, *VM* - ventromedial nucleus, *DM* - dorsomedial nucleus, *HD* - dorsal hypothalamic area, *MT* - mamillothalamic tract, *DHGG* - dorsal hypothalamic cell group, *HP* - posterior hypothalamic area, *CCG* - caudal cell group, *NSC* - neurosecretory cell, *NC* - nerve cell; *dark circles - DA NSC, open circles - 5-HT NSC, open cored circles - NA NSC, dark triangles - DA NC, open triangles - 5-HT NC, open cored triangles - NA NC*

pods have been found. These probably have an inhibitory effect on the endocrine cells.

The MA innervervation of hypothalamic peptidergic "Gomori-positive" neurosecretory cells (NSC) seems to be relatively poor in lower vertebrates as compared with reptiles, birds, and mammals (KONSTANTINOVA, 1971).

Synapses of a predominantly MA nature have been observed on the perikarya of peptidergic NSC in vertebrates (BARGMANN, 1965; POLENOV and SENCHIK, 1966), where monoamines can act as neurotransmitters with a probable inhibitory effect on the function of peptidergic NSC.

Thus, two kinds of hypothalamic MA NSC have been observed: (1) CSF-contacting MA NSC of an ependymal type and (2) MA NSC of a neuronal type, which are not in direct contact with CSF.

It seems reasonable to suggest that, in the course of the evolution of the hypothalamus, the system of bipolar MA NSC of the ependymal type, contacting the CSF, has been replaced by a system of multipolar MA NSC of the neuronal type with a more specialized and efficient action (Fig. 1).

References

BARGMANN, W.: Über Synapsen im endokrinen System. Nova Acta Leopoldina 30, 173, 199-206 (1965)

BARGMANN, W., LINDNER, E., ANDRES, K.H.: Über Synapsen an endokrinen Epithelzellen und die Definition sekretorischer Neurone. Untersuchungen am Zwischenlappen der Katzenhypophyse. Z. Zellforsch. 77, 282-298 (1967)

BAUMGARTEN, H.G.: Biogenic monoamines in the cyclostome and lower vertebrate brain. Prog. Histochem. Cytochem. 4, 1-90 (1972)

BJÖRKLUND, A., MOORE, R.Y., NOBIN, A., STENEVI, V.: The organization of tubero-hypophyseal and reticulo-infundibular catecholamine neuron system in the rat brain. Brain Res. 51, 171-191 (1973)

BJÖRKLUND, A., NOBIN, A.: Fluorescence histochemical and microspectro-fluorometric mapping of dopamine and noradrenaline cell groups in the rat diencephalon. Brain Res. 51, 193-205 (1973)

EKENGREN, B.: Aminergic nuclei in the hypothalamus of the roach *Leuciscus rutilus*. Cell Tissue Res. 159, 493-502 (1975)

KONSTANTINOVA, M.S.: The distribution of monoamines in the hypothalamus and hypophysis of vertebrates (Review in Russian). J. Evolut. Biochem. Physiol. 7, 213-218 (1971)

KONSTANTINOVA, M.S.: Monoamines in the liquor-contacting nerve cells in the hypothalamus of the lamprey, *Lampetra fluviatilis* L. Z. Zellforsch. 144, 549-557 (1973)

KONSTANTINOVA, M.S.: Monoamines in liquor-contacting nerve cells of the hypothalamus in vertebrates. (Review in Russian). J. Evolut. Biochem. Physiol. 11, 187-190 (1975)

OORDT, P.G.W.J. van, GOOS, H.T.Th., PEUTE, T., TERLOU, M.: Structural and functional aspects of two types of Gomori-negative neurosecretory centres in the caudal hypothalamus of amphibia. In: Neurosecretion - The Final Neuroendocrine Pathway. KNOWLES, F., VOLLRATH, L. (eds.) Berlin-Heidelberg-New York: Springer-Verlag 1974, pp. 182-192

POLENOV, A.L.: Morpho-functional principles of neurosecretory (peptidergic) and adrenergic regulating mechanisms of the hypothalamus. In: Proc. of the XIth All-Union Congr. of Pavlov Physiological Society (in Russian). CHERNIGOVSKY, V.N. (ed.). Leningrad: Nauka 1970, Vol. I, pp. 311-315

POLENOV, A.L., BELENKY, M.A., GARLOV, P.E.: KONSTANTINOVA, M.S.: The hypothalamo-hypophysial system in Acipenseridae. VI. The proximal neurosecretory contact region. Cell Tissue Res. 170, 129-144 (1976)

POLENOV, A.L., GARLOV, P.E., KONSTANTINOVA, M.S., BELENKY, M.A.: The hypothalamo-hypophysial system in Acipenseridae. II. Adrenergic structures of the hypophysial neuro-intermediate complex. Z. Zellforsch. 128, 470-481 (1972)

POLENOV, A.L., SENCHIK, J.I.: Synapses on neurosecretory cells of the supraoptic nucleus in white mice. Nature 211, 1423-1424 (1966)

SCHARRER, B.: Neurohumors and neurohormones: definition and terminolgy. J. Neuro visc. Rel. (Suppl.) 9, 1-20 (1969)

VIGH, B.: Das Paraventricularorgan und das zirkumventriculäre System des Gehirns. Studia Biologica Hungarica. Budapest: Akadémiai Kiadó 1971, Vol. X

Evolution of the Neurosecretory System in Crustacea

E. E. KULAKOVSKI
Zoologic Institute, Academy of Sciences of the USSR, Leningrad, USSR

At present, many data have accumulated that show the important role of the neurosecretory system (NSS) in control of different processes of metabolism, reproduction, sexual differentiation, ontogenetic development, and adaptive change of coloration in Crustacea with different levels of organization. The NSS coordinates intercommunication of different functions. Being functionally plastic, it influences the responses of animals to varying factors in the environment. Problems of neurohormonal control concern the intimate relations between elements of the NSS, their origin, interaction, and place among other integrating organism systems.

The question of evolution of the NSS in Crustacea acquires great importance for further successful study of neurosecretory phenomena in this large taxonomic division. Most of the data concerning the structure and function of the crustacean NSS elements have been obtained in the study of representatives of the subclass Malacostraca. Attempts to identify the NSS of the higher groups of crustaceans with that of the primitive ones without consideration of the phylogenetic development of this structure are very difficult. On the one hand, such a point of view may lead us to erroneous conclusions and, on the other hand, it creates many terminological difficulties. These problems are a serious obstacle in the study of the structure and function of the NSS. In order to remove these contradictions we suggest that the following main stages of the evolution of the NSS of crustaceans be distinguished.

A. The Group of Primitive Crustacea

The principal characteristic feature of the NSS of representatives of this group is the absence of the neuroendocrine complex of sinus gland and X-organ. The NSS is represented only by a number of separate groups of neurosecretory cells (NSC). These cells are located mainly in the supraesophageal ganglia. According to cytomorphologic properties, one may distinguish several types of NSC. The most important in a functional respect are the numerous NSC of the protocerebrum. They are gathered in two groups in the median part of brain. The NSC in each group are in different functional states. A characteristic feature of these NSC is an enlargement along the axons. This is visible at different stages of the neurosecretory cycle. The enlargement is located near the NSC. The collected axons of each group of NSC form the neurosecretory tract extending along the circumesophageal connective tissue. The neurosecretory material passes from the brain along these tracts for further discharge. In the optic ganglia there are no neurosecretory formations that might correspond to the X-organ or to the sinus gland.

B. The Highest Crustacea, Mysidacea

The most important part of the crustacean NSS, the complex of X-organ and sinus gland, first appears in Mysidacea. This complex is located in the eyestalk. It consists of only one group of NSC (X-organ) in the last proximal optic ganglion and the axonal terminals of these cells, which form the neurohemal organ (sinus gland). Along the axons of NSC of the X-organ there are enlargements. These enlargements are located near the sinus gland. Such axonal enlargements are not formed in the sinus gland itself. In the optic ganglia of Mysidacea there are several groups of NSC apart from the X-organ. These NSC have a marked secretory cycle, but they are not connected with the sinus gland. Neurohemal formations other than the sinus gland are absent in this group of Crustacea.

C. The Highest Crustacea, Decapoda

The X-organ-sinus gland complex reaches its maximal development in the most organized representatives of the highest crustaceans. Many different groups of NSC are connected with the sinus gland. They are located not only in the optic ganglia but also in other parts of the CNS. The sinus gland itself becomes larger. The enlarged axonal terminals accumulate within the sinus gland, and accessory neurohemal organs, the pericardial and postcommissural organs, appear.

The development of the crustacean NSS was paralleled by the development of their CNS. In this evolution one may observe the process of complication of the NSS, which consists of the centralization and specialization of its elements. This process is very complicated and many-sided. In each case it has its peculiar features. In our opinion, the general patterns of evolution of the NSS of crustaceans are those discussed and represented in the above schema.

Neurosecretion and Evolution of the Visceral Nervous System in Insects

V. J. A. NOVÁK and I. B. MUSKÓ
Department of Evolutionary Biology, MBÚ ČSAV, Praha, ČSSR and Institute of Biology, MTA, Tihany, Hungary

One of the most important findings in insect neurosecretion has been the discovery of the perisympathetic neurohemal organs in the median visceral system by RAABE (1965, 1966, etc.) and her co-workers (for review see RAABE, 1971; NOVÁK, 1975). Our study of the neurosecretory system in *Gryllotalpa gryllotalpa* L. (MUSKÓ and NOVÁK, 1973, 1976) has suggested a very general character for these organs in insect anatomy and their possible evolution. These questions are given special attention in the present paper.

The perisympathetic organs appear in the form of spindle-shaped thickenings of the transverse branches of the median visceral nerve, which rises from the upper anterior surface of each of the ganglia of the ventral nerve cord in *Gryllotalpa*. The organs contain a phloxinophil Gomori-negative neurosecretion. Histologic examination of the portion of the ganglia mentioned reveals, in each of them, a special group of cells beneath the neural lamella, from which the transverse branches and both the anterior and posterior tracts of the median visceral nerve arise (Fig. 1). Its cells, being about 100 in number, are mostly small rounded nerve cells. There are two exceptions. There is a large neuron in the middle of the group, the length of which is more than half the diameter of the group and the axon of which is evidently the main component of the posterior branch of the median visceral nerve (Plate I, C). There are also two moderately large neurosecretory perikarya with phloxinophilic cytoplasm on either side of the neuron, which are undoubtedly the source of the neurosecretion in the neurohemal organs (Fig. 1, Plate I, B, D). This group, by its compactness and three-dimensional shape, suggests at first sight a tiny ganglion incorporated into the larger one. This concept is reinforced by the study of histologic sections, which show distinct traces of a homogeneous envelope of varying thickness on most of the surface of this body. It stains in exactly the same way as the neural lamella of the large ganglion. The conclusion that it is a small ganglion of the median visceral nerve that has been incorporated into the large ventral nerve-cord ganglion is further supported by the fact that similar ganglia occur on the median visceral nerve of several groups of phylogenetically lower insects. This was shown by the co-workers of RAABE in their study of the perisympathetic organs, e.g., in the cockroach *Leucophaea maderae* etc. (BESSÉ, 1967). It then reappears in some Holometabola, even if only partially protruding from the large ganglion; the whole median visceral nerve is incorporated into one of the connectives, as in many beetles (GRILLOT, 1968; PROVANSAL and GRILLOT, 1972), or lies outside the connective, as in *Vespa crabro* (PROVANSAL, 1968) (Fig. 2).

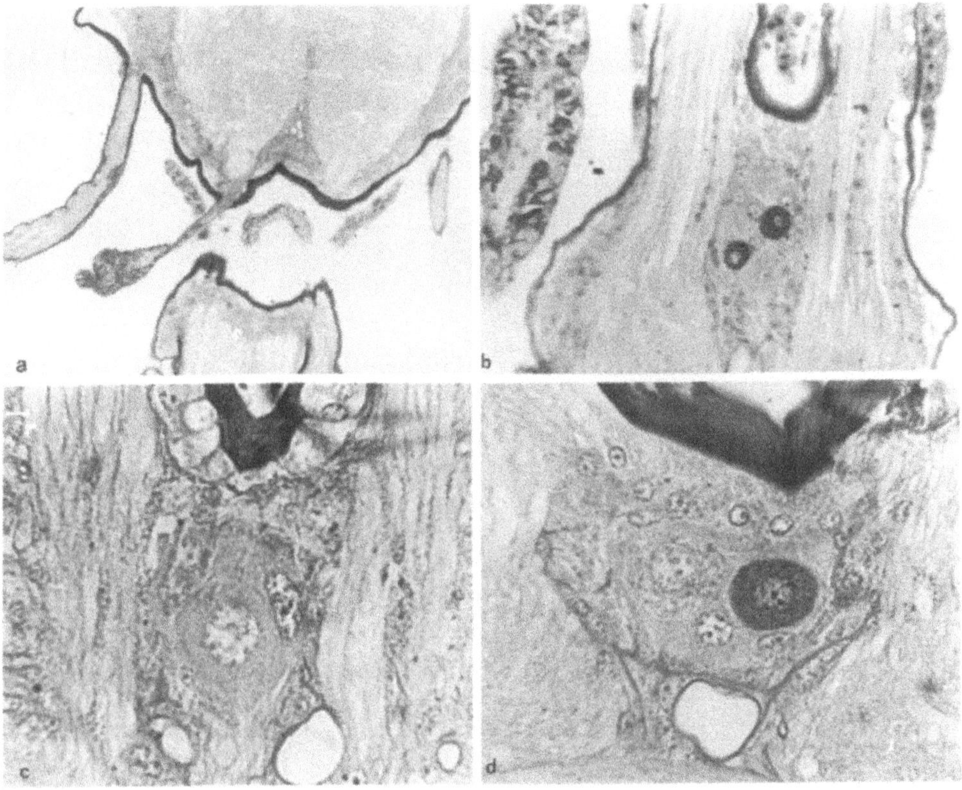

Plate I. Median visceral ganglion in *G. gryllotalpa* L., median sections, stained with Azan. For explanation see text and Figure 3. (a) posterior portion of metathoracic ganglion with incorporated median visceral ganglion and left perisympathetic neurohemal organ. × 240; (b) median visceral ganglion in abdominal ganglion, with two phloxinophil neurosecretory cells. × 640; (c) median visceral ganglion with large central neuron. × 2200; (d) median visceral ganglion with one of two phloxinophil neurosecretory cells. × 2200

It is interesting to note that in similar cases the ganglion itself, when exposed to the hemolymph circulation, becomes a secondary neurohemal organ with neurosecretion accumulating in it, either together with the primary perisympathetic organs as in *V. crabro*, or in it alone, after the disappearance of the primary perisympathetic organs (as in cockroaches and some beetles) (Fig. 2). This is probably why RAABE and her co-workers did not realize their true ganglionic character, calling them the median perisympathetic organ, even though their own histologic pictures clearly show their ganglionic character and their differentiation from the lateral organs (cf. PROVANSAL and GRILLOT, 1972, Fig. 3, p. 875).

It can thus be concluded that the phylogenetically older structure of the median visceral nerve, running independently from the ventral nerve cord, included a small ganglion in each thoracic and abdominal segment. The two systems approached each other

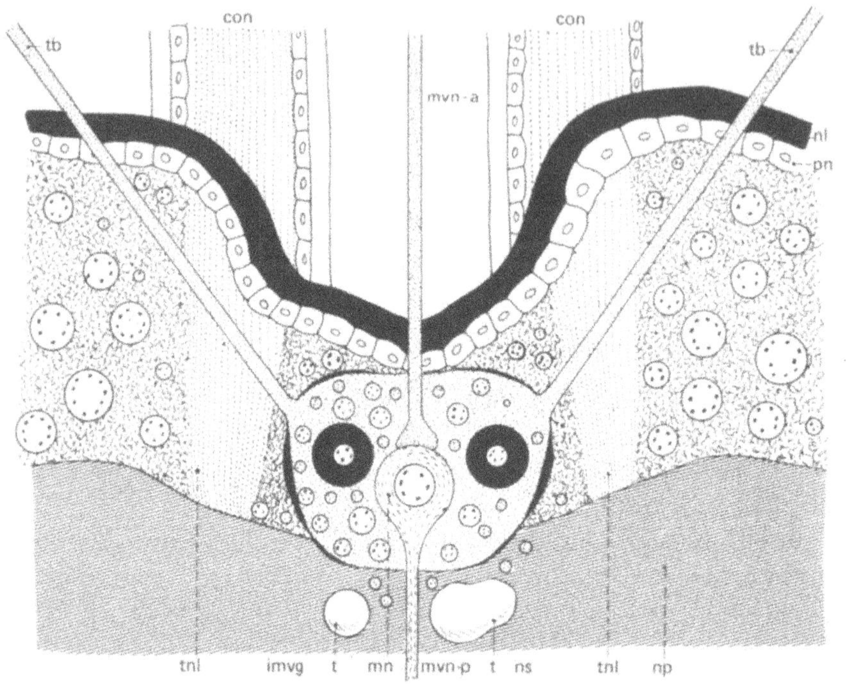

Fig. 1. Schematic histologic section of incorporated median visceral ganglion inside an abdominal ganglion of *G. gryllotalpa* L. (cf. Plate I). *con* - connective, *imvg* - incorporated median visceral ganglion, *mn* - median large neuron, *mvn-a* - anterior section of median visceral nerve, *mvn-p* - posterior section of same, *nl* - neural lamella, *np* - neuropil, *ns* - neurosecretory cell, *pn* - perineurium, *t* - trachea, *tb* - transverse branch of median visceral nerve, *tnl* - traces of neural lamella of incorporated ganglion

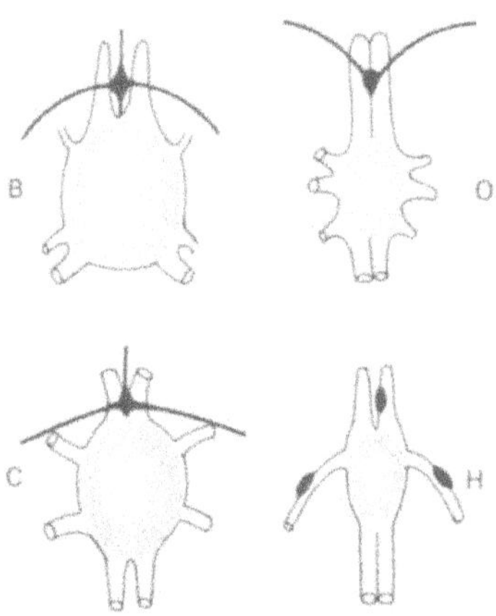

Fig. 2. Median visceral ganglion in four different insect orders (adapted from various papers by RAABE et al., cf. NOVÁK, 1975). *B* - Blattoptera, *O* - Odonata, *C* - Coleoptera, *H* - Hymenoptera

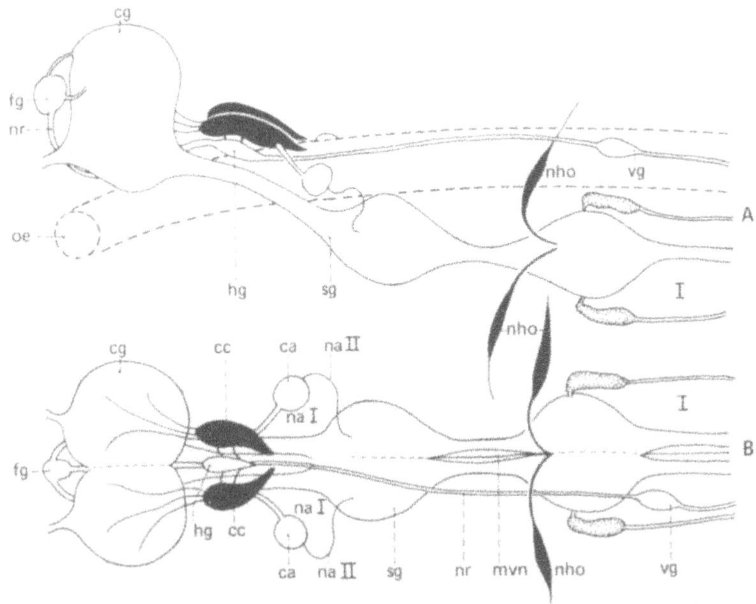

Fig. 3. Schema of insect nervous system: (A) median view, (B) lateral view; *ca* - corpora allata, *cg* - cerebral ganglion, *cc* - corpora cardiaca, *fg* - frontal ganglion, *hg* - hypocerebral ganglion, *vg* - visceral ganglion, na_1 - nervus allatus I, na_{II} - nervus allatus II, *nr* - nervus recurrens, *mvg* - median ventral ganglion, *mvn* - median ventral nerve, *nho* - perisympathetic neurohemal organs, *sg* - subesophageal ganglion, *I* - 1st thoracic ganglion of ventral nerve cord, *oe* - esophagus

only gradually, with the result that they are fused in different degrees in advanced insect orders. In this way, a hypothetical structure of the original innervation of each body segment can be deduced (Fig. 3).

Also, like the individual ganglia of the ventral nerve cord, the median visceral ganglia gradually changed their structure and integrated among themselves and/or with the underlying ventral nerve cord, to reach their present shape. This structure is more or less clearly recognizable in most thoracic and abdominal segments of most phylogentically newer insects (Fig. 4). It is less so, however, in the head segments, even though there exists here the possibility of a uniform morphologic origin. First of all, there are three visceral ganglia corresponding to the three orginal segments of the head, and thus three components of the cerebral ganglion: the frontal ganglion (protocerebrum), the hypocerebral ganglion (deuterocerebrum), and the visceral ganglion (tritocerebrum); the last may be separated into two in some cases, together with the corresponding part of the recurrent nerve. The corpora cardiaca are formed from the original three pairs of organs of the three components of the cerebral ganglion. They would thus correspond as serial homologues to the perisympathetic neurohemal organs of the subse-

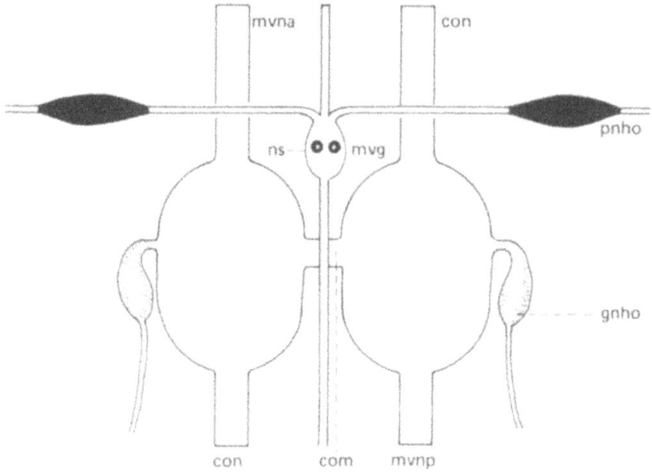

Fig. 4. Schematic structure of hypothetical original nervous and neurosecretory metameric units. *com* - commissure, *con* - connective, *gnho* - ganglionic neurohemal organ, *mvg* - median visceral ganglion, *mvna* - anterior portion of median visceral nerve, *mvnp* - posterior portion of same, *ns* - neurosecretory cells

quent ganglia of the ventral nerve cord. Their composite structure in locusts, as described by HIGHNAM (1961) and by DIVAKAR and NOVÁK (1973), together with the three pairs of nervi corporum cardiacarum, strongly support this conclusion.

The nervus allatus would then also represent a composite structure, its anterior portion (between the c. cardiacum and c. allatum) being a prolongation of some of the n. corporum cardiacarum, whereas its posterior section (between the c. allatum and subesophageal ganglion) would be the lateral branch of the median visceral system in the subesophageal ganglion. The separation of the esophageal (i.e., stomatogastric) sympathetic system from the median visceral one, irrespective of their common origin, may be seen as resulting from their separation by the esophagus (Fig. 3B).

In this way, the structure of the sympathetic nervous system could be fully understood on the basis of the same simple morphologic principles that apply in most other insect organs derived from annelidlike ancestors. Further evidence will be necessary to confirm this view, from which a number of important questions follow.

References

BESSÉ, N.: Neurosécrétion dans la chaine nerveuse ventrale de deux blattes, *Leucophaea maderae* et *Periplaneta americana*. Bull. Soc. Zool. Fr. 92, 73-86 (1967)

CHALAYE, D.: Neurosécrétion au niveau de la chaine nerveuse ventrale de *Locusta migratoria migratorioides*. Bull. Soc. Zool. Fr. 92, 87-108 (1967)
CHARLET, M.: Étude histologique de la pars intercerebralis de la larve d'*Aeschna cyanea Mull*. C. R. Acad. Sci. (Paris) 275, 1047-1050 (1972)
DIVAKAR, J., NOVÁK, V.J.A.: Anatomy and histology of the *corpora cardiaca* in the desert locust, *Schistocerca gregaria Forsk*. Acta Ent. Bohemoslov. 70, 145-149 (1973)
GRILLOT, J.P.: Description d'organes neurohémaux métamériques associés à la chaine nerveuse ventrale chez deux Coléoptères: *Chrysocarabus auronitens Fabr*. (Carabidae) et *Oryctes rhinoceros* L. (Scarabaeidae). C. R. Acad. Sci. (Paris) 267, 772-775 (1968)
HIGHNAM, K.C.: The histology of the neurosecretory system of the adult female desert locust, *Schistocerca gregaria*. Q. J. Microsc. Sci. 102, 27-38 (1961)
MUSKÓ, I., NOVÁK, V.J.A.: The structure and ultrastructure of the metameric neurohaemal organs in *Gryllotalpa gryllotalpa L*. Communicated at the VII Eur. Conf. Comp. Endocrinol., Buda-Pesth. Acta Biol. Hung. (1973)
MUSKÓ, I., NOVAK, V.J.A.: The perisympathetic and the ganglionic neurohaemal organs in *Gryllotalpa gryllotalpa L*. Acta Ent. Bohemoslov, 1976 (in press)
NOVÁK, V.J.A.: Insect Hormones, 4th ed. London: Chapman and Hall 1975, p. 600
PROVANSAL, A.: Mise en évidence d'organes neurohémaux métamériques associées à la chaine nerveuse ventrale chez *Vespa crabro L*. et *Vespula germanica Fabr*. C. R. Acad. Sci. (Paris) 267, 864-867 (1968)
PROVENSAL, A., GRILLOT, J.P.: Les organes périsympathiques des insectes holométaboles. I. Coléoptères. Ann. Sco. Ent. Fr. (N.S.) 8(4), 863-913 (1972)
RAABE, M.: Étude des phénomènes de neurosécrétion au niveau de la chaine nerveuse ventrale des phasmides. Bull. Soc. Zool. Fr. 90, 631-654 (1965)
RAABE, M.: Recherches sur le neurosécrétion dans la chaine nerveuse ventrale du phasme *Carausius morosus*: liaison entre l'activité des cellules B et C pigmentation. C. R. Acad. Sci. (Paris) 263, 408-411 (1966)
RAABE, M.: Neurosécrétion dans la chaine nerveuse ventrale des insectes et organes neurohémaux métamériques. Arch. Zool. Exp. Gén. 112, 679-694 (1971)

Pattern of Neuroendocrine Cell Complexes (Subunits) in Hypothalamic Nuclei: Neurobiological and Phylogenetic Concepts

A. OKSCHE
Department of Anatomy and Cytobiology, Justus Liebig University, Giessen, FRG

From neurohistological investigations of avian hypothalamo-hypophyseal systems, it can be concluded that the hypophysiotropic tuberal nuclei consist of cluster-like aggregations of differing neuroendocrine elements (OKSCHE et al., 1974). In further studies this concept of anatomical subunits was extended to parvocellular and magnocellular nuclei of the anterior hypothalamus (OKSCHE and FARNER, 1974; OKSCHE, 1976). It appears to be consistent with current immunohistological, microchemical, and electrophysiological findings concerning the functional organization of the hypothalamus (for review, see SÉTÁLÓ, 1976; PALKOVITS, 1976; DYER, 1976). These investigations have shown that neurons with certain immunochemical properties (e.g., LHRH- and vasopressin-reactive neurons) are distributed over extended hypothalamic regions (cf. KNOWLES and VOLLRATH, 1974). Although the problem of cross-reactions of closely related hypothalamic peptides has not been definitely solved, it should be realized that extensive hypothalamic areas contain cells producing immunoreactive materials. Not all of these neurons, however, are connected with one of the neurohemal areas. Therefore, from a functional standpoint, their secretions may be considered to be transmitter-like substances. Especially in birds, numerous nerve cells producing different types of elementary granules were observed outside the classical hypophysiotropic zone of the tuber and in the parvocellular preoptic, suprachiasmatic, and anterior hypothalamic regions (OKSCHE and FARNER, 1974). These structural elements may possibly represent a morphological correlate of recent neurochemical data indicating that the hypothalamus produces not only hypophysiotropic hormones but also other, as yet only partly identified, peptides with a wide range of biological properties (GUILLEMIN, 1976).

In our opinion the cluster-like subunits of hypothalamic nuclei consist not only of cells elaborating different types of neurohormones and neurotransmitter-like substances but also of steroid "receptors" (hormone concentrating elements), interneurons, intrinsic collaterals and afferents of differing origin. All of these elements are arranged in a patterned manner according to the general morphologic *Bauplan* of the hypothalamus. In this spatial arrangement, specialized zones of neuropil located between cell clusters may be essential for the propagation of excitation along certain channels and circuits (cf. OKSCHE, 1976). Since the reports by OKSCHE et al. (1974), OKSCHE and FARNER (1974),

---

[1]Dedicated to Professor Berta SCHARRER with sincere appreciation for her outstanding contributions to neuroendocrinology.

and OKSCHE (1976), systematic light- and electron-microscopic investigations on reptiles, birds, marsupials, and insectivores have supplied new evidence supporting the concept of anatomical and functional subunits of the classical hypothalamic nuclei. As mammals descended from mammal-like reptiles and birds from archosaurian (ruling) reptiles (cf. ROMER, 1966), special emphasis must be placed on the Reptilia. In terms of evolution and structural organization, the reptilian brain is more highly developed than the amphibian brain and offers the key for the comparison of avian and mammalian hypothalami. For this reason, previous studies on reptilian hypothalami (OKSCHE, 1976) were extended to additional families and species.[2]

The following chelonian, crocodilian, lacertilian, and ophidian species were used for neuroanatomical analysis of the reptilian hypothalamus:

ANAPSIDA, Testudines (Chelonia).

Cryptodira. Emydidae: *Clemmys leprosa, Cuora amboinensis, Geoemyda trijuga thermalis, Pseudemys ornata callirostris;* Testudinidae: *Testudo carbonaria, T. elegans.*

Pleurodira. Pelomedusidae: *Pelomedusa subrufa.*

ARCHOSAURIA, Crocodilia. Alligatoridae: *Caiman crocodylus.*

LEPIDOSAURIA, Squamata.

Sauria (Lacertilia). Gekkonidae: *Hemidactylus flaviviridis, Gekko gekko, Eublepharis* sp. Agamidae: *Uromastyx hardwickii, Calotes versicolor.* Scincidae: *Scincus scincus, Chalcides ocellatus.* Lacertidae: *Lacerta agilis, L. vivipara, Acanthodactylus* sp. Anguidae: *Anguis fragilis.* Varanidae: *Varanus exanthematicus.*

Serpentes (Ophidia). Colubridae: *Natrix natrix, Pytas korros.* Elapidae: *Naja naja, Bungarus multicinctus, B. fasciatus.*

Among the most conservative reptilian group, the chelonians, *Clemmys leprosa* can be considered a primitive turtle. In *Clemmys,* rostral and tuberal parvocellular neurons, poor in Nissl substance, are arranged in distinct periventricular rows (Fig. 1A-F). A sparse lateral accumulation of hypothalamic neurons is visible at the level of the paraventricular organ. The basal portion of the tuberal complex is formed by small, relatively undifferentiated neurons arranged in thin layers parallel to the infundibular recess. In conclusion, the general morphologic pattern of the chelonian hypothalamus is rather uniform; no striking differences exist between Cryptodira and Pleurodira, between the turtles of the Old and the New World, or between aquatic and terrestrial forms.

In many respects, the architecture of the lacertilian hypothalamus (Fig. 2C) resembles that of the chelonians (Fig. 2A). In several lacertilian families, e.g., Lacertidae, the aggregation

---

[2]Detailed observations will be published in Cell Tiss. Res.

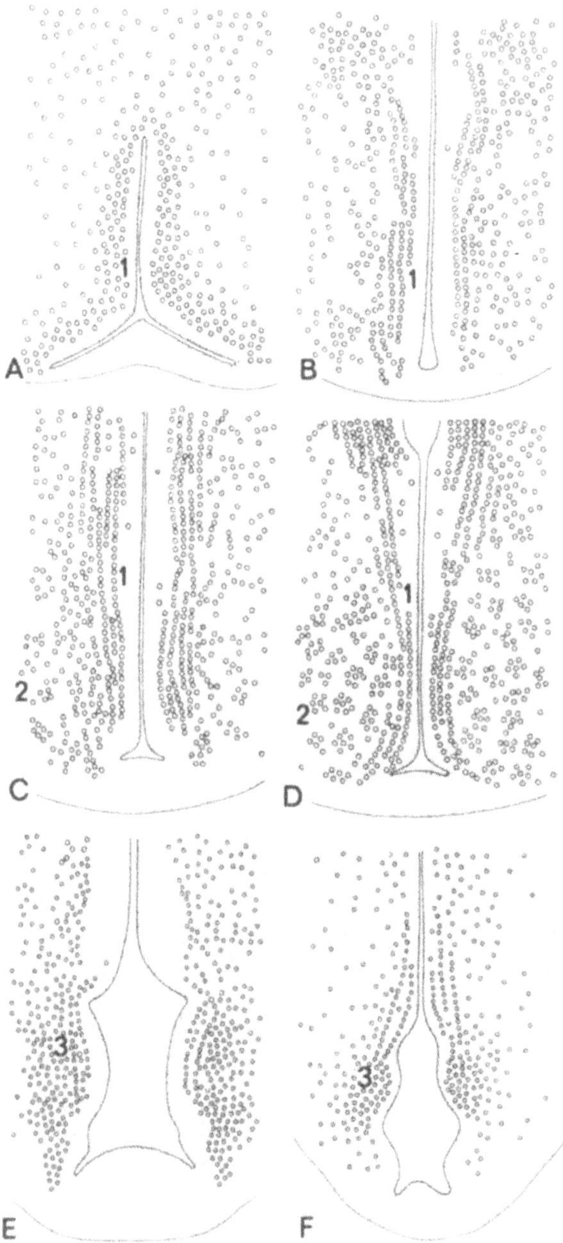

Fig. 1A-F. Morphologic pattern of neuronal arrangements, in the hypothalamus of the turtle, *Clemmys leprosa*. Diagrammatic representation. Note distinct periventricular rows *1* of nerve cells. (A-F) rostrocaudal sequence of cross sections (six different levels) through the hypothalamus. (A) preoptic region; (C,D) diffuse lateral accumulation of cells *2*; (E,F) basal tuberal nucleus *3*

of lateral hypothalamic neurons is rather inconspicuous. However, in the more advanced Varanidae (*V. exanthematicus*) a considerably more extensive development of the lateral hypothalamus is found. In general, the lateral hypothalamus appears to be essential for integration of different inputs and intrinsic hypothalamic functions.

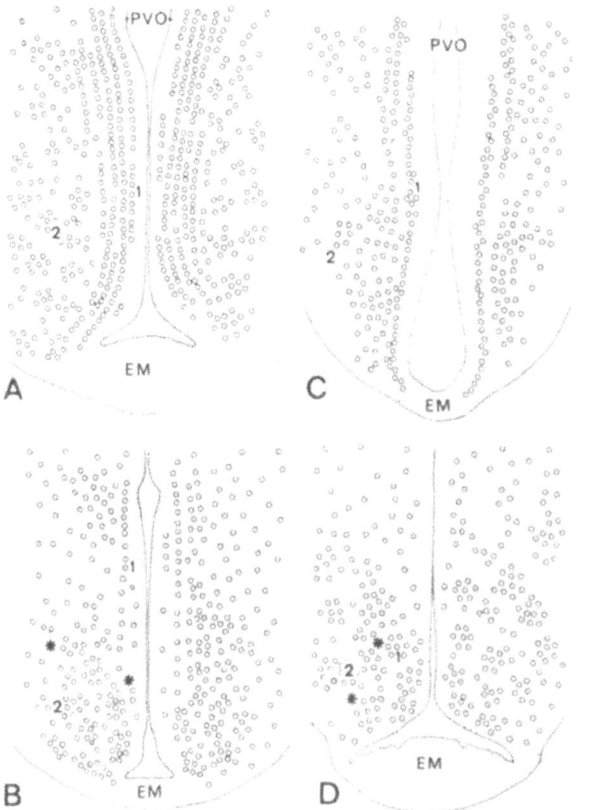

Fig. 2A-D. Differences in distribution pattern of tuberal neurons in turtles (A) *Geoemyda trijuga thermalis*; crocodiles (B) *Caiman crocodylus*; lizards (C) *Lacerta agilis*; and snakes (D) *Natrix natrix*. Diagrammatic representation (for microphotographs, see OKSCHE, 1976). PVO paraventricular organ; EM median eminence. In contrast to turtles and lizards, where periventricular rows of neurons *1* dominate (note haze-like appearance of a lateral group: *2*), cluster-like arrangement of neurons (*) is characteristic of medial *1* and lateral *2* tuberal nuclei of snakes (Colubridae, Elapidae). In *Caiman crocodylus*, the periventricular arrangement of neurons *1* is still visible; however, local proliferation results in formation of well-organized cell clusters (*) and lateral nuclear areas *2*

According to ROMER (1966), the Ophidia represent the latest form of reptiles. Snakes were derived from lizards, and a relation to the Varanoids most likely exists. Our investigation of the more primitive Hemophidia is still in progress, but in Colubridae and Elapidae examined in the present study, the hypothalamic architecture is characterized by (1) cluster-like groups of highly differentiated nerve cells encompassed by abundant zones of neuropil, and (2) distinct lateral hypothalamic nuclei (Fig. 2D). The general morphologic pattern of these ophidian hypothalami closely resembles the architecture of the avian hypothalamus (cf. OKSCHE and FARNER, 1974).

In terms of comparative anatomy, the Crocodilia "... have been among the least progressive of ruling reptiles; they are the only members of the archosaurian stock which survived" (ROMER, 1966). On the other hand, the ancestors of birds must be sought among Archosauria. In recent studies, our knowledge of the hypothalamus of *Caiman crocodylus* was considerably increased. Although a general morphologic pattern of periventricular neuronal arrangements is clearly visible, especially in younger animals, these groups of cells exhibit signs of local proliferation leading to well-organized cell clusters and formation of lateral nuclei (Fig. 2B). The cluster-like subunits consisting of smaller and larger neurons, partly rich in Nissl substance, are very distinct and separated by wide zones of neuropil. Electron microscopically, such neuropils display a highly organized, locally differing structure rich in axodendritic synapses. These synapses are very abundant in close vicinity to the clustered secretory tuberal neurons. An increasing body of evidence suggests that in crocodiles the hypothalamo-hypophyseal (e.g., gonadotropic) functions are far from primitive.

Unfortunately, in comparative neuroendocrinological research, investigations with reptiles have been much neglected. The outline of hypothalamic neuroanatomy presented in the present report may give an idea of trends in evolution that led to the complex avian and mammalian hypothalami. It should be noted that VIGH-TEICHMANN et al. (1976) have focused their attention on another evolutionary aspect of the reptilian hypothalamus. In turtles and lizards the hypothalamus is rich in secretory ciliated neurons, probably derivatives of the CSF-contacting neuron system. In snakes, these ciliated intramural neurons are not conspicuous.

Among the mammals, very distinct cluster-like arrangements of hypothalamic neurons can be observed in the opossum (*Didelphys virginiana*) and the hedgehog (*Erinaceus europaeus*). Again, zones of neuropil encompassing these clusters exhibit a most remarkable degree of ultrastructural organization (Fig. 3)[3]. The regional differences in the quantitative contribution of dendrites, axons, axodendritic synapses of different types and glial processes to this ultrastructural mosaic are striking. Morphometric analysis of these elements and spatial reconstructions of circumscribed neuropil formations could provide an anatomical basis for fundamental functional interpretations. However, this task is arduous and several of the methodological procedures must still be designed.

Along this line of hypothalamic microarchitecture, our collaboration with electrophysiologists has revealed a number of unsolved problems. In the guinea pig and the golden hamster, thermosensitive neurons were identified in a rostral (preoptic) hypothalamic area (WÜNNENBERG et al., 1976). These elements are located in close vicinity to a part of the gonadotropic system (for details, see KNOWLES and VOLLRATH, 1974). In the domestic mallard, a correlation between osmoregulatory and thermoregulatory functions has been observed; the region of the supraoptic and paraventricular nuclei appears to be essential for these functions (SIMON, personal communication). In connection with the above-mentioned physiological findings, one could hypothesize that the specific patterns of intrahypothalamic synapses establish the anatomical basis for functional isolation or interaction, convergence or divergence, and integration of external and internal information.

Further evidence for functionally linked subunits of hypothalamic nuclei results from our work with the arcuate nucleus of the male albino mouse. At the Sixth International Symposium on Neurosecretion, OKSCHE et al. (1974) quoted morphometric pilot studies performed by ZIMMERMANN and SCHNEIDER that indicate rhythmic changes

---

[3]Detailed observations will be published in Cell Tiss. Res.

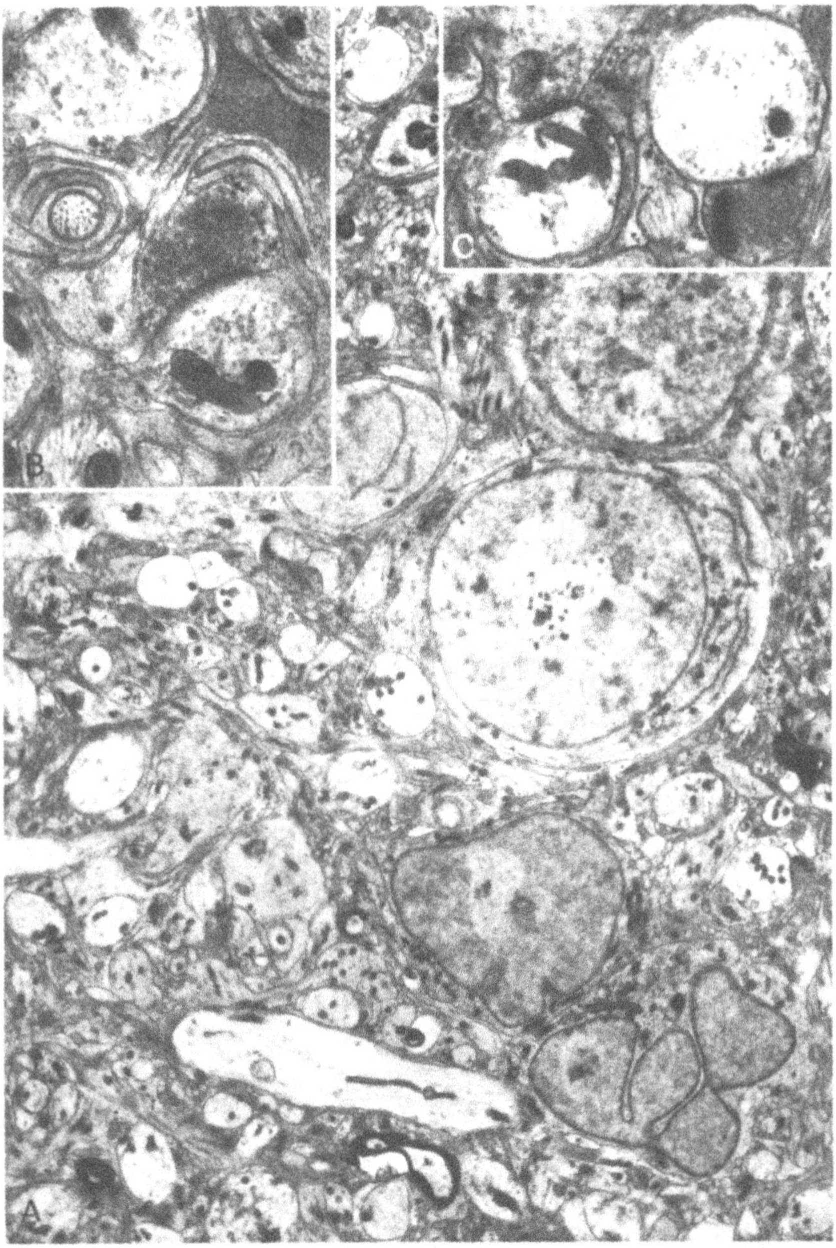

Fig. 3A-C. Cluster-like arrangement of tuberal neurons in opossum, *Didelphys virginiana*, encompassed by highly organized neuropil containing numerous axodendritic synapses (insets B, C). (A) × 4000; (B,C) × 10,000

in the activity of compartment-like subunits of the arcuate nucleus. This work has now been completed (SCHNEIDER, 1976). The preliminary results were confirmed in extensive studies with subsequent morphometric analysis and microspectrophotometric estimations of RNA concentrations in the cytoplasm. (For a detailed account of these findings, see SCHNEIDER, 1976.)

The evolution of the nervous system depends largely on rearrangement of the structural relationships of the basic cellular units that already exist in primitive nervous systems (LENTZ, 1968). The formation of functionally related cell clusters can be regarded as an important step in this rearrangement. In the vertebrate hypothalamus it leads to patterned entities of neuroendocrine cell complexes that form structural and functional subunits of the classical hypothalamic nuclei. This developmental process is closely correlated with the formation of corresponding zones of neuropil. Finally, the differentiation of specific synaptic patterns appears to be responsible for the increasing functional complexity within a pool of hypothalamic neurons. (For general and genetic aspects of cell patterning, see BRENNER, 1975.)

Ackowledgments. The investigations cited in this report were supported by research grants from the Deutsche Forschungsgemeinschaft to the author (Schwerpunktprogramm "Biologie der Zeitmessung"; Ok 1/22). The author is greatly indebted to Mrs. H. Dühring, Miss I. Lyncker, and Dr. R.L. Snipes for their help in preparing the manuscript, to Mrs. G. Möller and Miss. M. Langbein for excellent laboratory assistance, to Miss D. Vaihinger for her efficient graphic work, and to Professor H.O. Hofer, Delta Regional Primate Research Center, Tulane University, Covington, La., USA, and Dr. G. Merker, Department of Physiology, University of Giessen, for supplying valuable animal material.

References

BRENNER, S. (ed.): Cell patterning. Ciba Foundation Symposium 29 (new series). Amsterdam-Oxford-New York: Assoc. Sci. Publ. 1975

DYER, R.: Electrophysiology of hypophysiotrophic neurones. In: Symposium on Structural and Functional Organisation of the Hypothalamus. Endocrinology - Proceedings of the V Int. Congr. of Endocrinology, Hamburg, 1976. JAMES, V.H.T. (ed.). Amsterdam-Oxford: Excerpta Medica 1977, Vol. 1, pp. 117-120

GUILLEMIN, R.: Hypophysiotropic and organotropic peptides of the hypothalamus. The Second Geoffrey Harris Memorial Lecture. V Int. Congr. of Endocrinology, Hamburg, 1976

KNOWLES, F., VOLLRATH, L. (eds.): Neurosecretion - The Final Neuroendocrine Pathway. Berlin-Heidelberg-New York: Springer-Verlag 1974

LENTZ, Th.L.: Primitive Nervous Systems. New Haven-London: Yale Univ. Pr. 1968

OKSCHE, A.: The neuroanatomical basis of comparative neuroendocrinology. Gen. Comp. Endocrinol. 29, 225-239 (1976)

OKSCHE, A., FARNER, D.S.: Neurohistological studies of the hypothalamo-hypophysial system of *Zonotrichia leucophrys gambelii* (Aves, Passeriformes). With special attention to its role in the control of reproduction. Adv. Anat. Embryol. Cell Biol. 48 (4), 1-136 (1974)

OKSCHE, A., OEHMKE, H.J., HARTWIG, H.G.: A concept of neuroendocrine cell complexes. In: Neurosecretion - The Final Neuroendocrine Pathway. KNOWLES, F., VOLLRATH, L. (eds.). Berlin-Heidelberg-New York: Springer-Verlag 1974, pp. 154-164

PALKOVITS, M.: Biochemical neuroanatomy (review and considerations). In: Symposium on Structural and Functional Organisation of the Hypothalamus. Endocrinology - Proceedings of the V Int. Congr. of Endocrinology, Hamburg, 1976. JAMES, V.H.T. (ed.). Amsterdam-Oxford: Excerpta Medica 1977, Vol. 1, pp. 105-110

ROMER, A.S.: Vertebrate Paleontology. 3rd. ed. Chicago-London: Univ. of Chicago Pr. 1966

SCHNEIDER, A.: Reaktionsmuster von Neuronenkomplexen im *Nucleus arcuatus* der Albinomaus. Karyometrische und cytophotometrische Studien. Med. Inaug.-Diss., Justus Liebig-Universität Giessen, 1976

SÉTÁLÓ, G.: Anatomy, using new immunohistologic techniques. In: Symposium on Structural and Functional Organisation of the Hypothalamus. Endocrinology - Proceedings of the V Int. Congr. of Endocrinology, Hamburg, 1976. JAMES, V.H.T. (ed.). Amsterdam-Oxford: Excerpta Medica 1977, Vol. 1, pp. 100-104

SIMON, E.: Personal communication, cf. Annual Report 1975 of the 'Max-Planck-Institut für physiologische und klinische Forschung'. W.G. Kerckhoff-Institut, Bad Nauheim. In: Max-Planck-Gesellschaft, Jahrbuch 1975, pp. 225-227. Göttingen: Vandenhoek & Ruprecht 1975

VIGH-TEICHMANN, I., VIGH, B., AROS, B.: Ciliated neurons and different types of synapses in anterior hypothalamic nuclei of reptiles. Cell Tissue Res. 174, 139-160 (1976)

WÜNNENBERG, W., MERKER, G., SPEULDA, E.: Thermosensitivity of preoptic neurons in a hibernator (golden hamster) and a non-hibernator (guinea pig). Pflügers Arch. 363, 119-123 (1976)

Evolution of Perisympathetic Organs and Insect Phylogeny

A. PROVANSAL and J. P. GRILLOT
Equipe de Neuroendocrinologie des Insectes, Université P. & M. Curie, 12, rue Cuvier, 75230 Paris Cedex 05, France

The perisympathetic organs (PO) show a very important morphologic variability. They may be located on sympathetic or somatic nerves, close to or within the nervous ganglia (GRILLOT et al., 1971; RAABE et al., 1973). Nevertheless, they always correspond to neurosecretory cells of the ventral nerve cord and are associated with the ventral visceral nervous system. Their diversity requires a definition of morphologic types. These have been classified into three basic types, termed mediotransverse, median, and transverse. In each basic type primitive, intermediate, and evolved organs can be distinguished (GRILLOT et al., 1971; RAABE et al., 1973).

The study of PO evolution has been performed by comparative anatomy on the one hand (GRILLOT, 1976), and by ontogenetic studies on the other hand (PROVANSAL, 1971). Some points still remain hypothetical, but the general pattern has been traced. The evolution of the PO seems to parallel insect phylogeny, established according to BEY-BIENKO's classification (BEY-BIENKO, 1962). Thus, the most archaic organs are present in the lowest Pterygota, Ephemeroptera, and Odonata, which are in many respects archaic insects. Primitive insects like Dictyoptera, Orthoptera, and Phasmoptera have primitive organs. In evolved insects (Holometabola), evolved organs are present especially in Hymenoptera, Coleoptera, and Diptera; however, in Planipenna and Trichoptera, still primitive orders in some respects, the PO are less evolved. In some very evolved groups like Diptera, primitive forms still remain; their PO also belong to primitive types. In Hemiptera, a quite distinct group, the PO are very peculiar. PO evolution seems to parallel the evolution of the central and sympathetic nervous system.

References

BEY-BIENKO, G.Y.A.: On the general classification of Insects. Entomol. Rev. 41, 3 (1962)

GRILLOT, J.P.: Les organes périsympathiques des Insectes. Essai sur leur évolution. Données structurales et physiologiques chez les Coléoptères et Diptères. Ann. Sc. Nat. Zoologie (Paris) 18, 311 (1976)

GRILLOT, J.P., BAUDRY, N., PROVANSAL, A., RAABE, M.: Les organes périsympathiques des Insectes Ptérygotes. Les principaux types morphologiques. C. R. Acad. Sci. (D) (Paris) 273, 2126 (1971)

PROVANSAL, A.: Caractères particuliers des organes périsympathiques de la larve de *Diprion pini* L. (Hyménoptère, Symphite, Diprionidae). C. R. Acad. Sci. (D) (Paris) 273, 855 (1971)

RAABE, M., BAUDRY, N., GRILLOT, J.P., PROVANSAL, A.: The perisympathetic organs of Insects. In: Neurosecretion. The Final Neuroendocrine Pathway. VI Intern. Symp. Neuros., London, 1973. Berlin-Heidelberg-New York: Springer-Verlag 1974

Ontogenesis of Neurosecretory Systems

Correlation Between Synthesis and Release of CRF During Stress at Different Periods of Rat Postnatal Ontogenesis

I. A. DRJEVEZKAJA, L. K. KARAULOVA, A. M. KOROVINA, S. S. MOLDOVANOVA, and O. A. DANILOVA
Institute of Pedagogics, Stavropol, Sechenov Institute of Evolutionary Physiology and Biochemistry, Leningrad, USSR

A. Introduction

Reactivity to stressful agents of the hypothalamo-hypophyseal-adrenocortical system changes in the course of postnatal ontogenesis (PINCUS et al., 1954; MIKHAILOVA, 1963; BLOCK, 1965; GRAD et al., 1967). This may be due to changes in the synthesis and release of CRF and/or ACTH. The aim of this study was to estimate CRF activity of hypothalamic extracts and pituitary ACTH content in rats of various ages, under stress, such as prolonged swimming. These findings were compared with the morphology of the hypothalamic "Gomori-positive" peptidergic neurosecretory (NS) system.

B. Materials and Methods

Untrained male white rats were used. Each age-group (1, 2-3, 5-6, 10-12, and 18-24 months old) was divided into three subgroups: (1) control, (2) stress of short duration, and (3) stress of long duration. Swimming in water at 30-32°C was considered to be stress. Swimming for 10 min for young rats and 30 min for old ones was considered to be stress of short duration. Swimming for 30 min and for 120 min for young and old rats respectively was considered stress of long duration. Acetic acid extracts of hypothalamic tissue were assayed by the ascorbic acid level in the adrenals of the recipient rats (ARIMURA et al., 1967). Pituitary ACTH content was studied using the technique of SKEBEL'SKAYA (1964). Rats 6 and 12 months old were used for morphologic studies (4- and 3-month-old rats served as controls; 5- and 3-month-old rats were decapitated after swimming for 30 min). Hypothalamic brain areas and hypophyses were fixed in Bouin's fluid and stained by Gomori-Gabe's paraldehyde fuchsin. The supraoptic nucleus, median eminence, and hypophyseal posterior lobe were studied. The amount of NS material in the posterior lobe was evaluated in arbitrary units according to a 5-degree scale.

C. Results

Physical stress of immature 1-month-old rats after only 10 min led to a significant decrease of CRF activity in the hypothalamic extracts and to an almost complete release of ACTH from the adenohypophysis (Table 1). The changes were more profound after a prolonged stress. After stress of short duration rats 2-3 months

Table 1. CRF activity of hypothalamic extracts and pituitary ACTH content in rats after physical stress

Age (months)	Animal group	Number of rats	CRF activity[a]	Pituitary ACTH (mE/100 of dry tissue)
1	Control	5	154 ± 8[b]	5.3 ± 1.6
	Stress of short duration	5	65 ± 7	0.7 ± 0.25
	Stress of long duration	5	37 ± 4	0.1 ± 0.04
2-3	Control	6	175 ± 8	7.8 ± 0.5
	Stress of short duration	7	57 ± 7	0.31± 0.01
	Stress of long duration	5	90 ± 6	4.3 ± 0.9
5-6	Control	7	112 ± 2	6.9 ± 0.1
	Stress of short duration	10	201 ±23	0.6 ± 0.006
	Stress of long duration	5	33 ± 3	0.2 ± 0.003
10-12	Control	15	126 ± 7	7.6 ± 0.38
	Stress of short duration	5	130 ± 9	2.8 ± 0.6
	Stress of long duration	5	72 ±11	0.23± 0.006
18-24	Control	9	107 ± 7	6.7 ± 1.19
	Stress of short duration	10	147 ± 7	4.46± 3.6
	Stress of long duration	5	128 ± 6[c]	0.52± 0.22

[a]Changes in ascorbic acid content (mg%) in adrenal glands of recipient rats after injection of hypothalamic extracts

[b]Mean ± SEM

[c]Differences between all the subgroups within the age-groups are statistically significant except for this one value

old reacted similarly to those 1 month old, but after prolonged stress the amount of CRF and ACTH were partly restored. After short stress, rats 5-6 months old showed an almost twofold increase in hypothalamic CRF activity and a sharp decrease in pituitary ACTH content. Prolonged stress resulted in a decrease of both hypothalamic CRF activity and pituitary ACTH content. In rats 10-12 and 18-24 months old the reaction to stress was less pronounced.

Morphologically, a decrease in NS-material content and its concentration around the blood capillaries in the posterior lobe was seen in rats 5-6 months old after 30 min swimming (3.8 units versus 4.2 units in controls). Posterior lobes of 12-month-old rats were partly devoid of NS material even in controls (3.1 units). The reaction to swimming in this group was less pronounced than in the younger one. Moderate hyperemia of the external median eminence was noted in rats after swimming. After stress, some NS cells in the supraoptic nuclei appeared dark, due to increased stainability of the karyoplasm and cytoplasm. The amount of NS material increased in the proximal part of the NS-cell processes.

D. Discussion

The age difference in the reactivity of the CRF-ACTH system is evident from the above data. Immature rats react with a prompt release of stored CRF and ACTH progressing during stress the amount released exceeds the amount synthesized. It appears that in immature rats the negative feedback mechanism is underdeveloped, and hyperactivity of the hypothalamo-hypophyseal-adrenocortical system results. In rats 2-3 months old synthesis of CRF and ACTH is more pronounced. In rats 5-6 months old CRF synthesis exceeds release if stress duration is short. This might reflect maturity, both of the elements which synthesize CRF and of the negative feedback mechanisms. Delayed reaction of the CRF-ACTH system to stress in old rats might be due to a lowering of excitability and to inertia of CRF-synthesizing structures. When evaluating the amount of Gomori-positive NS material in the posterior lobes of rats after noxious stimuli, POLENOV (personal communication) also noticed a less-pronounced reaction to stress in old rats as compared with young animals.

In histologic preparations, only the hyperemia of the external median eminence might be correlated with the increased CRF release. Although the release of neurohormones from the posterior lobe in young stressed rats was seen to parallel the release of CRF from the hypothalami, this correlation is probably not causal. The decreased amount of NS material in the posterior lobes reflects peptide-neurohormone release through the para-adenohypophyseal path, as is well known in various stress conditions (POLENOV, 1968). The appearance of dark NS cells in the supraoptic nucleus might be connected with previous high activity due to increased demand for vasopressin and, less probably, for CRF.

References

ARIMURA, A., SAITO, T., SCHALLY, A.V.: Assays for corticotropin-releasing factor (CRF) using rats treated with morphine, chlorpromazine, dexamethasone, and nembutal. Endocrinology 81, 235-245 (1967)

BLOCK, L.N.: Age changes of the adenohypophysis-adrenal cortex system. Thesis, Khar'kow, 1965

GRAD, B., KRAL, A.V., PAYNE, R.C., BERENSON, J.: Plasma and urinary corticoids in young and old persons. J. Gerontol. 22, 66-71 (1967)

MIKHAILOVA, N.N.: Reaction of the hypophysis and adrenal cortex of young rats to stress factors and the role of the nervous system in this reaction. Thesis, Moscow, 1963

PINCUS, G., ROMANOFF, L.P., CARLO, J.: Excretion of urinary steroids by men and women of various ages. J. Gerontol. 9, 113-117 (1954)
POLENOV, A.L.: Hypothalamic neurosecretion. Leningrad: Nauka 1968
SKEBEL'SKAYA, Yu.B.: ACTH content in the rat embryo hypophysis. Probl. Endocrinol. 10, 74-77 (1964)

Time of Cell Origin in Mouse Supraoptic Nucleus

N. D. GRACHEVA and O. A. DANILOVA

Central Research Roentgenoradiologic Institute, Ministry of Health of the USSR and Sechenov Institute of Evolutionary Physiology and Biochemistry, Academy of Sciences of the USSR, Leningrad, USSR

The advantages of autoradiographic study of neurocytogenesis utilizing ^{3}H-thymidine have already been established (ANGEVINE and SIDMAN, 1961; FUJITA and MIYAKE, 1962; etc.). Recently IFFT (1972), and SHIMADA and NAKAMURA (1973) studied the time of final division of matrix cells before their migration to the hypothalamic nuclei, using tritiated thymidine autoradiography. To the authors' knowledge there are only single autoradiographic studies on the development of the supraoptic nucleus (SON) in mice.

The present report concerns only the time of final division of the cells making up the SON in mouse hypothalamus. In this study double labeling with ^{3}H- and ^{14}C-thymidine was applied to determine the time of the cell's origin. ^{3}H-thymidine (^{3}H-TH) was given to 23 pregnant mice of CH_3Black or C_3HA strains on one of the 9th to 19th days of gestation. After 12, 24, or 48 h, the same animals were injected with ^{14}C-thymidine (^{14}C-TH). Eight pregnant mice were killed 1 h after the second injection of the label to fix the embryos on the 11th and 14-19th days of gestation. The 15 other pregnant mice were allowed to survive and the offspring examined on the 1st, 10th, or 30th days after birth. Brains were fixed in Carnoy's solution, embedded in paraffin and sectioned serially in a coronal or sagittal plane at 5 µm and processed for autoradiography with type-R nuclear emulsion. Photographs of the SON in the serial sections were taken under × 120 magnification. Subsequently, the brain sections were examined systematically with an ocular grid under × 900 magnification. ^{3}H- and ^{14}C-labeled cells in the field of the grid were dotted in situ in the photograph from which the drawings were made.

From the 11th to the 15th embryonic days, the hypothalamic region consisted of a thick matrix layer bordering the third ventricle and recessus opticus. The matrix cells were double labeled. Later, the matrix layer had become thinner; it disappeared on the 19th embryonic day. The first groups of the cells were seen only in the caudal regions of the future SON on the 15th embryonic day.

To clarify the gradient of the time of cell origin in the SON, maps of ^{3}H- and ^{14}C-labeled cells (^{3}H-cells and ^{14}C-cells) were arranged according to the time of ^{3}H- and ^{14}C-TH injections and to the levels in a brain rostrocaudally (Fig. 1). Moreover, the intervals between the injections allowed the ^{3}H-labeled fraction of the matrix cells to complete first divisions before the injection of the second label to give ^{3}H-cells for the brain struc-

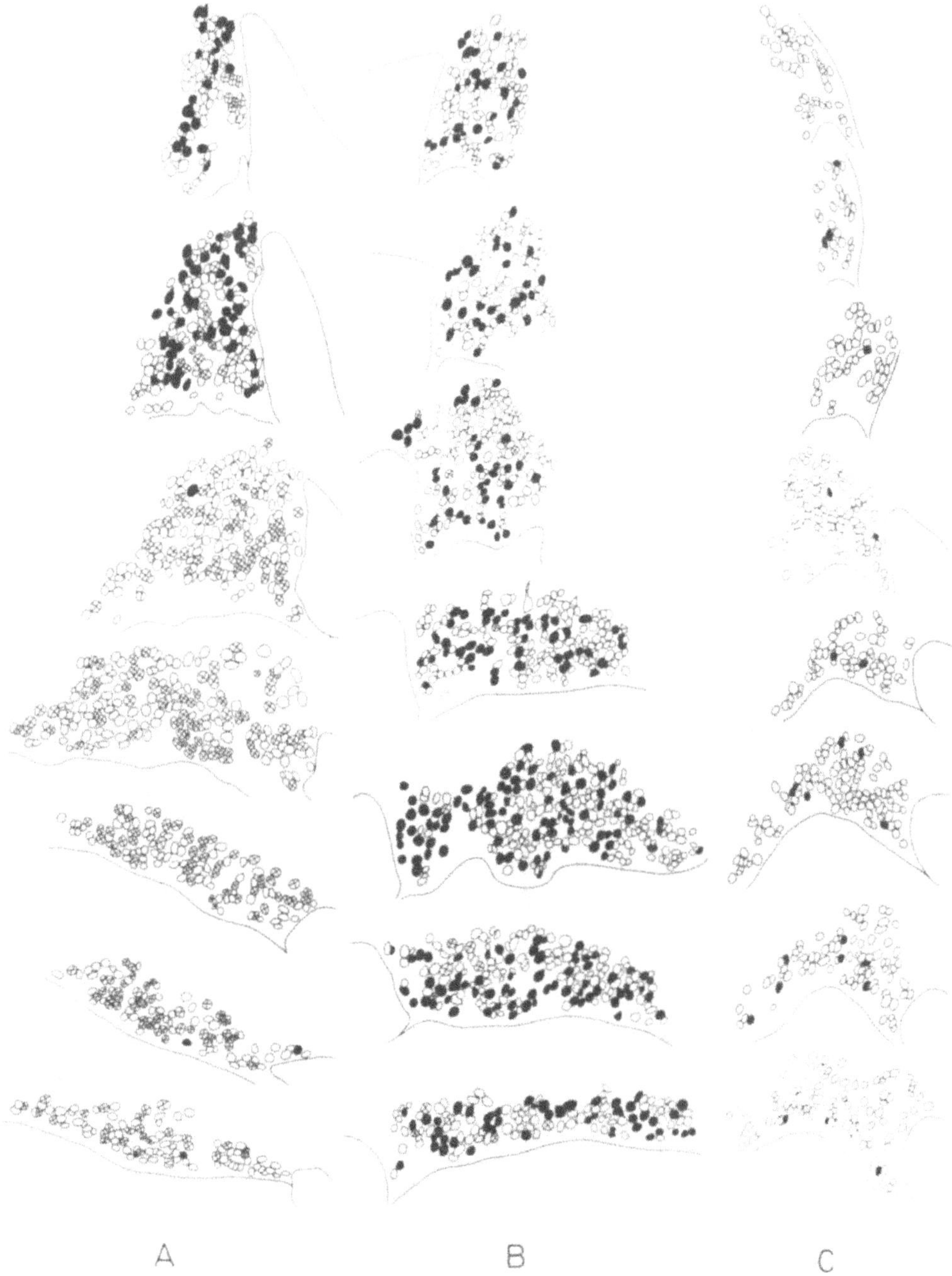

Fig. 1. Drawings of serial sections through mouse SON. Note distribution of ^{3}H-cells (black) and ^{14}C-cells (cross) in animals injected with ^{3}H-TH and ^{14}C-TH on days (A) 11-12, (B) 12-13, (C) 13-14 of gestation and killed on first postnatal day. Rostrocaudal direction from bottom to top

tures. All the cells of the subsequent generations were additionally labeled with ^{14}C and were classified as cells that originated later than ^{3}H-cells.

On days 9 and 10 of gestation, ^{3}H- and ^{14}C-TH were injected, the mice were examined postnatally, and a few lightly labeled cells were found in the SON, i.e., the cell migration into the nucleus had not yet started.

When the labels were given on days 10-11 of pregnancy, only ^{14}C-cells were found in the SON. When the labels were given on days 11-12 of pregnancy, ^{3}H-cells (27.6-40%) were localized in the caudodorsal parts of the SON (Fig. 1A), and a few lightly labeled ^{3}H-cells appeared in some sections of the ventrorostral regions of the SON, in which chiefly ^{14}C-cells were found. ^{3}H-cells of the caudodorsal regions were heavily labeled: 18-37 silver grains over the nuclei.

When ^{3}H- and ^{14}C-TH were given on days 12-13 of pregnancy, ^{3}H-cells were distributed in all the parts of the SON with the gradient of labeled-cell number from 23% to 54% in the caudorostral direction (Fig. 1B). From the 13th embryonic day, the production of the cells for the SON was strongly reduced and the labeled cells were regularly distributed in all the caudorostral parts (Fig. 1C). The injection of the labels with 12, 24, or 48 h interval did not change the general picture of the labeled-cell distribution after day 13 of embryonic life.

The smallest number of ^{3}H-cells arose on days 14 and 16 of gestation and the latest ^{3}H-cells migrated into the SON on day 17 of embryonic life. However, when ^{3}H- and ^{14}C-TH were injected on days 17-18 of gestation, a few ^{14}C-cells were found in the SON of the postnatal mice, i.e., the migration of the single cells could take place on day 18 of gestation.

When a single injection of ^{3}H-TH was given on day 19 of embryonic life and the mice examined postnatally, not all of the cells in the SON were labeled. The described labeled cells were classified as neurosecretory cells (NSC).

The mean numbers of reduced silver grains were counted over the nuclei of ^{3}H-cells to estimate the quantity of matrix-cell generation required to form the SON during histogenesis. ^{3}H-cells formed on day 12 of gestation were found to have mean grain counts lower than those arisen on days 11 and 13 of embryonic life (Fig. 2). The fact was confirmed by histograms of the distribution of the cells according to the number of grains over the nuclei (Fig. 3). The histograms of the cells formed on days 11 and 13 of gestation (Fig. 3A, C) had both modes differing by a factor of two, which testified to the existence of the two subsequent generations among the cells of the current day. ^{3}H-cells of the 12th embryonic day had a histogram (Fig. 3C) with one (lesser) mode, i.e., the cells arising on the 12th embryonic day were the second generation of the current day. This fact was confirmed by the experiment with a 12 h interval between injections of the labels on day 12 of gestation, in which almost all

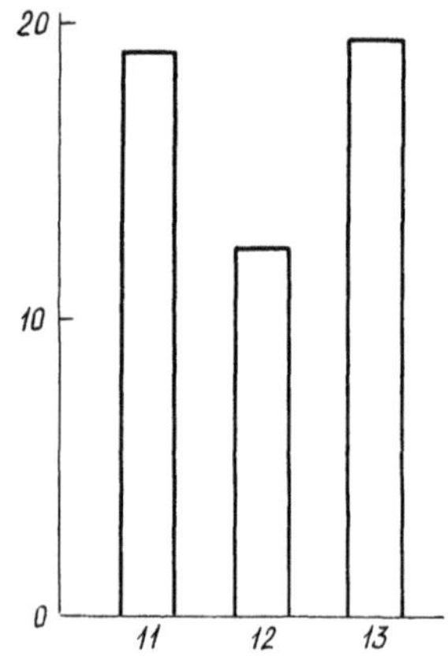

Fig. 2. Mean grain counts over NSC of SON in postnatal mice. *Ordinate* - mean grain counts, *abscissa* - age on day of ^{3}H-TH injection

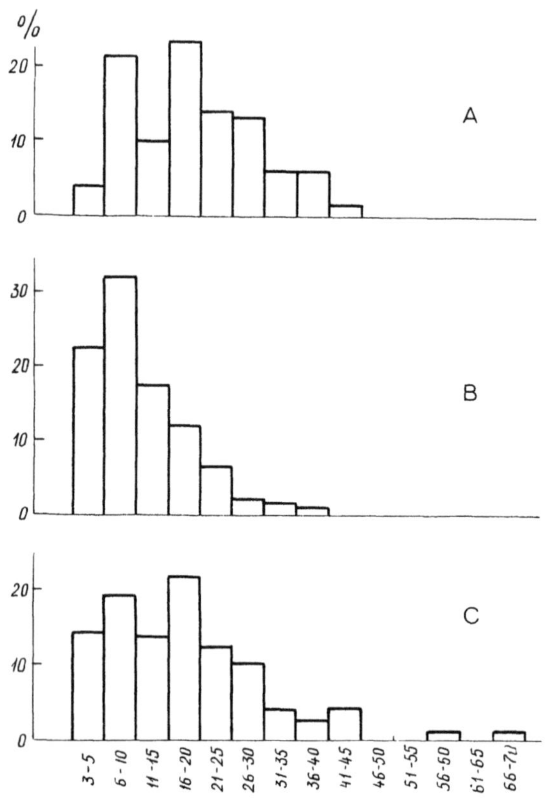

Fig. 3A-C. Histograms of cell distribution according to number of grains over nuclei of SON in postnatal mice. Note cells arisen on day (A) 11, (B) 12, and (C) 13 of embryonic life in animals killed on first postnatal day. *Ordinate* - number of cells (percentage), *abscissa* - number of grains

the cells became additionally labeled with carbon-14. Thus, from days 11 to 13 of gestation the cells of six subsequent generations took part in histogenesis of the SON, but there was a pause at the early part of day 12, as all the cells repeated the division during the current day before the migration into the SON.

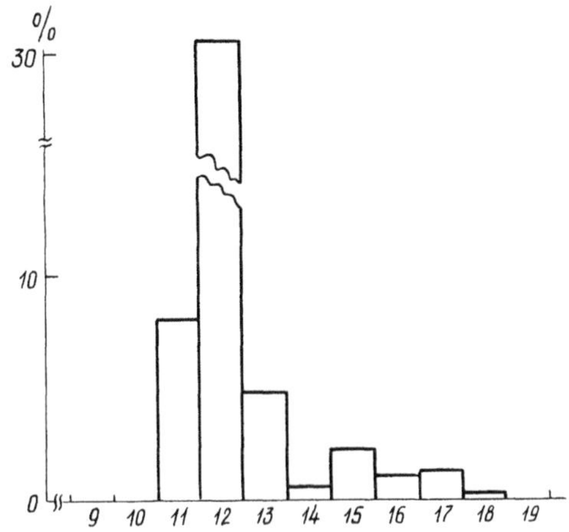

Fig. 4. Time of origin of NSC in mouse SON as found in postnatal animals injected with ^{3}H-TH and ^{14}C-TH on designated days of gestation with intervals 12, 24, or 48 h between injections. *Ordinate* - percentage of cells labeled, *abscissa* - age on day of injection

Some ^{3}H-cells deserve special attention because they had many more silver grains over their nuclei than the control cells (elongated right arm of the histograms, Fig. 3). It is supposed that some matrix cells that had migrated into the SON after DNA synthesis avoided the subsequent mitosis, and the existence of polyploid cells among the NSC of the SON might be expected.

The data obtained allow us to conclude that, during embryogenesis, mouse SON is formed from day 11 to 17 of gestation with most NSC being formed on days 11-13 (Fig. 4). It is also clear that a dorsocaudal-ventrorostral gradient exists at the time of cellular origin in mouse SON, and is very pronounced during the early stages of histogenesis. In other words, in order to form the SON the NSC arose 4 days earlier than the structure of the nucleus itself was built.

When the SON was filled principally with NSC, some glial cells began to migrate into the nucleus on day 14 of gestation. The glioblasts were doubly labeled and divided mitotically; this means that they continued proliferating. The repeated divisions of the glial cells were confirmed by the fact that almost all of them had lost the label by day 30 after birth, as occurs in the other parts of the developing nervous system (GRACHEVA, 1973, 1975).

Thus, the application of double labeling with ^{3}H- and ^{14}C-TH allowed us to estimate more precisely the time of spatial formation of the SON during histogenesis and to define the time sequence of migration of the NSC and glioblasts.

References

ANGEVINE, J.D., SIDMAN, R.L.: Autoradiographic study of cell migration during histogenesis of cerebral cortex in the mouse. Nature (London) 192, 766-768 (1961)

FUJITA, S., MIYAKE, S.: Selective labelling of cell groups and its application to cell identification. Exptl. Cell Res. 28, 158-161 (1962)
GRACHEVA, N.D.: Terms of appearance and ways of migration of cells in histogenesis of the cerebral cortex. Archiv Anat., Histol. and Embryol. (Leningrad) 65, 21-30 (1973)
GRACHEVA, N.D.: The terms of appearance of cells in histogenesis of the spinal cord. Archiv Anat., Histol. and Embryol. (Leningrad) 68, 22-28 (1975)
IFFT, J.D.: An autoradiographic study of the time of final division of neurons in rat hypothalamic nuclei. J. Comp. Neurol. 144, 193-204 (1972)
SHIMADA, M., NAKAMURA, T.: Time of neuron origin in mouse hypothalamic nuclei. Exp. Neurol. 41, 163-173 (1973)

Effect of Extirpation of the Cervical Sympathetic Ganglia on Development of the Neurosecretory Peptidergic and Parvocellular Nuclei of Rat Hypothalamus During Postnatal Ontogenesis

L.M. LEPEKHINA
Sechenov Institute of Evolutionary Physiology and Biochemistry, Academy of Sciences of the USSR, Leningrad, USSR

Extirpation of the cervical sympathetic ganglia (CSG) results in retardation of the growth of young rats (EAYRS and TAYLOR, 1951; LEPEKHINA, 1975). Our purpose was to show the hypothalamic nuclei (supraoptic - SO, paraventricular - PV, suprachiasmatic - SCH, ventromedial - VM, dorsomedial - DM, arcuate - ARC) in which morphologic changes occur after extirpation of CSG in young rats, and to show how these changes are correlated with growth retardation. Twenty intact and twenty-six operated animals were studied during the course of 5 months of postnatal ontogenesis. A karyo- and cytometric study was made on the 10th, 20th, and 30th days after birth as well as at the ages of 2, 3, and 5 months. The results were treated statistically on the computer. Bilateral extirpation of the CSG was made within the first 5 days after birth.

The operated rats show retardation in the development of PV and DM neurons at the age of 10 days, of SO neurons at the age of 20 days, and SCH neurons at the age of 2 months. Both nuclei and cytoplasm are of smaller size and do not reach a normal size even in adult rats. In operated rats, retention of neurosecretion is observed in SO neurons and even more in PV neurons. Degenerative changes are most considerable in SO neurons. No deviation from normal development was found in VM or ARC neurons of operated rats. Thus, the retardation of growth in young rats after CSG extirpation is accompanied by retardation of the development of the SO, PV, and DM nuclei of the hypothalamus.

References

EAYRS, J.T., TAYLOR, S.H.: J. Anat. (Lond.) 85, 330-337 (1951)
LEPEKHINA, L.M.: Bull. Exp. Biol. & Med. 79, 498-500 (1975) (in Russian)

Hypothalamic Control of the Development of Endocrine Functions in the Human Fetus

S. E. LEVINA
Institute of Developmental Biology, Academy of Sciences of the USSR, Moscow, USSR

Human fetal endocrine development has been examined during the past 15 years, but data related to neuroendocrine regulation in fetal life are sparse in literature. To investigate the problem, we have compared the radioimmunologically determined concentrations of TSH, FSH, LH, and GH in the plasma with those in the cerebral liquor in 54 fetuses 15-35 weeks old, which had been dead for 2-10 h. Cerebral liquor was obtained by syringe from the undissected cerebral ventricles without any admixture of blood.

Hypophyses of those fetuses were divided into symmetrical halves and incubated in vitro for 24 h. To half of the hypophyses we added the basal hypothalamus of the same fetuses, to the other half a similar piece of fetal brain cortex ("control"). The levels of the release of five hypophyseal hormones into the media (TSH, FSH, LH, GH, and ACTH) were also examined radioimmunologically and the data were compared with the hormonal concentrations in the plasma and cerebral liquor.

The results indicate very high plasma concentrations in fetuses as compared with those in adults. GH-concentrations have been found from 24.5 ± 6.99 to 47.7 ± 7.86 ng/ml of fetal plasma, equal in both sexes. The results also show that the concentrations of three glycoprotein tropins depend on fetal sex (Figs. 1, 2): during the second half of prenatal life the mean TSH concentration in females is 2.83 ± 0.114 ng/ml and in males 2.14 ± 0.347 ($p < 0.01$); concentrations of FSH in females are from 6.18 ± 2.263 to 8.75 ± 2.055 ng/ml and in males from 1.37 ± 0.524 to 2.59 ± 1.118 ng/ml (sex differences are significant); lastly, for LH the respective means are from 25.5 ± 5.63 to 30.9 ± 4.73 ng/ml and from 20.7 to 26.6 ± 5.69 ng/ml (LEVINA, 1976). Thus the patterns of GTH sex-dependent secretion are similar in fetuses and in adults though without cyclicity in female fetuses (LEVINA, 1974).

All hormones examined have been discovered in the cerebral liquor in concentrations in general a little lower than in plasma. The comparison of the concentrations makes it possible to find evidence for additional features of neuroendocrine sexual differentiation developing from the middle of prenatal life. Significant positive correlations have been observed between plasma levels of FSH and LH ($r = 0.69$) only in females. On the other hand they are established between plasma and cerebral liquor levels for TSH ($r = 0.66$), for FSH ($r = 0.82$) and for LH ($r = 0.89$) only in males (Figs. 1, 2).

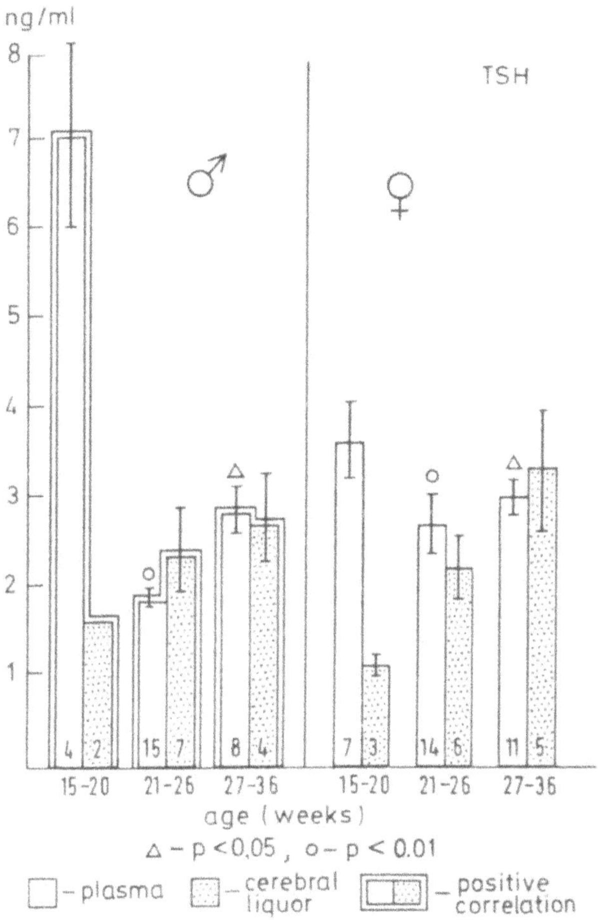

Fig. 1. Concentration of TSH in the plasma and cerebral liquor in fetuses of both sexes and various ages. Numbers at the bottom of columns mean numbers of fetuses studied

The question arises: to what degree does the sexual differentiation of the hypophyseal secretion depend on the hypothalamic influences? The incubation of the hypophysis of the same fetuses in vitro indicates that under experimental conditions the addition of the basal hypothalamus alters the hormonal release into the media from the second trimester of prenatal life. At the beginning of the second trimester the secretion levels decrease slightly as compared with controls: for ACTH ($p < 0.05$), for TSH ($p < 0.01$) and to a smaller degree for GH ($p < 0.1$). By the end of the second trimester these inhibiting hypothalamic influences become reduced and later, for some hormones, turn to stimulating action.

For ACTH the stimulating effect of hypothalamic addition appears from the middle of prenatal life, for GTH it is pronounced during the third quarter (for LH $p < 0.05$) and the effect decreases towards birth; for TSH release stimulation ($p < 0.05$) starts in the last third of prenatal life (Fig. 3). GH release stimulation is not observed under the experimental conditions until the 35th week; probably it begins only postnatally (LEVINA, 1976).

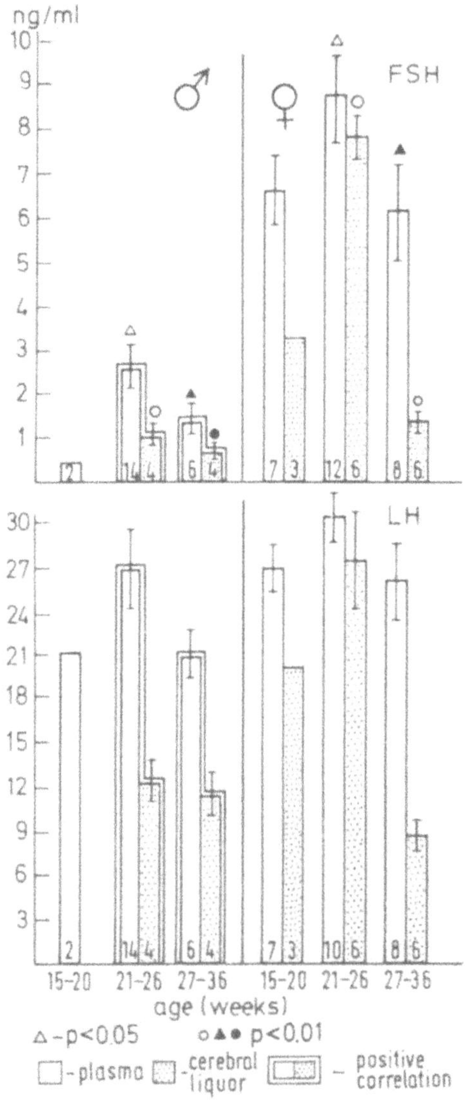

Fig. 2. Concentrations of FSH and LH in the plasma and cerebral liquor in fetuses of both sexes and various ages. Designations as in Fig. 1

One can see that there are sexual differences in the hypothalamic influences on both GTH and TSH release (Fig. 3) into the medium. Thus higher levels of all three glycoproteid tropins in plasma of fetal females compared with fetal males depend at least partly on sexual differentiation of hypothalamic control of hypophyseal secretion. It is of interest to note that these findings relate only to glycoprotein hypophyseal hormones, possibly supporting the suggestion of their common ancestor cistron.

Correlation analysis of the results disclose additional features of early sexual differentiation of fetal hypothalamic activity. Significant correlations between TSH plasma concentration and the TSH secretion level induced by the added hypothalamus are found during the period examined in females ($r = 0.53$); and be-

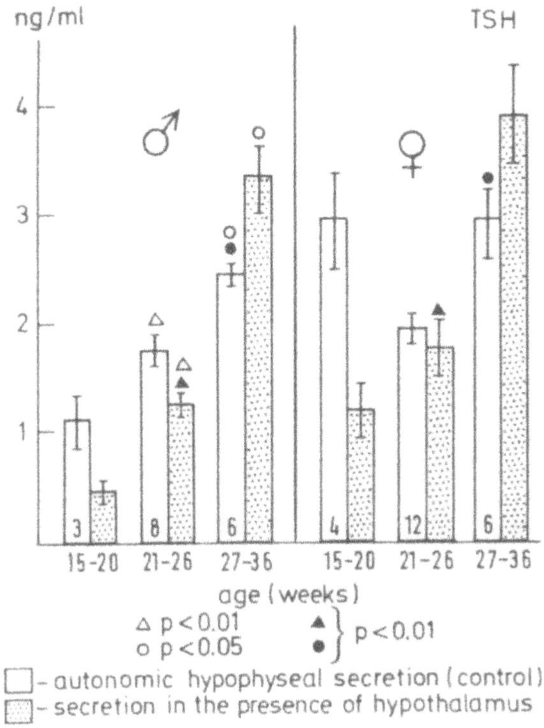

Fig. 3. Influence of hypothalamic addition on TSH secretion level of the fetal hypophysis in vitro in various ages and both sexes. Designations as at Fig. 1

tween the ACTH and TSH secretion levels in controls during the last third of prenatal life (r = 0.89) also in females. In males there are significant correlations between LH plasma concentration and the LH secretion level in both controls (r = 0.82) and in preparations with hypothalamus added (r = 0.84) and also between the ACTH secretion levels in controls and with hypothalamus added (r = 0.80). Finally in both sexes we can see significant correlations between FSH plasma concentration and FSH secretion level in controls (r = 0.67) and with hypothalamus added (r = 0.61), as well as between TSH and GH secretion levels in controls (r = 0.36).

These results indicate (1) that sexual differentiation of neuroendocrine regulation takes place at a very early period (it is already present by the middle of prenatal life) and affects many facets of hypothalamo-hypophyseal function. The investigation has also shown (2) the existence of early interrelationships (also present by the middle of prenatal life) in the functions of fetal endocrines.

In our opinion the data also show (3) the early development of selective permeability of the fetal blood-brain barrier in relation to hypophyseal hormones which is different both between male and female and in various periods of pregnancy.

(4) The hormones observed in cerebral liquor are probably not postmortem artifacts. Their role is not clear so far, but nega-

tive short feedbacks are not yet formed by them in prenatal life as there are no negative correlations between concentrations of any given hormone in the plasma and cerebral liquor of the fetuses. ZH added to the media (Ing/ml) instead of the hypothalamus also did not alter the levels of hypophyseal ZH secretion as compared with controls.

References

LEVINA, S.E.: Essays on Sexual Development in Early Development of Higher Vertebrates (in Russian). Moscow: Nauka 1974

LEVINA, S.E.: Endocrine Development in Human Prenatal Life (in Russian). Moscow: Medicina 1976

Hypothalamic Control of Glucocorticoid Activity. The Adrenal Gland of the Fetal Rat

M. S. MITSKEVICH and O. N. RUMYANTSEVA
Laboratory of Hormonal Regulations, Institute of Developmental Biology, Academy of Sciences of the USSR, Moscow, USSR

To inhibit different links in the fetal hypothalamo-hypophyseal-adrenal system (HHAS), metopirone, hydrocortisone, and dexamethasone were used. Each of these substances was shown to inhibit the glucocorticoid activity of adrenal glands. This effect was accompanied by a change in the glycogen content of the liver and adrenal glands of rat fetuses.

We have previously studied the role of hypothalamo-hypophyseal control in the development and hormonal activity of fetal adrenal glands. The study performed on encephalectomized and decapitated fetuses showed that, in the absence of hypothalamus or hypophysis, a significant decrease in glucocorticoid function of the fetal adrenals takes place (MITSKEVICH and RUMYANTSEVA, 1972).

Further studies of the HHAS activity were aimed at elucidating its role in the control of physiologic processes that depend on glucocorticoid action. A change of glycogen content in the liver and adrenals served as a criterion. Accumulation of glycogen in the fetal liver is known to be under the control of the fetal adrenal glucocorticoids (JACQUOT, 1959).

It has also been shown (in adult animals) that glycogen present in the adrenal gland seems to be related to steroidogenesis; stress and ACTH-activation of adrenals produce a marked decrease in the level of glycogen in the gland (NOBLE and PAPAGEORGE, 1955). It has been established in our investigations of the glycogen content in the liver and adrenal glands of rat fetuses that encephalectomy and decapitation cause a marked change in the glycogen content of the liver and adrenals. In the liver, glycogen concentration was consistently decreased, while in the adrenals it was increased, as compared to the control (RUMYANTSEVA and MITSKEVICH, 1974). These data indicate that HHAS is involved in the control of glycogen content in fetal tissue. However, since decapitation and encephalectomy are a severe interference, probably causing various undesirable side disturbances, thus affecting the end result, it seemed desirable to verify the data obtained by additional means. For this purpose we have undertaken an investigation of fetal HHAS activity using metopirone, hydrocortisone, and dexamethasone - drugs that block the system by affecting its different links. Metopirone acts at the adrenal level, but only the end-product synthesis (that of corticosterone and cortisol) is blocked. A decrease in the blood corticoid level causes (by a feedback mechanism) an increase of the amount of circulating ACTH, which in turn produces hypertrophy of the adrenals. Hydrocortisone acting at the hypophyseal level suppresses the adrenocorticotropic function, and this leads to the cessation of glucocorticoid synthesis in the adrenals.

Dexamethasone is most likely to act directly on the hypothalamus (DUPOUY, 1974) causing, via the latter, the suppression of the adrenocorticotropic function of the hypophysis and consequently, the suppression of the glucocorticoid function of the adrenals.

A. Materials and Methods

The experiments were carried out on 19 rat fetuses 5 days old. Metopirone was twice injected into pregnant females in a dose of 50 µg in 0.6 ml saline. Immediately after metopirone injection, 2 ml isotonic glucose solution (50 g/l) were injected into the same females. Hydrocortisone acetate in a dose of 0.3 mg, as well as dexamethasone in a dose of 0.13 mg in 0.1 ml saline were given as a single injection directly into the fetuses. The fetuses were fixed on the second day; the adrenals and liver were used for subsequent histochemical and biochemical determination of glycogen.

B. Results and Discussion

A reliable increase in the weight of the adrenal glands as compared to the control was observed in rat fetuses subjected to metopirone. The amount of glycogen in the adrenals was found to be similar to that in the adrenal glands of the control fetuses. A consistent (2.5 times) decrease in the glycogen content of the liver was also observed (Fig. 1).

Uniform results were obtained in the experiments with hydrocortisone and dexamethasone injection. As Figure 2 shows, the weight of the adrenal glands was no different from that of the control.

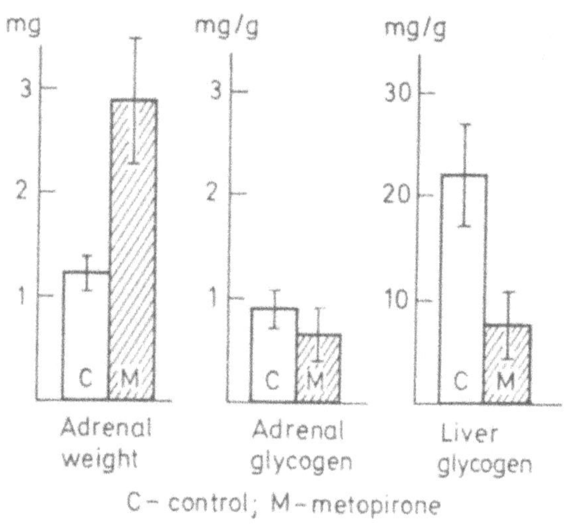

Fig. 1

Fig. 2

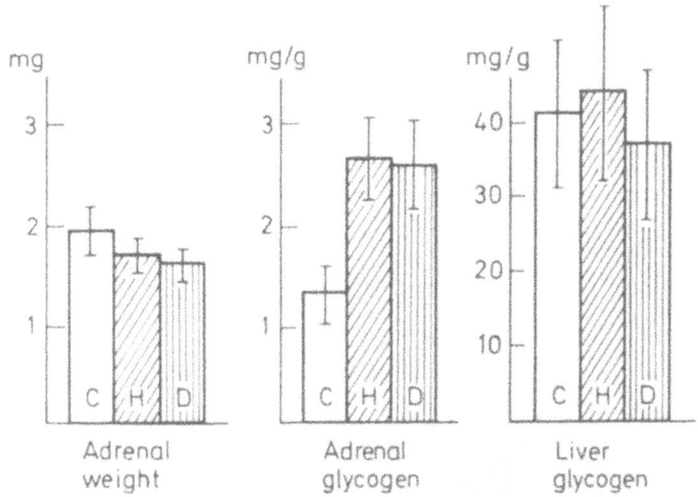

C-control; H-hydrocortisone; D-dexamethasone

At the same time, the amount of glycogen in the adrenals was twice as high as that in the control, while in the liver it remained at the level of the control fetuses.

Thus, the results obtained reflect the specific action of each of the three substances tested. Metopirone-induced decrease of the glycogen level in the fetal liver is accounted for by glucocorticoid deficiency. Glycogen concentration in the adrenals remains at the same level as in the control, which can be explained by the fact that, although no end products of steroidogenesis are formed, the activity of the adrenal cortex does not in fact differ from the control.

Hydrocortisone and dexamethasone, although differing as to the site of their action on the HHAS, both inhibit steroidogenesis in the adrenals and cause an increase of glycogen content in them. The fact that the glycogen concentration in the liver remained unchanged shows that the quantities of the substances (glucocortocoids) injected were insufficient to maintain the same glycogen concentration in the liver as that in the control fetuses. The fact that the above-mentioned changes in the glycogen level are achieved by blocking any link of HHAS of rat fetuses points to the ability of this system as a whole to control certain physiologic functions in the last days of rat prenatal development.

References

DUPOUY, J.P.: Sites of the negative feedback action of corticocosteroids on the hypothalamo-hypophysial system of the rat fetus. Neuroendocrinology 16(3-4), 148-155 (1974)

JACQUOT, R.: Recherches sur le contrôle endocrinien de l'accumulation de glycogène dans le foie chez le foetus de rat. J. Physiol. (Paris) 51, 655-692 (1959)

MITSKEVICH, M.S., RUMYANTSEVA, O.N.: A possible role of the hypothalamus in the control of adrenocortical and thyroid functions during the foetal life. Ontogenez (USSR) 3, 376-384 (1972)
NOBLE, N.L., PAPAGEORGE, E.: Loss of adrenal glycogen in the rat following stress or treatment with various hormones. Endocrinology 57, 492-497 (1955)
RUMYANTSEVA, O.N., MITSKEVICH, M.S.: Glycogen content in the suprarenals and liver of rat foetuses with special reference to the level of adrenocorticotropic function. Ontogenez (USSR) 5(4), 372-380 (1974)

Morphofunctional Characteristics of the Hypothalamo-Hypophyseal Neurosecretory System (HHNS) in Round Goby, *Gobius melanostomus* Pallas, in Early Ontogenesis

E. B. MOISEYEVA
Azov Black Sea Research Institute of Marine Fisheries and Oceanography, Kerch, USSR

The development of the HHNS was studied in fry born in aquaria, from 1 to 60 days after hatching. Fixations of fish were done every 3-5 days. In newly hatched fry, certain parts of the HHNS were already formed. In the adenohypophysis (A), pro-, meso-, and meta-A are distinguished; chromophil cells are absent. In distal parts of the neurohypophysis (NH) there is some compact PAS-negative, Gomori-positive substance. However, the nucleus-preopticus neurosecretory cells and the preopticohypophyseal tract are not seen; neither are the nucleus-lateralis-tuberis cells. Individual capillaries are present in the NH of fry from the 1st day of life. Their number increases with age, indicating the possibility of release of neurosecretory material into the blood. In 7-10 days acidophilic cells of the meso-A associated with growth regulation are differentiated. At 15 days one sees acidophilic cells of the pro-A and, at 20-25 days, basophilic cells of the meso-A, which have a thyrotropic function. Before the beginning of morphologic differentiation of acidophilic and basophilic cells of the meso-A the contacts of the Gomori-positive fibers with corresponding cell types appear in the region of these cells. This fact suggests participation of Gomori-positive neurosecretion in the differentiation of adenohypophyseal cells. As fry develop, the amount of neurosecretory substance in the NH increases, as does the number of axoadenar contacts within the A. They are mostly found in the zone of basophilic cells. Since the first capillaries are observed in the meso-A only in 45-day-old gobies, it seems that neuronal adenocriny is one of the principal ways by which neurohormonal factors influence the A glandular cells of the round goby during its early ontogenesis.

Embryonization of Development and Differentiation of the Neurosecretory System in Insect Embryogenesis

E. N. POLIVANOVA
Institute of Evolutionary Morphology and Ecology of Animals, Academy of Sciences of the USSR
Leningrad, USSR

According to current concepts, the embryonization of development in Arthropoda in general and in insects in particular has great significance for the evolution of this invertebrate group (EZHICOV, 1936; GHILAROV, 1949, 1970). A profound embryonization of insect development is demonstrated by the early onset of a functioning endocrine system in embryogenesis of insects with incomplete metamorphosis, and by embryonic molting cycles. An investigation of the embryos of *Eurygaster integriceps* (Insecta, Hemiptera) has revealed that in the ontogenesis of this insect, some elements of the neurosecretory system disposed in the medial part of the protocerebrum start functioning earlier than other endocrine organs. Large fuchsinophilic D-type cells with fine-granular neurosecretion appear in embryos early in the second half of the developmental period. Before the beginning of cuticle secretion of the future larva, the second type of fuchsinophilic cells (A-cells) appears in the medial part of the protocerebrum. Shortly before hatching, the fuchsinophilic neurosecretion is found in the wall of the aorta. The functional activity of the neurosecretory system in embryos is evidenced by the possibility of inhibition of the release of neurosecretory material under the influence of low temperatures or juvenile-hormone analogs.

References

EZHIKOV, I.I.: Zool. Anz. 114, 141-152 (1936)
GHILAROV, M.S.: Specificity of the soil as habitat and its role in insect evolution. P.-H. Acad. Sci. USSR, 276 (1949)
GHILAROV, M.S.: Regularities in adaptation of arthropods to the terrestrial life. P.-H. Nauka, 279 (1970)

Nuclear Volume Changes in Cells of the Nucleus arcuatus (NA) During Prenatal Development in Man

S. V. VLADIMIROV
Institute of Human Morphology, Academy of Medical Sciences, Moscow, USSR

It is known that the adenohypophyseal function begins during embryonic life. It is not known whether a functional relationship between the hypothalamus and hypophysis exists in fetuses, or at what time this relationship is established. The present study was undertaken in order to elucidate this problem. The extent of development and cell differentiation of the nucleus arcuatus (NA) was detected by karyometric methods. A total of 60 fetuses, from 11 to 31 weeks old (males and females) were studied. The hypothalami of full-term infants were investigated to obtain data for comparison. Adjacent sagittal paraffin sections were stained with cresyl violet and Gomori's CHP. Nuclear volumes were measured on 100 nuclei from each NA, projected onto paper, and the average volume was calculated for each fetus. The mean nuclear volume of NA neurons in both males and females increases steadily from 11 to 19 weeks. However, the mean nuclear volume decreases at 20-21 weeks. Thus, the average nuclear volume in 18-19 week-old fetuses amounts to 138 and 142 μm^3, but that of 20-21 week-old fetuses is 81 and 192 μm^3, in females and males respectively. After this time the nuclei of cells of the NA show a marked growth; by 24-25 weeks the average nuclear volume (192 μm^3) reaches that of full-term infants (189 μm^3). Consequently, by 20 weeks of embryogenesis the NA is formed as a separate hypothalamic structure. After this, the process of cell differentiation continues to increase and the average nuclear volume reaches a maximum at 24-25 weeks. It is suggested that the specific function of NA of human fetuses begins by 24-25 weeks.

Investigations on the Development of the Hypothalamo-Hypophyseal Neurosecretory System During Ontogenesis in the Chick, *Gallus gallus* L.

H. WAND-KABISCH and H. LUPPA

Department of Cell Biology and Regulation, Section of Biosciences, Karl Marx University, Leipzig, GDR

Precise observations on the development of the classic neurosecretory system in ontogenesis are especially interesting in view of the importance of the neurohypophyseal system in intrinsic brain functions.

Embryos of the White Leghorn breed (*Gallus gallus* L.) were studied between the 7th and 21st day of incubation (i-day). Also, recently hatched chicks were studied up to the 4th week of postnatal development. The presence of neurophysin was demonstrated by the pseudoisocyanin chloride method (STERBA, 1961). The occurrence of neurophysin in the classic neurosecretory system is shown in the following figures: On the 11th i-day (Fig. 1) the first fluorescing granules of neurophysin appear in the neural lobe; the hypothalamic nuclear regions are still unstained. Figure 2 (12th i-day) shows the paraventricular nucleus in a sagittal section with first traces of neurophysin in the neurosecretory perikarya. On the 14th i-day (Fig. 3) neurophysin is more clearly visible in the perikarya: the neurophysin-containing cells of the hypothalamic periventricular region are widely scattered. On the 16th i-day a distinct progress in the differentiation of the classic neurosecretory system takes place. At this stage, the paraventricular nucleus displays a well developed periventricular portion (Fig. 4). The neurophysin-containing neurons increase in number and show varying concentrations of neurosecretory material. The first axonal processes with fine beads are visible. On the 21st i-day (the day of hatching), the neurophysin concentration has increased further; the neurosecretory nuclei exhibit their final extension, and the median eminence reveals an accumulation of neurophysin in its internal part. Figure 5 shows the typical pyramid-like structure of the ventral part of the supraoptic nucleus, as known from adult animals. Differences in intensity of fluorescence refer to individual secretion cycles of the cells. A comparison with chicks two weeks old demonstrates that the classic neurosecretory system passes through further maturation after hatching. Figure 6 shows cells of the lateral part of the paraventricular nucleus of a

→

Fig. 1. 11th i-day, neural lobe. × 240

Fig. 2. 12th i-day, paraventricular nucleus, sagittal section. × 240

Fig. 3. 14th i-day, paraventricular region. × 255

Fig. 4. 16th i-day, paraventricular nucleus. × 240

Fig. 5. 21st i-day, supraoptic nucleus, ventral part. × 225

Fig. 6. 2 week old chick, paraventricular nucleus, lateral part. × 255

Fig. 7. 2 week old chick, cranial neurophysin-containing fibers. × 255

Fig. 8. 2 week old chick, neural lobe. × 175

For explanations, see text

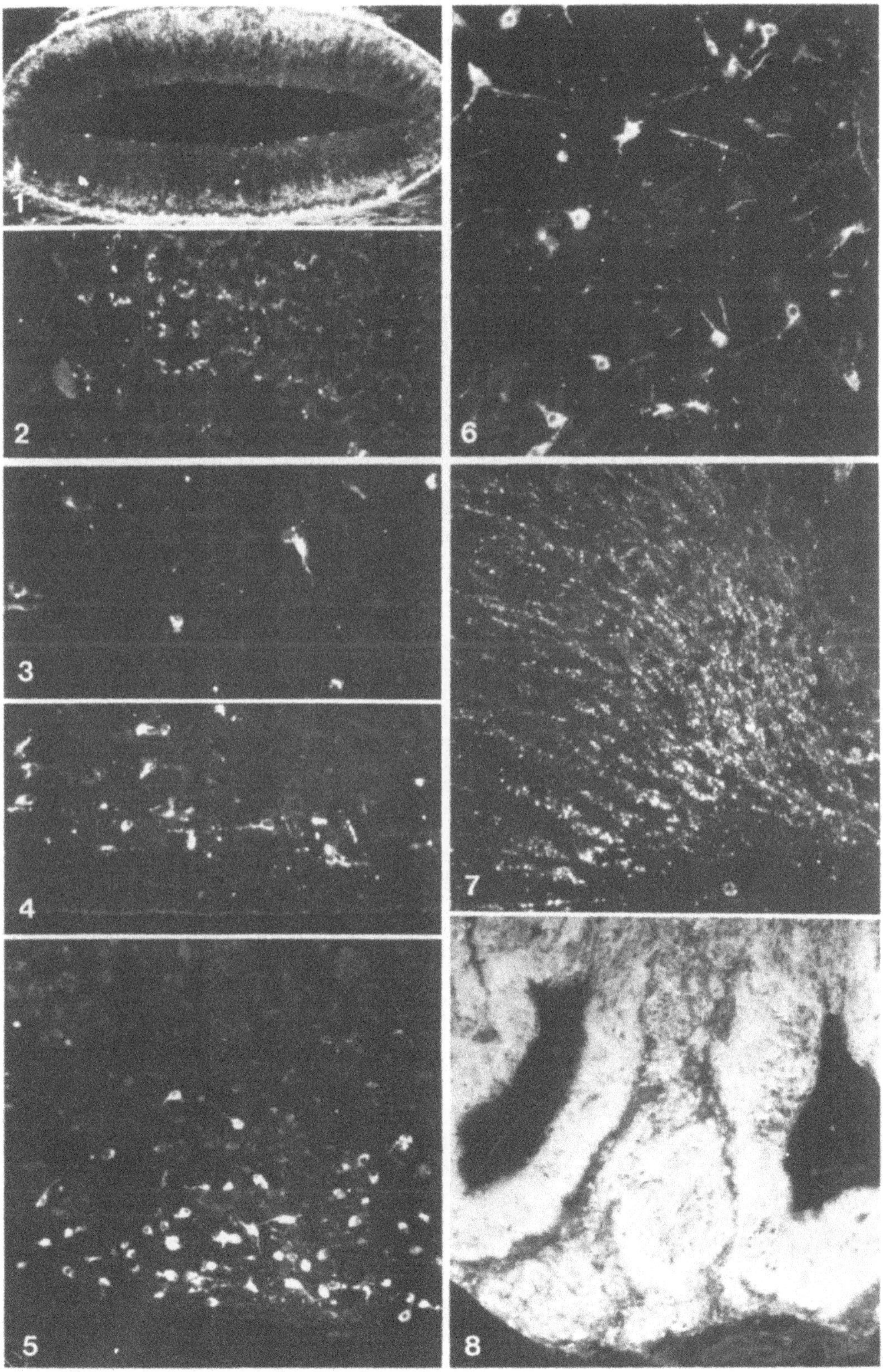
1
2
3
4
5
6
7
8

chick 14 days old. Now the cell processes and nerve fibers in the neuropil are marked distinctly. There is an accumulation of neurophysin-containing fibers between the paraventricular and supraoptic nuclei in the cranial portion of the hypothalamus (Fig. 7). The neural lobe reveals an accumulation of neurophysin, a picture that resembles the situation in the adult stages (Fig. 8).

The time lag of 48 h between the detection of the first osmiophilic granules in the electron microscope (WECHSLER, 1967; FIORONI and WECHSLER, 1968) and the occurrence of pseudoisocyanine fluorescence may be explained on the basis of methodical differences. However, the identity of the electrondense bodies and of neurosecretory elementary granules has not been shown. Furthermore, a false interpretation of the presence of primary lysosomes, which are already observable in the matrix cells, must be considered. On the other hand, a picture with positive fluorescence seems to be a good criterion for the detection of neurophysin in the cell because the technique is based upon the staining of the carrier proteins of the neurohormones (STERBA, 1964). The evidence for simultaneous occurrence of peptide neurohormones is to be expected from immunocytochemical investigations.

References

FIORONI, P., WECHSLER, W.: Elektronenmikroskopischer Nachweis neurosekretorischer Elementargranula im *Processus infundibularis* von Hühnerembryonen. Naturwissenschaften 55, 497-498 (1968)

STERBA, G.: Über eine sehr spezifische Methode zum Nachweis von Neurosekret. Acta Biol. Med. Germ. 7, 228-231 (1961)

STERBA, G.: Grundlagen des histochemischen und biochemischen Nachweises von Neurosekret (= Trägerprotein der Oxytocine) mit Pseudoisozyaninen. Acta Histochem. 17, 268-292 (1964)

WECHSLER, W.: Developmental analysis of the fine structure of different nerve cell types. Exp. Biol. Med. 1, 153-169 (1967)

Regularities in the Development of Nucleus praeopticus (Np) in Acipenseridae

I. V. YAKOVLEVA and N. A. EFIMOVA
Sechenov Institute of Evolutionary Physiology and Biochemistry of the Academy of Sciences of the USSR, Leningrad, USSR

Early stages in the development of the elements of the peptidergic preoptico-hypophyseal system (PHS), especially those of neurosecretory cells (NSC), have not been studied sufficiently (see YAKOVLEVA, 1974). Only isolated electron-microscopic observations on Teleostei have been reported (FOLLENIUS, 1965). The development of the structures of the PHS in Acipenseridae at early stages of postembryonic ontogenesis has been studied light microscopically (see YAKOVLEVA, 1974) and electron microscopically (EFIMOVA, 1970; YAKOVLEVA et al., 1974; EFIMOVA et al., 1975, 1976). Some new details are given in the present paper.

Prelarvae (stage I-III), larvae (stage IV) (after YAKOVLEVA, 1952), small fry of sturgeon *Acipenser güldenstädti* Brandt, and sexually immature (1-2 years old) sterlet *A. ruthenus* L. served as the materials for the present study.

In I-II stage prelarvae after hatching an extensive matrix zone with numerous mitoses, undifferentiated cells (u-cells) and type-II NSC are observed in the Np region. Side by side with these cell elements small, "young", poorly differentiated type-I NSC occur in the dorsal part of the Np in stage-III prelarvae and stage-IV larvae.

The u-cells are the smallest in the Np. They contain round nuclei and a narrow rim of cytoplasm. The latter has many ribosomes and polysomes, and single cisternae of rough endoplasmic reticulum (RER). Golgi complex is weakly developed. Transitional forms exist between the u-cells and the small young type-I and -II NSC. The perikarya and nuclei of type-I NSC are larger than those of type II. The RER and Golgi complex of type I are more developed than those of type II. Type-I NSC contain a moderate number of large (d = 110-250 nm) neurosecretory granules. Type-II NSC, on the other hand, possess many small (d = 60-170 nm) secretory granules. Terminal swellings of dendrites of type-II NSC penetrate into the cavity of the third ventricle. The dendrites on type-I NSC are weakly expressed. The nature of type-II NSC is not quite clear.

In fry, side by side with young type-I NSC, large differentiated type-I light and dark NSC are seen in the dorsal part of the Np. In sterlet 1-2 years old, pyknomorphous degenerated type-I NSC occur. In both fry and animals 1-2 years old, the u-cells are concentrated near the matrix zone, in the ventral part of the Np, in the vicinity of the recessus praeopticus.

Type-I light NSC are large and have a relatively light karyoplasm and cytoplasm, and moderately widened cisternae of the RER.

Type-I dark NSC are smaller and have more osmiophilic karyoplasm and cytoplasm than the light NSC; the cisternae of the RER are wider and polysomes are more densely arranged, compared with those of the light cells. Pyknomorphous type-I NSC are the smallest. Their strong osmiophilic bodies and nuclei are of irregular angular shape. The cisternae of the RER are much wider.

Thus, some transitional forms representing different generations of these cells are observed during development of type-I NSC. They are as follows: the bases of development are a matrix cell, a u-cell, a specifically differentiated small young type-I NSC, a highly differentiated large type-I NSC (light and dark) and a degenerated NSC. Distinct dorsoventral and mediolateral gradients in the development of the NSC have been revealed in the Np. Moreover, these NSC develop heterochronically. A matrix zone and u-cells occurs constantly within the Np in Acipenseridae. In animals older than 1 year, the matrix zone is found only in the ventral part, in close vicinity to the recessus praeopticus. The presence of the matrix zone suggests that type-I NSC have a source for their renewal, and that the Np in Acipenseridae are able to regenerate physiologically (see POLENOV et al., 1972). Different age populations of type-I NSC persist from the moment of their appearance in the Np, in all age groups of Acipenseridae. For this reason, type-I NSC of different sizes and in different functional states are constantly seen within the Np in adult animals (POLENOV et al., 1972). Thus, heteromorphism of the definitive Np is due to asynchronous development of type-I NSC within the Np. This makes possible a different degree of differentiation of the cells composing the Np and asynchronous onset of specific functioning of each cell.

References

EFIMOVA, N.A.: The Ultrastructure of the Neurosecretory Cells of the Preoptic Nucleus in Sterlet. Abstracts. XIIIth Conference of Postgraduates. Leningrad 1970, pp. 19-21

EFIMOVA, N.A., SENCHIK, Yu.I., YAKOVLEVA, I.V.: Electron microscope studies of neurosecretory cells of the sturgeon fry nucleus preopticus. Tsitologiia (Leningrad) 17, 620-627 (1975)

EFIMOVA, N.A., YAKOVLEVA, I.V., SENCHIK, Yu.I.: Peculiarities of the Ultrastructure and Development of Preoptic Nucleus Neurosecretory Cells in the Sturgeon Larvae. Abstracts of CnNIORKh Conference. Guriev 1976, pp. 113-114

FOLLENIUS, E.: Bases structurales et ultrastructurales des corrélations hypothalamo-hypophysaires chez quelques Poissons Téléostéens. Ann. Sci. Nat. Zool. 12, Ser.7, 1-150 (1965)

POLENOV, A.L., CHETVERUKHIN, V.K., YAKOVLEVA, I.V.: The role of ependyma of the recessus praeopticus in formation and physiological regeneration of the Nucleus praeopticus in lower vertebrates. Z. Mikrosk. Anat. Forsch. 85, 513-532 (1972)

YAKOVLEVA, I.V.: Histogenesis of the sturgeon thyroid gland and the hypophysis with special reference to the larva stage of development. Thesis. Leningrad 1952

YAKOVLEVA, I.V.: Development of the elements of hypothalamo-hypophysial neurosecretory system in early ontogenesis of vertebrates. In: Hormonal Factors of Individual Development. ASTAUROV, B.L. (ed.). Moscow: Nauka 1974, pp. 45-60

YAKOVLEVA, I.V., EFIMOVA, N.A., SENCHIK, Yu.I.: The characteristics of ultrastructures of neurosecretory cells at different stages of differentiation from the Nucleus praeopticus of juvenile sterlet (*Acipenser ruthenus* L.). Ontogenesis (Moscow) 5, 180-186 (1974)

Structure and Function of Neurosecretory Systems in the Brain of Vertebrates

Neurosecretion in Vertebrates

G. STERBA
Department of Cell Biology and Regulation, Section of Biosciences, Karl Marx University, Leipzig, GDR

The impetus emanating from a scientific event is not only determined by the quality of the papers read and the discussions held but is also dependent on the atmosphere in which a scientific exchange can develop. I believe that the Seventh International Symposium on Neurosecretion in Leningrad has confirmed this experience. All of us will remember with pleasure the open-mindedness of all participants and the enthusiastic curiosity of our younger colleagues. Seldom has respect for scientific achievement been so clearly perceptible as in the last few days.

Regarding vertebrates, our symposium has focused on the evolution of neurosecretory systems and the morphofunctional analysis of the exohypothalamic parts of the classic neurosecretory system. In contrast to the two preceding symposia in Kiel (1969) and London (1973), the complexes of "hypophysiotropic neurosecretion" and "monoaminergic mechanisms" were treated sporadically, a fact that partly mirrors the trend of international interest in the field of neurosecretion. As had already appeared in outline in London, we are in a stage that is characterized by a pronounced change of interest towards the interactions of the classic neurosecretory system with other neuronal systems. Due to this development, the subject of neurosecretion is newly oriented as to its contents, and this makes clear both the state of independence of the relevant researches and its role as a mediator between neuroendocrinology and neurobiology. The individual tasks resulting from this require that progress made both in neuroendocrinologic and in neurobiologic fields are also taken into consideration. Methodologically, the new tasks can only be accomplished if we avail ourselves of electrophysiologic, biochemical, and pharmacologic techniques to a greater extent. This does not imply that the experts in neurosecretion preferentially trained in anatomy and histology necessarily have to become physiologists, biochemists, or pharmacologists, but more and more cooperation with specialists in other disciplines is absolutely necessary for research in the field of neurosecretion. When considering my own studies along with these remarks, the emphasis placed on the evolution of the neurosecretory systems can be understood as an endeavor to review the foundations of our research in a new stage of orientation. Professor POLENOV and his colleagues have been successfully concerned with this study. Their results have shown us that we possess rather distinct ideas about the descending part of the classic neurosecretory system. They show that, in the individual groups of vertebrates, a uniform basic principle with relatively slight variations is realized. On the other hand, the symposium has given suggestions that some findings that have been considered well established have to be studied anew. This includes the question of the turnover of hormones and neurophysins in the neurons, the capacity of neurophysins to bind hormones in vivo, the axonal transport of the neurophysin vesicles, as well as problems of embryogenesis and aging.

The second predominant subject is the exohypothalamic subsystem and the inclusion of the classic neurosecretory system in cerebral functions; data, largely concurring, were reported particularly in the second part of the symposium. Helped by the perfection of immunohistologic and ultrahistochemical techniques, results were achieved in this field that break new ground and will, therefore, command our attention in the next few years. One may predict that, within the foreseeable future, several brain atlases with exact cartographic details of the exohypothalamic-neurosecretory fiber connections can be expected, and that the synapses of these fibers with other neurons will gain general neurobiologic importance as a model for peptidergic synapses.

Mention should be made of the fact that such central questions as the consolidation of memory and the generation of emotions were contributed to the discussions about the exohypothalamic part of the classic neurosecretory system. With this, however, the development already indicated above has reached a stage of particular topicality with respect to man. For example, their diffuse arrangement precludes a systematic analysis of the peptidergic synapses of the system with electrophysiologic methods, i.e., an analysis of the synaptic functions of the hormones of the posterior lobe.

Finally, I should like to comment briefly on nomenclature. In my opinion it is necessary to specify the term "peptidergic" for the classic neurosecretory system of vertebrates. The immunohistologic methods permit statements as to whether oxytocin, vasopressin, or another hormone of the posterior lobe is formed in a neuronal structural unit. Therefore, it would be only natural to follow an old suggestion made by BARGMANN (1967) and to speak of oxytocinergic, vasopressinergic, vasotocinergic etc. neurons, fibers, terminals, and synapses. It is considerably more difficult to find a collective name that gives a clear definition of the peptidergic neurons of the classic posterior-lobe system to distinguish them from other peptidergic neurons. All hormones of the posterior lobe are homologs of oxytocin. Therefore, we have decided to use the collective name "oxytocinergic." We are aware that its use can lead to misunderstanding and that a better term should be found. We think it useful to study this problem further, and we ask you for suitable suggestions that will help us to agree upon a uniform nomenclature at the next symposium.

Fat Ingestion as a Stimulus of Vasopressin (ADH) Release

JU. O. ABELSON
Sechenov Institute of Evolutionary Physiology and Biochemistry of the USSR Academy of Sciences, Leningrad, USSR

ADH release as a response to fat ingestion was first suggested by ZAKS et al., who observed an acute decrease of water diuresis in dogs and rats after administration of sunflower oil or butter (GZGZYAN and ZAKS, 1967; ABELSON and ZAKS, 1969; ABELSON, 1969). An increase in urine osmolality, prevention of the antidiuretic reaction by ethanol, and some other facts indicated the ADH-induced nature of that antidiuresis, but direct evidence was absent until now. In the present study the effect of fat on urine flow was investigated in rats with inherited hypothalamic diabetes insipidus (DI rats, Brattleboro strain). Whereas in Wistar rats the phenomenon of "fat antidiuresis" can be reliably reproduced in most of the cases (ABELSON, 1969), only some DI rats were found to be responsive to fat. Thus, 1 ml of sunflower oil administered into the stomach did not produce an antidiuretic effect in 12 of 19 DI rats; in the other seven, urine output during a 90-min collection period decreased by only $48.1 \pm 3.5\%$. No changes in urine osmolality were observed in the course of the antidiuretic reaction. At the same time, creatinine excretion diminished, indicating a decrease in glomerular filtration rate. Ethanol failed to prevent the antidiuresis. Since the antidiuretic effect after fat ingestion in DI rats can be observed rather rarely as compared to non-DI rats, it may be concluded that, in normal animals, administration of moderate amounts of fat is followed by ADH release. The role of the neurohormone in this situation remains to be established.

References

ABELSON, Ju.O.: J. Evol. Biochem. a. Physiol., 5, 335 (1969)
ABELSON, Ju.O., ZAKS, M.G.: Sechenov Physiol. J. USSR, 55, 368 (1969)
GZGZYAN, D.M., ZAKS, M.G.: Sechenov Physiol. J. USSR, 53, 711 (1967)
(all papers in Russian)

Comparative Light- and Electron-Microscopic Investigations of Neurosecretory Cells

A. ÁBRAHAM and A. STAMMER
Zoologic Institute of Attila József University, 6722 Szeged, Hungary

We carried out investigations on the neurosecretory cells of the earthworm (*Lumbricus terrestris*), the water beetle (*Dytiscus marginalis*), the carp (*Cyprinus carpio*), and the horseshoe bat (*Rhinolophus ferrum-equinum*). We investigated the supraesophageal and abdominal ganglia of the earthworm and water beetle, and the preoptic, supraoptic, and paraventricular nuclei of the carp and horseshoe bat. The light-microscopic investigations were carried out on impregnated and stained sections. The material for the electron-microscopic investigations was fixed in 1% osmium tetroxide buffered with veronalacetate and embedded in Araldite, cut with an LKB ultramicrotome, and examined with electron microscopes of various types. In the supraesophageal ganglion of the earthworm, the unipolar neurosecretory cells are peripherally chamferred, passing centrally into the processes. The consistent-sized homogenous secretory granules fill the cytoplasm completely. In the axons, both secretory and synaptic vesicles occur. The former are dense and large (1400 Å), the latter are clear and small (300 Å). In the large neurosecretory cells of the water beetle, very different-sized secretory granules are homogeneously dark. The secretory granules appeared in the neuropil both inside and outside the axons. The preoptic nuclei of the carp are longitudinal bodies under the ependyma of the third ventricle. Their unipolar cells are stained very darkly with chrome-hematoxylin. In the axons the neurosecretory material is arranged in longitudinal clots. In the paraventricular nucleus of the horseshoe bat the cells are multipolar, the granules uniform, and in the processes they are arranged in lines. The supraoptic nuclei are demarcated bodies close to the brain surface. Their multipolar cells are large, and full of small granules. This system is particularly characterized by the large roundish secretion bodies lying alongside the small granules. In the organization of the neurosecretory cells of annelids and insects, the common origin is easily visible. The preoptic, supraoptic, and paraventricular nuclei of fish and bats represent newer acquisitions in phylogenesis.

Extravascular Spaces in the Pituitary of Teleostei Revealed by Use of Horseradish Peroxidase

M. ABRAHAM, M. KIESELSTEIN, and S. LISSON-BEGON
The Hebrew University of Jerusalem and the Hospital for Chronic Diseases, Jerusalem, Israel

Specimens of *Mugil cephalus*, *M. capito*, and *Cyprinus carpio* were injected with horseradish peroxidase (HRP) (10 mg/100 g body wt.) and killed after 3.5 h. Their pituitaries were fixed, incubated in TRIS-buffered diaminobenzidine and H_2O_2 and studied under the electron microscope. Peroxidase molecules spread through the pituitary tissue and exposed, in both the adenohypophysis (AH) and the neurohypophysis (NH), an elaborately interconnected system of spaces, suggesting the probable pathway of metabolite exchange between the circulatory system and the cells. These spaces, stained black with HRP, are important in elucidating the relationship between epithelial stellate-cell, neurosecretory, glial, and vascular elements of the gland.

Details of the structure and possible function of the main components of this system of spaces are discussed below:

1. The pericapillary spaces (PCS) are not limited to the immediate surroundings of the capillaries (Figs. 1, 5, 7). They extend from the capillary region proper, and often form links between neighboring capillaries. In freshwater specimens of euryhaline species, with a high prolactin-cell activity, the PCS in the rostral pars distalis are more developed than those in seawater specimens. At the periphery of the pituitary where the capillaries run close to the surface of the gland, their PCS are interconnected by an unbroken space around the gland (Fig. 5). Externally, this space is bounded by a thin sheet of connective-tissue cells.

2. The interlobular spaces (ILS) between the NH and the AH, 180-350 nm in width, are linked with the PCS (Fig. 7). The ILS, interposed at the AH-NH interface, and usually described as "basement" membranes and regarded as a barrier, are actually part of the extravascular space system, and so may act as a connection rather than as an obstacle between axons and epithelial cells. Occasionally, the NS axons traverse the ILS from the NH to the AH, thus interrupting the continuity of the ILS. The latter may act as a storage and/or distribution system of NS hormones to a large number of cells immediately adjacent to the AH-NH interface. Along the ILS, "synaptoid" swellings and vesicles are encountered at the NH side, suggesting the discharge of NS hormones into the ILS.

3. The pericellular (Figs. 1 and 2) and periaxonal (Fig. 4) spaces. In the AH, the pericellular spaces often enlarge and form secretory "lakes" (Fig. 2), with exocytotic figures at the region of contact between cell border and lake. Secretory lakes are abundant on the periphery of the AH in freshwater *M. cephalus*.

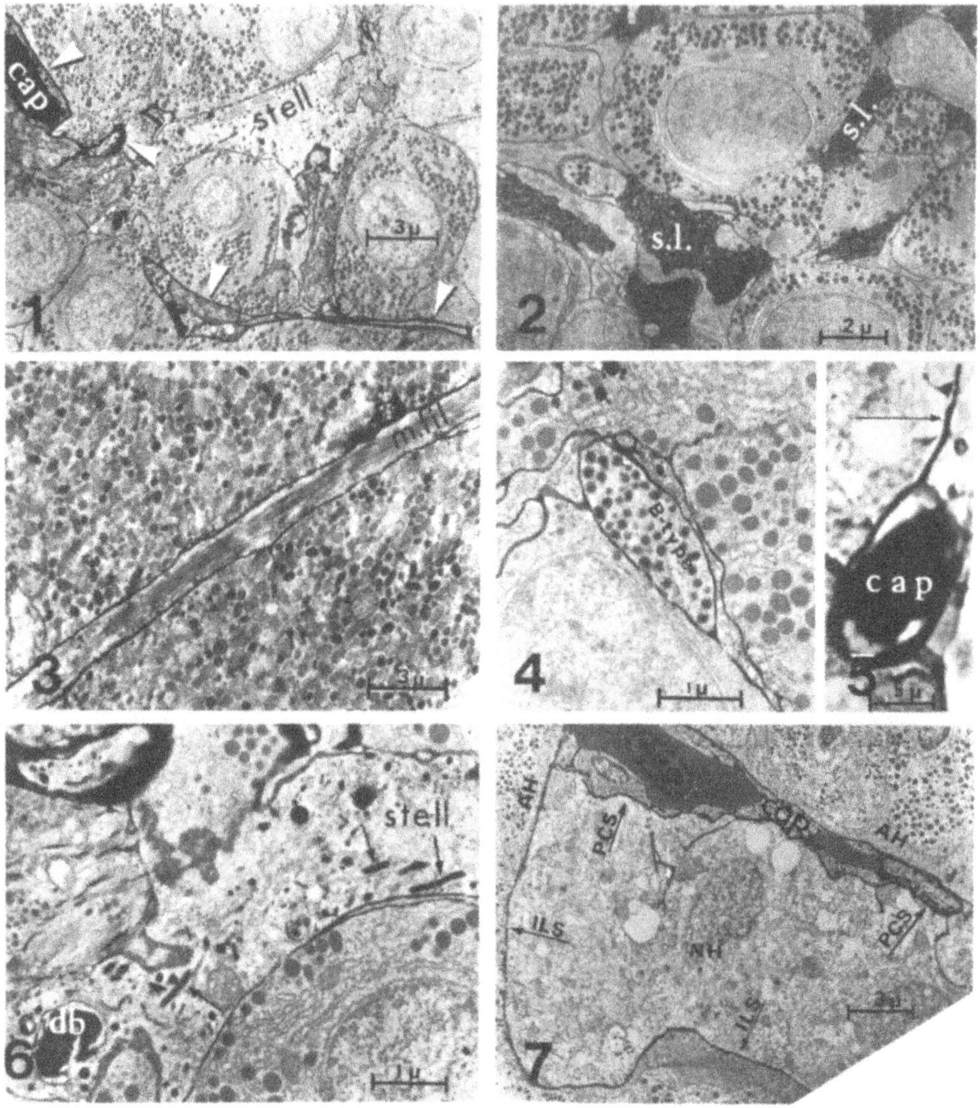

Fig. 1. Capillary (*cap*) and pericapillary spaces (*arrowheads*) from caudal pars distalis of *M. cephalus*; *stell* - stellate cell

Fig. 2. Prolactin cells with pericellular spaces and secretory lakes (*s.l.*) from freshwater specimen of *M. cephalus*

Fig. 3. Extension of fibrillar pituicyte between axonal swellings of NH of *M. cephalus*; *m. fil* - microfilaments

Fig. 4. *B-type* NS axon between AH cells of *M. cephalus*

Fig. 5. Circumpituitary spaces (*arrow*) connected to pericapillary spaces at periphery of pituitary, close to its surface; *M. cephalus*

Fig. 6. Stellate cell (*stell*) with two kinds of phagosomes; rounded (*db*) and tubular (*arrows*); *M. cephalus*

Fig. 7. Interlobular spaces (*ILS*) connected to pericapillary spaces (*PCS*) in rostral pars distalis of *C. carpio*; *AH* - adenohypophysis, *NH* - neurohypophysis, *cap* - capillary

4. The peristellate cell spaces (Figs. 1 and 6) and the periglial spaces (Fig. 3). The stellate cells are found throughout the AH, with the possible exception of the pars intermedia. They extend in slender projections between the epithelial cells, forming small intercellular canaliculi that connect secretory cells and pericapillary spaces. Recently, intercellular structures that may act as spacing junctions were found (ABRAHAM, LAVI and LOTAN, unpublished) at the meeting point of the intercellular canaliculi and the pericapillary spaces in the rostral pars distalis of *Aphanius dispar*.

Phagocytotic activity enables the stellate cells to accumulate in their cytoplasm numerous structures containing HRP (Figs. 1 and 6). These dark-stained phagosomes are of two kinds: (1) large rounded or irrregular bodies, and (2) tubular profiles often reaching a length of 1 μ in a section plane. The amount of peroxidase-positive particles increases in the vicinity of the pericapillary spaces. The stellate cells are strategically placed between the secretory cells, capillaries, and NS axons that have penetrated into the AH. They may be involved with neuroendocrine regulation and/or transport. They may also have a protective function.

There is a parallelism in structure and possibly in function between the stellate cells of the AH and the pituicytes of the NH. Two types of pituicytes were found: (1) phagocytotic pituicytes, which may have a function corresponding to that of the stellate cells with phagosomes, and (2) fibrillar pituicytes, which extend between the axonal swellings of the neural lobe. These extensions are very long, and it is possible that their external borders form a connecting system between the axonal swellings and the ILS. The large number of microfilaments within these pituicytes may enable the latter to move, thus facilitating the propulsion of the material that accumulates in the periglial spaces towards the ILS, and hence to the capillaries.

Some Neuroendocrine Aspects of Tanycyte Histophysiology

I. G. AKMAYEV, O. V. FIDELINA, A. P. POPOV, and I. F. EGOROVA
Institute for Experimental Endocrinology and Hormone Chemistry, Moscow, USSR

Much attention is presently focused on the specialized ependyma of brain ventricles in connection with some features suggesting its implication in neuroendocrine function (KNOWLES, 1972). The latter applies especially to the tanycyte ependyma of the floor and ventrolateral walls of the third ventricle. The relationship between the tanycytes on the one hand and the hypophyseal adrenocorticotrophic function and the gonadal hormones on the other has been the subject of our enzyme-histochemical and ultrastructural investigations in recent years.

Enzyme-histochemical studies revealed a negative correlation between tanycyte metabolic and hypophyseal adrenocorticotrophic activities (AKMAYEV and FIDELINA, 1974). It was noteworthy that the activity of certain redox enzymes in male rats increased following sustained dexamethasone treatment, and diminished after bilateral adrenalectomy. The relationship between the tanycytes and hypophyseal-adrenocorticotrophic activity was later studied with the same experimental models at the ultrastructural level. The results of this ultrastructural investigation are consistent with the previously established fact. They also attest to selective β-tanycyte involvement in these correlations. Among the rat tanycytes, the authors distinguish several types differing in topographic and metabolic features, and designate them by letters of the Greek alphabet (AKMAYEV et al., 1973). Their localization within the ependyma of the third ventricle and conventional designations are represented in Figure 1.

Long-term (8 days) dexamethasone administration (5 μg/100 g daily) resulted in enhanced β-tanycyte activity, evidenced by activation of the Golgi apparatus, and an increase of polyribosomes and lipid inclusions. Activation of the Golgi complex was manifested by a significant increase in the number of vesicles, among which two sharply differentiated types were distinguished: 40-50 nm vesicles with smooth contours and moderately dense core (type I, Fig. 2a) and 40-90 nm coated vesicles with an electron-lucent center (type II, Fig. 2b). After bilateral adrenalectomy (10, 14, 22 days), the changes in the β-tanycytes were of a different character. In the Golgi area the number of type I vesicles decreased. The number of lipid inclusions did not exceed the control level. Vesicles resembling catecholamine vesicles in appearance and size (type III, Fig. 2c) were demonstrated with appreciably greater frequency. The number of vesicles distinguished by an extremely peculiar appearance increased most markedly (type IV, Fig. 2d). Such vesicles resembled irregular rosettelike structures 50-140 nm in size, with a small amount of dense material between the light center and the limiting membrane. These structures were described by WITTKOWSKI (1972), who considered them

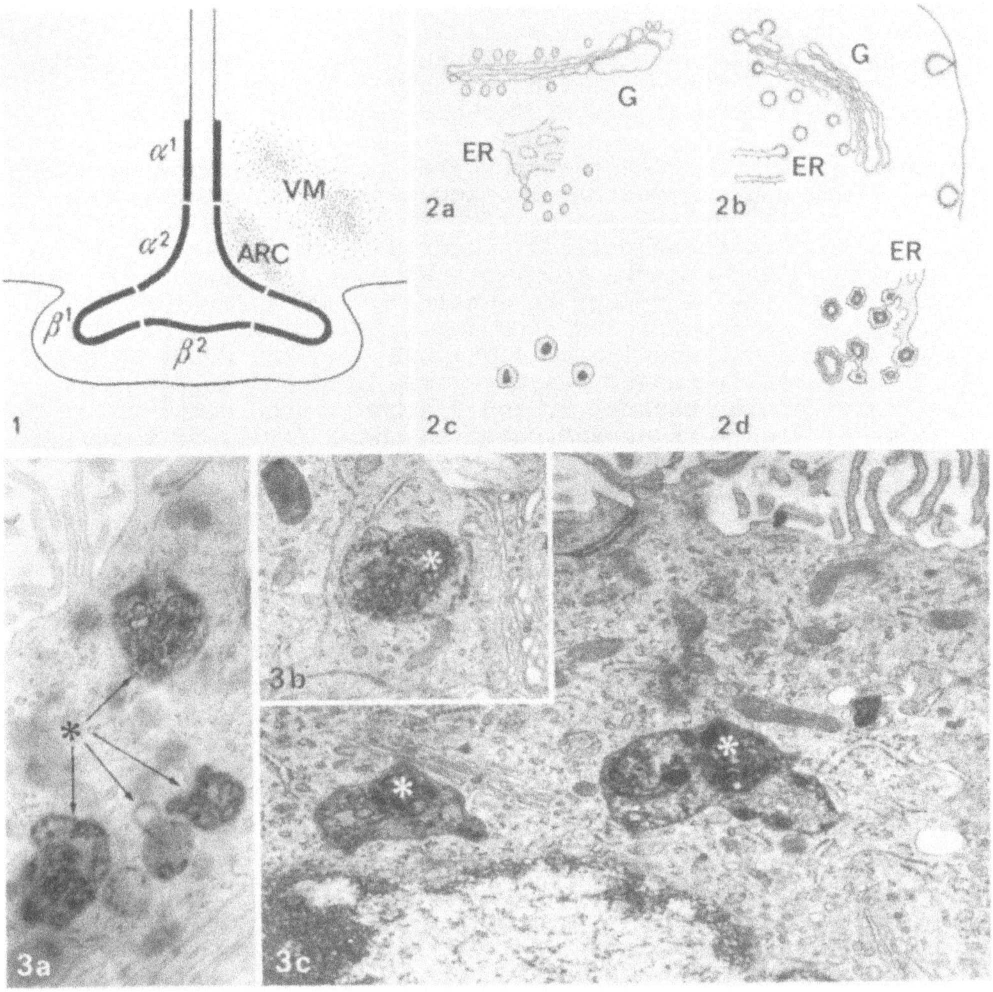

Fig. 1. Scheme representing topography of types of rat tanycytes. *ARC* - arcuate nucleus, *VM* - ventromedial nucleus
Fig. 2a-d. Different vesicle types (I-IV) in rat β-tanycytes. *G* - Golgi complex, *ER* -endoplasmic reticulum
Fig. 3a-c. Lysosomelike structures (*) in rat α^2-tanycytes. Electron micrographs. × 9000 (Fig. 3a,b), × 14,000 (Fig. 3c)

a probable secretory product of the median-eminence tanycytes. It is possible that their increased amount in adrenalectomized rats is indicative of a delayed transport of the secretion. On the other hand, activation of the Golgi apparatus in long-term dexamethasone administration may point to enhanced transport (or secretory) activity of the β-tanycyte. The authors believe that the correlation between β-tanycytes and hypophyseal-corticotrophic activities is regulated by a feedback mechanism and provide evidence for the existence of a coupling servomechanism between the β-tanycytes and the hypophyseal-adrenocortical system. It is therefore logical to suppose that the β-tanycytes contribute to the inhibiting control of ACTH secretion. The mechanism of this control is still not clear and may be explained in two possible ways: either β-tanycytes secrete some factor that suppresses ACTH secretion, or they exert an inhibiting effect through intensification of their transport activity.

The relationship between the tanycytes and the gonadal hormones was studied in early postnatal ontogenesis, when the hypothalamic nerve structures are hypersensitive to the circulating hormones, i.e., in the "critical period" of sexual differentiation of the hypothalamus. The authors took into account the suggestion that tanycytes may act as receptors sensitive to the level of gonadal hormones in the CSF (KNOWLES and ANAND KUMAR, 1969). The activity of some dehydrogenases (GDH, LDH, G-6-PD, GPDH, $NADH_2$-DH) in the different types of tanycytes was studied in young male and female rats on days 3, 5, and 7 after birth. Clear-cut differences between females and males in the activity of these enzymes were revealed in the β^1-tanycytes. The authors suppose that the differences are due to the occurrence in these cells of corresponding receptors for the gonadal hormones and point to the involvement of tanycytes in the mechanisms of sexual differentiation of the hypothalamus. Attention was also drawn to the increase of aldehydefuchsin-stained lysosomelike structures in α^1- and α^2-tanycytes of female and male rats at the age of 1-3 weeks of postnatal life (Fig. 3). A modified Gomori aldehydefuchsin technique was used to identify these structures in semithin epoxy sections (STOECKEL et al., 1972).

References

AKMAYEV, I.G., FIDELINA, O.V.: Morphological aspects of the hypothalamic-hypophyseal system. V. The tanycytes: their relation to the hypophyseal adrenocorticotrophic function. An enzyme-histochemical study. Cell Tissue Res. 152, 403-410 (1974)

AKMAYEV, I.G., FIDELINA, O.V. KABOLOVA, Z.A., POPOV, A.P., SCHITKOVA, T.A.: Morphological aspects of the hypothalamic-hypophyseal system. IV. Medial basal hypothalamus. An experimental morphological study. Z. Zellforsch. 137, 493-512 (1973)

KNOWLES, Sir F.: Ependyma of the third ventricle in relation to pituitary function. Prog. Brain Res. 38, 255-270 (1972)

KNOWLES, Sir F., ANAND KUMAR, T.C.: Structural changes, related to reproduction, in the hypothalamus and in the pars tuberalis of the *Rhesus* monkey. Philos. Trans. R. Soc. Lond.(Biol.) 256, 357-375 (1969)

STOECKEL, M.E., PORTE, A., DELLMANN, H.-D.: Selective staining of neurosecretory material in semithin epoxy sections by Gomori's aldehyde fuchsin. Stain Technol. 47, 81-85 (1972)

WITTKOWSKI, W.: Zur Ultrastruktur der Gefäßfortsätze von Ependym- und Gliazellen im Infundibulum der Ratte. Z. Zellforsch. 130, 58-69 (1972)

Adrenergic Regulation of Hypothalamic Neurosecretory Functions

B. V. ALESHIN
Institute of Endocrinology and Hormone Chemistry, Kharkov, USSR

It may now be regarded as certain that the mediobasal hypothalamus controls the hormonopoietic functions ofthe anterior pituitary (at least in mammals and humans). The small neurosecretory cells of the mediobasal hypothalamus produce specific oligopeptide adenohypophysiotropic hormones. However, the reactions associated with an increase or decrease of one or another anterior-pituitary hormone secretion are often accompanied by marked changes in the functional activity of the large "Gomori-positive" cells of the anterior hypothalamus. In particular, intensification of the hypophyseal thyrotropic function, observed after thyroidectomy or cervical sympathectomy, in many cases coincides with an obvious decrease in the secretory activity of the supraoptic nucleus cells. In contrast, after an increase of antidiuretic hormone secretion (elicited, for example, by administration of hypertonic saline solutions) and hence, a rise in the Gomori-positive cell activity, the hypophyseal thyrotropic function decreases, and the thyroid shows signs of depression (ALESHIN, 1971, 1974). On the other hand, intensification of the hypophyseal adrenocorticotropic function (for example in response to stress or superior cervical sympathetic ganglia (GCS) stimulation) occurs simultaneously with a pronounced increase in the secretory activity of the supraoptic nucleus cells. These observations would support the hypothesis of a participation of this magnocellular nucleus in the regulation of adenohypophyseal hormonopoiesis by suppression of the pituitary thyrotropic function and stimulation of the adrenocorticotropic function. However, the Gomori-positive neurosecretory cells, the main function of which is control of the water metabolism and maintenance of the organism's osmotic balance, do not participate directly in regulation of the anterior pituitary. Hence, involvement of Gomori-positive cells in the reactions controlled by the mediobasal hypothalamus suggests that both neurosecretory hypothalamic formations (the adenohypophysiotropic area of the mediobasal hypothalamus and the magnocellular nuclei of the anterior hypothalamus) are influenced by the same regulatory mechanisms.

Since the neurons of the mediobasal hypothalamus are adrenergic, the principal role in the regulation of adenohypophysiotropic hormone release should belong to the catecholamines. In experiments performed on male adult rabbits we have found a small but consistent rise in the noradrenaline concentration of the hypothalamus in all cases of increased thyrotropin production and secretion by the anterior pituitary (see reports of CHUPRINOVA et al., also of OUS and ALESHIN, in this volume). Our findings permit us to assume that this catecholamine stimulates release of thyrotropin-releasing hormone (thyroliberin) by the mediobasal hypothalamus; this is in accordance with the results of the direct effect of noradrenaline on the hypothalamus. This catecholamine in vitro stimulates the explanted hypothalamus to increased release of thyrotropin-releasing hormone (GRIMM and REICHLIN, 1973).

At the same time, noradrenaline acts as a depressant on the hypothalamic regulation of the pituitary adrenocorticotropic function (GANONG, 1972). Indeed, an increase of pituitary adrenocorticotropic hormone secretion was associated with a decrease in the hypothalamic noradrenaline level. The results of our experiments indicate that noradrenaline stimulates thyroliberin release by the mediobasal hypothalamus, whereas decrease of this catecholamine level in the hypothalamus favors discharge of corticotropin-releasing hormone (corticoliberin).

The presence of numerous noradrenergic synapses on the perikarya and dendrites of Gomori-positive cells (POLENOV and SENCHIK, 1966) would indicate that fluctuations in the hypothalamic noradrenaline level not only influence the adenohypophsiotropic hormone release via the mediobasal hypothalamus, but must also be reflected in the functioning of the anterior hypothalamic neurosecretory magnocellular nuclei. In previous studies from our laboratory we have shown that the secretory activity of the supraoptic nucleus cells increases markedly in response to stimulation of the GCS and decreases following cervical sympathectomy (ALESHIN, 1971). It seems that these findings permit us to ascribe to the sympathetic impulses a stimulating effect on Gomori-positive cells of the anterior hypothalamus. However, the subsequent analysis of these responses revealed that impulses deriving from GCS do not reach the hypothalamic neurosecretory formations directly. The effects on the Gomori-positive cells in response to interventions applied to the GCS are mediated by hypothalamic noradrenergic mechanisms. The source of the hypothalamic noradrenergic neurons is the mesencephalic reticular formation (BJÖRKLUND et al., 1970; HÖKFELT and FUXE, 1972). Impulses sent by GCS affect the latter. Therefore, stimulation of the GCS is followed by a pronounced rise in the total catecholamine content (not only noradrenaline, but also adrenaline) in the midbrain and hypothalamus. Adrenaline is absent from the brain of rabbits under normal conditions, and probably appears there as a result of conversion of some noradrenaline under these conditions. Hence, the influence of sympathetic impulses on the hypothalamus consists of intensification of the biosynthesis of catecholamines. Besides, with the appearance of adrenaline in the rabbit's hypothalamus, the effects elicited in it by noradrenaline decrease.

As stimulation of GCS results in increased activity of the supraoptic nucleus neurosecretory cells, and in the appearance of adrenaline in the hypothalamus under such conditions, it would seem that the effect of this stimulation on the Gomori-positive cells ought to be ascribed to the latter. However, depletion of hypothalamic catecholamines (after administration of reserpine or chlorpromazine) in our experiments was followed not by a decrease but, on the contrary, by a distinct increase in the secretory activity of the Gomori-positive cells. Since the appearance of adrenaline in the hypothalamus is followed by a weakening of the noradrenaline effects, the activation of Gomori-positive cells under these conditions means that noradrenaline exerts an inhibitory influence on them.

With the decrease of noradrenaline influence resulting from the appearance of adrenaline in the hypothalamus, or following depletion of the latter of catecholamines present in it, the Gomori-positive cells display a high activity, since the inhibitory effect of noradrenaline on them diminishes.

The high cholinesterase content of the anterior hypothalamic neurons is evidence that the Gomori-positive cells belong to the cholinergic ones and as such are stimulated by acetylcholine (ABRAHAMS et al., 1957; KOELLE, 1961). Hence, a decrease of the inhibiting effect of noradrenaline is associated with a rise of Gomori-positive cell activity as a result of developing prevalence of the acetylcholine stimulating effect.

Thus, the association of the secretory activity of supraoptic nucleus neurons with the regulation of the pituitary thyrotropic function is not the result of any inhibitory effect of the Gomori-positive cells on thyrotropin production and secretion by the anterior pituitary. In fact, this association is a secondary consequence of the increase of noradrenaline concentration in the hypothalamus. The rise of the noradrenaline level that occurs in these circumstances simultaneously promotes thyroliberin release by the neurosecretory cells of the mediobasal hypothalamus, and inhibits the function of the supraoptic nucleus. The physiologic value of such additional involvement of the Gomori-positive cells in reactions controlled by the mediobasal hypothalamus could consist in the modulating effect that the Gomori-positive cells supposedly exert on the release of adenohypophysiotropic hormones by the mediobasal hypothalamic cells HEDGE and SMELIK, 1969). The Gomori-positive cells of the anterior hypothalamus are in turn influenced by the mediobasal hypothalamus. Thus, destruction of the ventromedial nucleus in our previous experiments elicited a marked rise in the secretory activity of the supraoptic nucleus cells (ALESHIN et al., 1974). This response depends on the structure of the ventromedial nucleus, in which the small neurosecretory cells are coupled with numerous adrenergic neurons (BROWNSTEIN et al., 1974). Elimination of the latter after destruction of ventromedial nucleus results in a decrease of the hypothalamic catecholamine level, thus causing a rise of the Gomori-positive cell activity.

Finally, the Gomori-positive cells of the anterior hypothalamus intervene in the regulation of adenohypophyseal hormonopoiesis in that the course of developing responses is strongly dependent both on the degree of hydration of the cytoplasm and on the correlation between the intracellular and extracellular fluid (i.e., on the processes controlled by the Gomori-positive cells of the anterior hypothalamus) in the peripheral effector glands ("target glands"), which are the final links of the developing response.

Transmission of hypothalamic efferent impulses first through the hypothalamic adenohypophysiotropic hormones and then through adenohypophyseal crinotropic hormones, thus produces control of the thyroid, gonads, and adrenal cortex (glucocorticoid and androgenic functions of the latter). Such a mode of hypothalamic regulatory impulse transmission may be designated as *transhypophyseal* or, more exactly, *transadenohypophyseal*. In contrast to the glands mentioned above, the other endocrine organs are not directly dependent on the pituitary, and therefore their control by the hypothalamus must be ensured not by the transadenohypophyseal, but some other mechanism.

As mentioned above, the neurosecretory cells of the mediobasal hypothalamus lie in close contact with adrenergic neurons of the usual type. Some of the latter send their axons in the complex of descending fibers of "Schütz's bundle" via the brain stem to the vagal nuclei, and further to the sympathetic nuclei of the spinal cord. Therefore, the regulatory signals, sent by the mediobasal hypothalamus (in particular, by its ventromedial-arcuate complex), may be transmitted to controlled effector organs both transadenohypophyseally (i.e., humorally via the adenohypophysiotropic hormones, produced by small neurosecretory cells) and along the neural pathways via the sympathetic and parasympathetic effector innervation (hence, without participation of pituitary, i.e., *parahypophyseally*).

The possibility of dual control (transadenohypophyseal and parahypophyseal) of the hypothalamic regulating effects is due to the evolutionary development of neurosecretory cells as a peculiar specialization of nerve cells. In general, all nerve cells are able to synthesize protein substances (SMITH, 1971). As a rule, the forming protein granules are carriers on which the mediators accumulate. But if, in the course of subsequent evolution, the capability for biosynthesis of protein substances becomes dominant, and the granule-carriers acquire the ability to exert stimulating or inhibiting effects on other functions or systems of the organism (i.e., hormonal properties) (PEARSE, 1968), then the Gomori-positive cells of the anterior hypothalamus at first develop as cholinergic neurons, and only later begin to produce neurosecretory substances (PRIJMAK and HAJOS, 1971). These features of the Gomori-positive cells permit us to characterize them as *"peptidocholinergic"*. In a similar way, the neurosecretory cells of mediobasal hypothalamus by their form, structure, volume, and location are so identical with the adjacent adrenergic neurons of the adenohypophysiotropic area of the mediobasal hypothalamus, that the evidence suggests that they may be regarded as developing from the latter. A characteristic of adrenergic neurons is the presence of the so-called "dense-core vesicles," or granules covered with a membrane and with an accumulation of catecholamines on their protein core. Transformation of adrenergic neurons into the neurosecretory cells could consist of the protein core, which is of indifferent physiologic aspect in ordinary adrenergic neurons, gradually becoming an oligopeptide hormone. It would follow that the neurosecretory cells of the mediobasal hypothalamus producing oligopeptide-adenohypophysiotropic hormones are *peptidoadrenergic neurons*.

The physiologic validity of the transformation of cholinergic and adrenergic neurons of the hypothalamus into peptidocholinergic and peptideadrenergic neurosecretory cells respectively resides in the fact that the transmission of hypothalamic stimuli via hormones ensures marked amplification of the initial nervous impulses and, moreover, favors generalization and prolongation in time of the effects elicited by these impulses.

References

ABRAHAMS, V.C., KOELLE, G.B., SMART, F.: Histochemical demonstration of cholinesterases in the hypothalamus of the dog. J. Physiol. (Lond.) 139, 137-144 (1957)

ALESHIN, B.V.: Histophysiology of the Hypothalamo-Hypophysial System (in Russian). Moscow: Medicina 1971

ALESHIN, B.V.: The mechanisms of hypothalamic regulations of the adenohypophysial functions (in Russian). Adv. Physiol. Sci. 5 (1), 48-81 (1974)

ALESHIN, B.V., DEMIDENKO, N.S., MAMINA, V.V.: Reactions of neurosecretory nuclei of the hypothalamus to destruction of some of them (in Russian). Histol. Embryol. 66 (10), 29-33 (1974)

BJÖRKLUND, A., FALCK, B., HROMEK, F., OWMAN, C., WEST, K.A.: Identification and terminal distribution of the tubero-hypophyseal monoamine fibre systems in the rat by means of stereotaxic and microspectrofluorimetric techniques. Brain Res. 17, 1-23 (1970)

BROWNSTEIN, M.J., PALKOVITS, M., SAAVEDRA, J.M., BASSINI, R.M., UTIGER, R.D.: Thyrotropin-releasing hormone in specific nuclei of rat brain. Science 185 (4147), 267-269 (1974)

GANONG, W.F.: Evidence for a central noradrenergic system that inhibits ACTH secretion. In: Brain-Endocrine Interactions. KNIGGE, K.M., SCOTT, D.E., WEINDL, A. (eds.). Basle: Karger 1972, pp. 254-266

GRIMM, Y., REICHLIN, S.: Thyrotropin-releasing hormone (TRH): neurotransmitter regulation of secretion by mouse hypothalamic tissue in vitro. Endocrinology 93, 626-631 (1973)

HEDGE, G.A., SMELIK, P.G.: The action of dexamethasone and vasopressin on hypothalamic CRF production and release. Neuroendocrinology 4, 242-253 (1969)

HÖKFELT, T., FUXE, K.: On the morphology and the neuroendocrine role of the hypothalamic catecholamine neurons. In: Brain-Endocrine Interactions. KNIGGE, K.M., SCOTT, D.E., WEINDL, A. (eds.). Basle: Karger 1972, pp. 181-223

KOELLE, G.B.: A proposal dual neurohumoral role of acetylcholine: its functions at the pre- and postsynaptic sites. Nature 190 (4772), 208-211 (1961)

PEARSE, A.G.E.: Common cytochemical and ultrastructural characteristics of cells producing polypeptide hormones (the APUD series) and their relevance to thyroid and ultimobranchial C cells and calcitonin. Proc. R. Soc. Lond. (Biol.) 170, 71-80 (1968)

POLENOV, A.L., SENCHIK, J.I.: Synapses on neurosecretory cells of the supraoptic nucleus in white mice. Nature 211 (5056), 1423-1424 (1966)

PRIJMAK, E.Ch., HAJOS, F.: Ultrastructure of neurosecretory cells and synapses in the supraoptic nucleus of the rat in early postnatal development (in Russian). Ontogenes 2 (3), 246-251 (1971)

SMITH, A.D.: Summing up: Some implications of the neuron as a secreting cell. Philos. Trans. R. Soc. Lond. (Biol.) 261, 423-437 (1971)

Fine Organization of Smooth Endoplasmic Reticulum in Neurosecretory Axons of Rat Neurohypophysis

G. ALONSO[1], A. RAMBOURG[2], and I. ASSENMACHER[1]
[1]Laboratoire de Neuroendocrinologie, ERA 85 du CNRS, Université de Montpellier II – Pl. E.-Bataillon, 34000 Montpellier, France. [2]Départment de Biologie, CEN de Saclay, 91190 Gif-sur-Yvette, France

The smooth endoplasmic reticulum (SER) was studied in thin (0.5-1 µm) sections of rat neurohypophysis after double impregnation of the tissue blocks with uranyl acetate and an aqueous solution of copper and lead citrate (THIERRY and RAMBOURG, in press).

In the neurosecretory axons of the infundibular stalk, the SER appeared as elongated tubules running parallel to the main axis of the axon, and presenting oblique anastomoses. Numerous neurosecretory granules seemed to lie in close relationship with these tubular elements. In the axonal swellings of the posthypophysis, the SER formed an irregular network of anastomosing tubules. These tubules generally showed an irregular diameter with many dilatations. In some Herring bodies the SER tubules were arranged in a three-dimensional system with polygonal meshes that enclosed many neurosecretory granules or mitochondria. In the terminal part of the axon, the SER tubule frequently appeared to make contacts with the axonal plasma membrane. In some terminals, which characteristically included polymorphic dense bodies, the network of tubules was very dense with fine meshes. At this level there were numerous microvesicles facing the basal membrane, and many of them were seen to bulge at the tip of the thinner tubules of the network.

Many questions arise concerning the role of such a continuous tubular system inside the axoplasm of neurosecretory neurons. The close association of the SER with granules or microvesicles strongly suggests an exchange of macromolecules between these cell organelles at any level of the axon.

Reference

THIERRY, G., RAMBOURG, A.A.: New staining technique for studying thick sections in the electron microscope. J. Microsc. (Oxf.) Biol. Cell (in press)

Effects of Different Salinities on the Neurohypophysis and Blood Osmolarity in *Acipenser ruthenus* L.

YU. V. ALTUFYEV and G. F. METALLOV
Sechenov Institute of Evolutionary Physiology and Biochemistry of the USSR Academy of Sciences, Leningrad, USSR

The neurohypophysis (Nh) of adult male and female *A. ruthenus* L. has been studied in chronic (15‰) and acute (22‰ and 32‰) experiments. The animals were maintained in water with the ionic composition of the Caspian Sea. The amount of neurosecretory material (NSM) in the Nh was estimated visually. The Nh of the fish is characterized by considerable hyperemia during all stages of the acute experiments with a lethal end, after 80 min in 32‰ and 5.5 h in 22‰ salinity. In group 1 (32‰) the Nh of the fish contained 3.8-4.1 units NSM (fluctuation 0.3 units). The average content of NSM in controls was 4 units. Blood osmolarity (BO) in group 1 increased from 315 to 395 mos*M*. In group 2 (22‰) 3.4-4.8 units NSM was found in the Nh (fluctuation 1.4), and 4 units in control. A tendency towards decreasing NSM content for 1-3 h was observed in group 2. An increase of BO from 265 to 395 mos*M* was visible in group 2, as was the case in group 1, though a tendency to decrease was noted for 1-3 h. Three phases of changes in the functional state of the Nh and BO were shown in group 3 (15‰). In phase 1 (up to 3 h) a considerable rise of both NSM content (up to 4.1 units versus 3.6 units in control) and BO (up to 320 versus 190 mos*M* in control) was seen. In phase 2 (6-12 h) a sharp decrease in the NSM content of the Nh (up to 2.5 units) was found. This provides circumstantial evidence that a large amount of neurohormone is discharged from the Nh into the blood circulation. In phase 3 (2-4 days) an increase in NSM content (up to 4.5 units) occurs; there is also a return to a normal level of blood osmolarity (185 mos*M*) on the second day and, later, stabilization. Different degrees of depressed release of neurohormones from the Nh under an extreme (32‰) and a strong (22‰) osmotic load is demonstrated. Release of the neurohormones providing water-salt homeostasis takes place under a bearable load (15‰).

Effects of Indomethacin on the Hypothalamo-Hypophyseal Neurosecretory System

V. I. ARHIPENKO, L. V. GERBILSKY, L. F. KOS, T. K. TRUDOVA, and V. K. STOBETSKAYA
Department of Histology, Medical Institute, Dnepropetrovsk, USSR

Four groups of animals were investigated: intact rats, water-deprived rats, rats given indomethacin, and rats initially given indomethacin and then transferred to water-deprived conditions while continuing to receive indomethacin. Some animals were investigated 3 days after being water deprived. The percentage ratio of cells of various functional activity in the supraoptic and paraventricular nuclei of the hypothalamus, the volume of the cell nuclei, and the RNP and neurosecretion content in the perikarya and in neurosecretory fibers of the median eminence and posterior lobe of the hypophysis have all been determined. The content of the sudanophilic substance in the zona glomerulosa of the adrenal cortex was investigated simultaneously. It was established that the administration of indomethacin in the dosage given (0.5 mg/100 g body wt.) inhibits the functional activity of the hypothalamo-hypophyseal system and of the zona glomerulosa of the adrenal cortex in normal water-regimen conditions. The administration of indomethacin for 3 days prior to water deprivation considerably inhibits the development of the response of the hypothalamo-hypophyseal system and of the zona glomerulosa of the adrenal cortex. It may be concluded that the inhibition of prostaglandin synthesis by indomethacin appreciably influences the functional condition of the neurosecretory cells of the hypothalamo-hypophyseal system and the gland cells of the zona glomerulosa of the adrenal cortex both in conditions of normal water intake and during water deprivation. Thus, an important role of the prostaglandins in the regulation of neurosecretory cells and cells of the zona glomerulosa of the adrenal cortex is shown.

Functional Morphology of the Peptidergic Hypothalamo-Hypophyseal Neurosecretory System of Rat in Postnatal Ontogenesis After Exposure to Aromatic Hydrocarbons

G. Z. BAKHTIZINA
Scientific Research Institute of Hygiene and Occupational Diseases, Ufa, USSR

The hypothalamo-hypophyseal neurosecretory system (HHNS) of intact and benzene- and xylol-poisoned rats on the 15th day of postnatal life shows changes neither in the content of the neurosecretory material (NSM), nor in the size of the cell nuclei, nucleoli, or cytoplasm. The relative temporal refractoriness of the HHNS in this period suggests that the system has not achieved a complete functional maturity by this time. The quantity and distribution of NSM in the neurosecretory centers and in the neurohypophysis of poisoned 1-month-old rats was distinctly different from that observed in the controls of the same age and mature rats. The decrease of secretory activity of the HHNS parallels that of the sex glands. A delay in the development of sex function was noted in experimental rats. Long-term poisoning in sexually mature rats was accompanied by obvious activation of the HHNS. An evident increase of nuclear volumes of cells in the arcuate and ventromedial nuclei compared with the cells of the suprachiasmatic nucleus was seen in the sexually mature animals. The data obtained speak for a selective sensitivity of the studied magnocellular and parvocellular nuclei to changes in the circulatory level of sex steroids. The effects of benzene and xylol cause various changes in the functional activity of the HHNS and in the sex glands at different stages of postnatal ontogenesis, and the changes found in the HHNS seem to be of an adaptive nature.

Pituitary Gonadotropic Activity and Ovarian Function After Deafferentation of the Mediobasal Hypothalamus (MBH) in the Rat

V. G. BARANOV, O. N. SAVCHENKO, M. V. PROPP, O. A. DANILOVA, L. N. MASLOVA, and G. S. STEPANOV

Pavlov Institute of Physiology, Sechenov Institute of Evolutionary Physiology and Biochemistry, Farm Animal Breeding and Genetics Institute, Leningrad, and Institute of Cytology and Genetics, Novosibirsk, USSR

Deafferentation of the MBH (DA rats) led to permanent estrus in 4 out of 40 operated rats. In most DA rats, permanent diestrus (13 rats) or irregular cycles with a predominant diestrus were established. Ovary weight in DA rats was one-half that of intact controls (IC rats). Four weeks after deafferentation, plasma progesterone (2.78 ng/ml in IC rats and 0.43 ng/ml in DA rats), plasma estradiol (42.0 pg/ml in IC rats and 21.0 pg/ml in DA rats) and plasma LH (4.99 ng/ml in IC rats and 1.15 ng/ml in DA rats) were statistically significantly diminished. The level of pituitary LH in permanently estrous DA rats was the same as in IC rats and twice as great as in the other DA rats. Sections were studied after staining with paraldehyde-fuchsin-azan. We found no correlation between ovarian function and (1) types of lesions produced by sectioning the afferents to the ventromedial nucleus, (2) the severity of destruction (if any) of the "Gormori-positive" neurosecretory elements, or (3) the quantity of Gomori-positive neurosecretory material in these elements. It is noteworthy that pituitary LH content was twice that of normal, regardless of whether the suprachiasmatic area was inside or outside the isolated area.

If this area was damaged in the course of deafferentation (as in permanent-estrus rats), pituitary LH did not show any elevation, but plasma sex hormones and ovary weight in these rats were significantly lower than normal. Destruction of the retrochiasmatic area in DA rats resulted in especially high values of pituitary LH (up to 20.4 µg/hypophysis). In DA rats with incomplete isolation of the MBH at the level of the median eminence, predominant rather than permanent diestrus was established. LH-RH content measured by radioimmunoassay in another group of DA rats showed a fall to one-tenth in the median eminence and arcuate nucleus and a twofold increase outside the isolated MBH, in the preoptic area. This agrees with recent data (WEINER et al., 1975; BROWNSTEIN et al., 1976). It seems that deafferentation leading to permanent or predominant diestrus was associated with the blockade of LH secretion, due to diminished release of LH-RH from the hypothalamus. Destruction of the suprachiasmatic area led to permanent estrus and to disturbances both of release and synthesis of LH. We suggest that the structures of MBH alone are insufficient to control the cyclic or even the tonic release of LH. Even a small portion of intact MBH tissue may serve as a path for the fibers bearing stimulatory impulses to the "isolated" MBH. The possibility of regeneration of neurosecretory fibers must also be taken into consideration (DANILOVA and POLENOV, 1977).

References

BROWNSTEIN, M.J., ARIMURA, A., SCHALLY, A.V., PALKOVITS, M., KIZER, Y.S.: The effect of surgical isolation of the hypothalamus on its luteinising hormone releasing hormone content. Endocrinology 98, 662-665 (1976)

DANILOVA, O.A., POLENOV, A.L.: "Gomori-positive" neurosecretion in the rat after deafferentation of the medial basal hypothalamus. Cell Tiss. Res. 176, 121-130 (1977)

WEINER, R., PATTOU, E., KERDELHUE, B., KORDON, C.: Differential effects of hypothalamic deafferentation upon luteinizing hormone-releasing hormone in the median eminence and organum vasculosum of the lamina terminalis. Endocrinology 97, 1597-1600 (1975)

Median Eminence (ME) of Hypophysectomized Rats: Structure and Ultrastructure

M. A. BELENKY and N. BOGDANOVIĆ-STOŠIĆ

Institute of Evolutionary Physiology and Biochemistry of the USSR Academy of Sciences, Leningrad, and University of Belgrade, Yugoslavia

The accumulation of PAF+ material near the primary portal capillaries in the ME of hypophysectomized animals is well known. Thin PAF+ fibers are recognizable on the 5th-6th postoperative day. There are distinct clusters of these fibers around the blood vessels in the subependymal region and also between ependymal (tanycyte) perikarya in the caudal part of the ME. Some fibers reach the third ventricle. The amount of PAF+ material gradually increases in all these regions of the ME during the first month after operation. By use of electron microscopy at least three morphologic types of nerve terminals were recognized in the ME of rats operated two months before. Peptidergic types A_1 and A_2 have elementary granules 120-190 nm and 100-150 nm in diameter, respectively. B-type fibers, very likely of monaminergic nature, show granules 80-100 nm in diameter. The percentage of A_2, B, and C terminals (containing only synaptic vesicles) is approximately equal in the rostral and caudal parts of the ME (A_2 = 29.3%; B = 40.1%; C = 30.6%), A_1 terminals being more frequent in the latter. A_1 terminals are mainly seen on the bases of the primary capillary loops and near the portal veins in the rostral part of the ME. These terminals are usually enveloped by a thin glial sheath and a basement membrane. In the caudal part of the ME A_1 terminals are also situated along the capillary loops. Many A_2 and B-type terminals' fibers seem to grow in between tanycyte perikarya and to make direct contact with the third ventricle in the most caudal part of the ME. It appears that A_1 fibers grow into the outer zone of the ME in the course of postoperative recovery, while A_2 and B-type fibers normally exist in this zone. Their distinct appearance is perhaps primarily the result of the accumulation of peptide hypophysiotropic neurohormones and monoamines, which is due to the disturbed portal circulation and neuroendocrine relationships.

The Supraoptico-Hypophyseal Neurosecretory System, Plasma Antidiuretic Activity, and Concentrating Ability of Kidneys in the Desert Rodent Big Gerbil (*Rhombomys opimus*)

M. A. BELIKOVA, L. N. IVANOVA, N. N. MELIDI, N. I. NASLEDOVA, and M. N. YURISOVA
Institute of Cytology and Genetics, USSR Academy of Sciences, Siberian Department, Novosibirsk, USSR

Peculiarities of the osmoregulating system in the big gerbil were studied under conditions of normal salt-water regimen and dehydration (of 7 and 23 days duration). In control animals there was found a low content of neurosecretory substance (NSS) in perikarya of neurosecretory cells and its moderate accumulation along the full length of neurosecretory fibers and in the hypophysis of the hypothalamo-hypophyseal neurosecretory system (HHNS). Water deficiency induced a progressive reduction of NNS throughout the system, especially in the nucleus paraventricularis and neurohypophysis. Cytometric analysis showed an increase in nuclear and nucleolar volumes in cells of supraoptic and paraventricular nuclei. Thus, dehydration activates both the synthesis of the NSS and release of neurohormone from the system. However, the degree of activation of the HHNS during dehydration was moderate, and no increase in plasma antidiuretic activity was seen. At the same time, the osmotic concentration of the urine was high. These peculiarities suggest that in desert rodents, in the process of adaptive evolution, significant changes both in the HHNS and in the effector link of the osmoregulating system have taken place. However, the resistance of the big gerbil to dehydration was mainly conditioned by renal-function reorganization directed to an increase in efficiency of its concentrating mechanism.

Ultrastructure of the Nucleus arcuatus (NARC) in Normal and Hypophysectomized Rats

N. BOGDANOVIC-STOŠIĆ, M. A. BELENKY, and A. L. POLENOV

Institute of Evolutionary Physiology and Biochemistry of the USSR, Academy of Sciences, Leningrad, and University of Belgrade, Yugoslavia

Four morphologic types of nerve cells (NC), with intermediate transitional forms, have been distinguished in NARC. A few dense-core vesicles 80-110 nm in diameter are the common feature for all cell types. These NC contain numerous mitochondria, Golgi complexes, and polysomes; lysosomes, multivesicular bodies, and nematosomes are also frequent. Rough endoplasmic reticulum (RER) is moderately developed. Type-1 NC have oval light nuclei and light cytoplasm. The cisternae of the RER are scarce and frequently narrow and short. RER and Golgi complexes are more numerous in type-2 NC. The cisternae are wider and frequently lie parallel to each other. Some of them are devoid of ribosomes. Type-3 NC have darker indented nuclei and dark cytoplasm. RER is usually dilated and well developed. Polysomes are frequent. Type-4 NC are similar to the so-called pyknomorphous elements described in the magnocellular hypothalamic nuclei. Both the nucleus and the neuroplasm have a marked electron density. RER and Golgi complexes are considerably dilated and frequently irregular in outline. Some degenerating mitochondria are seen. The percentage of various cell types in normal rats is 1, 54%; 2, 23.8%; 3, 21.5%; 4, 0.8%. All NC of NARC are somewhat hypertrophic in rats 2 months after hypophysectomy. The number of lysosomes and dense-core vesicles increases. The percentage of type-3 NC is slightly higher (up to 25%) than in normal animals, while that of type-4 NC is markedly increased (up to 13.6%). All the cell types in the NARC of both normal and hypophysectomized rats probably represent various functional transitional stages of a single cell type. It seems likely that these NC are primarily concerned with the production of monoamines and their discharge into the portal circulation. The changes in NARC are mainly due to the disturbed neuroendocrine interaction and the normal release of different biologically active substances into the primary portal capillaries of the median eminence.

Functional Morphology of the Neurohormonal System in Myocardial Infarction

N. K. BOGDANOVITSCH
Institute of Human Morphology, Academy of Med. Sciences of the USSR, Moscow, USSR

It is known that the hormones of neurosecretory cells (ADH vasopressin) and adrenal cortex (gluco- and mineralocorticoids) have a direct influence on blood vessels and the myocardium. In the present research the morphologic state of the hypothalamohypophyseal neurosecretory system (HHNS) and the adrenal cortex (AC) of 80 men who died at different periods after the onset of myocardial infarction (1 day-1,5 months) were studied. In one-third of the cases, sodium and potassium in the blood (plasma and erythrocytes) were examined in the course of the disease. Our research shows that myocardial infarction is accompanied by strong activation of the HHNS and AC. It is displayed: (1) in a tendency to reduced noradrenaline content in the hypothalamus (biochemical research in 12 cases); (2) in a rise of neurosecretory activity (especially of the supraoptic nucleus, SON) shown by morphometric, morphologic, and histoenzymologic tests; and (3) in a hypertrophy of corticotropic cells, with an increase of histamine concentration in the gland (as judged by the number of mast cells in the adeno- and neurohypophysis). In the AC, an increase of synthetic and secretory function, with an increased activity of steroidogenic enzymes (3β-ol, NADP) and a predominance of dark cells with prominent cytoplasmic RNA, were observed. If myocardial infarction was complicated by decompensation (20 cases), a high activity of the HHNS was found, with multiple small vacuoles in the secretory cells of the SON. Their appearance clearly corresponded to the rise of Na^+ and the fall of K^+ in the erythrocytes. In the above cases one invariably saw a hypertrophy of the zona glomerulosa of the AC which produces aldosterone. No exhaustion of the neurohormonal system was observed in myocardial infarction.

The Functional Morphology of the Hypothalamo-Hypophyseal Neurosecretory System (HHNS) After Direct and Reflex Stimulation of the Hypothalamus in Cats

E. A. BORISOVA and S. I. TEPLOV
A. L. Polenov Neurosurgical Research Institute, Leningrad, USSR

The functional morphology of the HHNS was investigated in physiologically acute experiments on cats under chloralose anesthesia. Stimulation (with vasoconstrictory effect) of the sympathetic trunk, vagus nerve, and supraoptic nuclei (NSO) was used. Stimulation of the preoptic zone, which caused vasodilatation, was performed as a control experiment. Other control animals were under adequate experimental conditions but were not stimulated. The microscopic preparations were stained by paraldehyde fuchsin, and light microscopy was performed. In control animals after preoptic stimulation, moderate signs of HHNS activity were observed in the NSO and paraventricular nuclei (NPV). The anesthesia and operation caused the release of neurosecretory material (NSM) from the posterior lobe. After stimulation of the NSO and the sympathetic trunk, the quantity of NSM in the posterior lobe was greater than that found after vagal stimulation. The stressor type of activation was observed after vagal stimulation. No changes were observed in the NPV after sympathetic and unilateral NSO stimulation. In these experiments, only the NSO was activated, the size of nucleoli of neurosecretory cells being increased. There were more light cells with intensive NSM synthesis and release in experimental animals than in controls. The infundibular part of the neurohypophysis contained the greatest amount of NSM. After unilateral NSO stimulation the activation of NSO was observed mostly on the side of stimulation. The reaction of the bilateral accessory neurosecretory cells was similar to that of the NSO, but less pronounced. In all cases where peripheral vasoconstriction was observed, the activation of NSO was evident. Since NSO is the main site of vasopressin synthesis, our data suggest vasopressin participation in vasoconstrictor mechanisms.

Ultrastructural Changes in the Hypothalamus and Neurohypophysis of Rats After Chronic Morphine Treatment

J. W. BOROWICZ, A. DANIELEWICZ-KOTOWICZ, and B. GAJKOWSKA
Polish Academy of Sciences, Medical Research Center, 00-748 Warsaw, 3, Dworkowa Str., Poland

Ultrastructural changes in neurons of the supraoptic and paraventricular nuclei, and in fibers of the neurohypophysis of the rat were observed after 60 days of administration of morphine hydrochloride in a dose of 5 mg/kg body wt. In the neurons of the supraoptic and paraventricular nuclei a decrease of secretory activity was observed, manifested morphologically by the decrease of the number of secretory granules. At the same time, the Golgi apparatus was well developed; in its vicinity one could observe numerous coated vesicles, multivesicular bodies, and lysosomes. In the fibers of the neurohypophysis the accumulation of neurosecretory granules was smaller than normal. Numerous fibers contained an abundance of lysosomelike structures and multilamellar bodies. These occurrences are indicative of the digestion of neurosecretory granules. In addition, many neurosecretory fibers showed degenerative changes, manifested by an irregular shape of the fibers, the disappearance of the tubular system, and the absence of secretory granules. Twelve days after morphine withdrawal, the neurons of the supraoptic and paraventricular nuclei and fibers of neurohypophysis revealed a normal appearance. On the basis of these studies it may be assumed that chronic administration of morphine causes great damage to nervous structures in the hypothalamo-hypophyseal system, which is a cause of decreased neurosecretion. However, these changes appear to regress after morphine withdrawal.

Granulolysis, a Possible Intracellular Regulatory Mechanism of Neurosecretion in the Hypothalamo-Posthypophyseal System of the Rat

J. A. BOUDIER and D. PICARD
ERA-CNRS n° 322, Laboratoire d'Histologie I, Faculté de Médecine, Marseille, France

Granulolysis occurs in neurosecretory (NS) neurons in conditions related to drastic changes in the amount and distribution of neurosecretory granules (NSG). After hypophysectomy as well as after inhibition of axonal transport by colchicine injection at the onset of rehydration in previously water-deprived rats, NSG accumulate in perikarya of the supraoptic nucleus (NSO); granulolysis takes place in both situations mainly by a process of sequestration of granules in autophagic vacuoles formed by smooth endoplasmic reticulum (SER); the process is particularly active in the proximal segment of the axons, whereas it is rather inefficient in perikarya; true crinophagy (i.e., membrane fusion between lysosomes and NSG) occurs seldom, and only in perikarya.

When dehydrated rats are allowed to drink freely, intense autophagic activity takes place within a few minutes, and during the first hours of rehydration. Some of the few NSG still present in the depleted posthypophysis are sequestered, but autophagic vacuoles formed by hypertrophied SER along axons and in endings devoid of NSG are seen to contain various cytoplasmic components, including clusters of microvesicles.

In conclusion, (1) In the NS neuron as a whole, widespread autophagic processes are important for maintenance of the steady-state level and turnover of cell components in general, e.g., when a high level of activity is suddenly lowered; (2) Quantitative regulation of NSG by granulolysis is but a particular aspect of the general regulatory process for which the lysosomal apparatus, including axonal SER, is responsible; (3) The rapidity of the onset of autophagy in the case of rehydration raises the question of its triggering mechanism.

Immunohistochemistry of the Hypothalamo-Neurohypophyseal System in the Common Spiny Mouse, *Acomys cahirinus**

M. CASTEL and J. HOCHMAN
Department of Zoology, Hebrew University of Jerusalem, Israel

Previous studies on desert-dwelling spiny mice of the genus *Acomys* indicated that these murids have a particularly efficient hypothalamic-neurohypophyseal system (HNS) and are able to replenish vasopressin stores that are taxed during dehydration (CASTEL) and ABRAHAM, 1969, 1972). It seemed of interest to apply current immunohistochemical techniques, using antivasopressin, to the HNS of *Acomys*; the present study deals with its ultrastructural aspects. The unlabeled-antibody-peroxidase technique of STERNBERGER (1974) was employed, both at the light- and electron-microscopic levels. Further details concerning preparation of tissues have been described by CASTEL and HOCHMAN (1976).

Antibodies to synthetic lysine vasopressin (LVP) were raised in rabbits by repeated injections of LVP, coupled to bovine-serum albumin (BSA), into multiple subcutaneous sites. The presence of antibodies to LVP in the rabbit serum was verified by conventional immunologic methods and by an antidiuretic bioassay to measure the extent of inactivation of standard solutions of vasopressin by the antiserum. Moreover, preliminary experiments showed that intraperitoneal injection of this antiserum into *Acomys* is able to evoke a prolonged diuresis, an unusual phenomenon in a desert-dwelling rodent. Prior to immunohistochemical staining, antibodies to BSA present in the primary antiserum were precipitated.

Immunoreactive neurosecretory granules (NSG) covered with peroxidase-antiperoxidase (PAP) molecules, were found throughout the HNS of *Acomys*. In the neuronal perikarya of the supraoptic nucleus (NSO) numerous immunoreactive granules were observed (Fig. 1), far exceeding those seen in similar studies of the NSO in albino mice and rats. The NSO also contained axons and small Herring bodies rich in immunoreactive NSG. In the median eminence (ME) PAP-covered NSG were found in axons and in Herring bodies, both in the main HN tract coursing through the inner zone of the ME and in the collaterals directed towards the portal capillaries in the external zone of the ME. In the neurohypophysis most of the axons, Herring bodies and NS terminals were replete with immunoreactive NSG (Fig. 2). In Herring bodies throughout the HNS and in NS terminals of the neural lobe, PAP molecules (presumably denoting specific staining of vasopressin) were found both within the granules and between them (Fig. 3). Although cytoplasmic PAP may be a diffusion artefact, it is possible that an extracellular pool of hormone does indeed exist (THORN, 1970), especially at sites of hormone release.

---

*This research was supported by the Israel-United States Binational Science Foundation (BSF), grant 200.

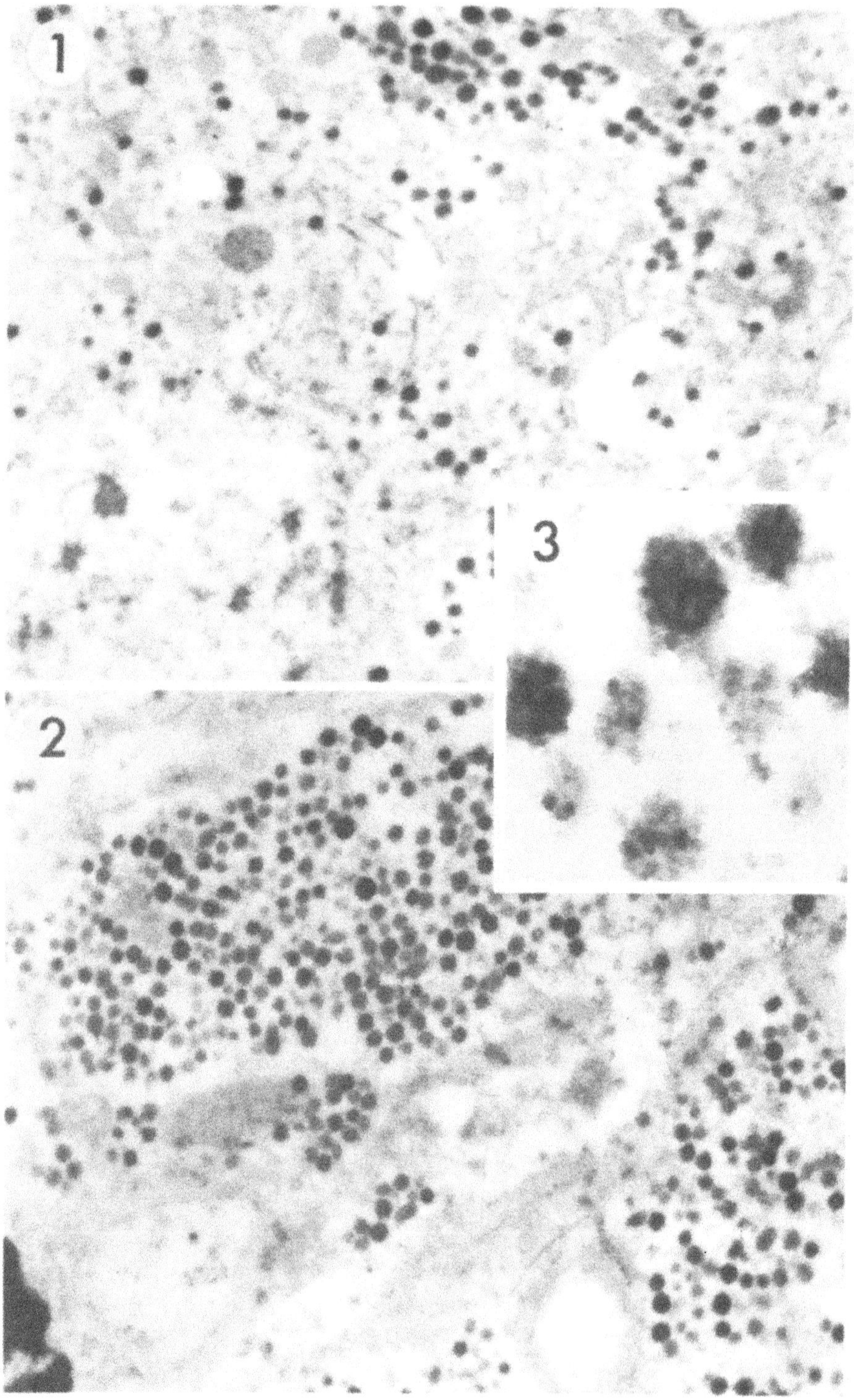
1
2
3

Fig. 1. Portion of NS cell from NSO of *Acomys*. Within cytoplasm numerous NSG immunoreactive to antivasopressin are seen. Nucleus at *lower left*. × 18,000
Fig. 2. NSG immunoreactive to antivasopressin in neurohypophysis of *Acomys*. At *lower left* small portion of endothelial nucleus is seen. × 18,000
Fig. 3. High magnification of immunoreactive NSG in neurohypophysis. Note characteristic PAP molecules covering NSG. Some extragranular PAP molecules are also seen. × 80,000

Our findings essentially bear out previous ultrastructural immunohistochemical reports on the rodent HNS (LECLERC and PELLETIER, 1974; SILVERMAN and ZIMMERMAN, 1975) and also present a new aspect: abundant immunoreactive vasopressin in the perikarya of the NSO in *Acomys*. In the laboratory species studied thus far, perikaryal immunoreactivity at the ultrastructural level has been sparse or absent. The presence of numerous presumably mature NSG that are immunoreactive to antivasopressin in the NSO of *Acomys* may indicate an adaptation to chronically arid conditions.

References

CASTEL, M., ABRAHAM, M.: Effects of a dry diet on the hypothalamic-neurohypophysial system in spiny mice as compared to albino rat and mouse. Gen. Comp. Endocrinol. 12 (2), 231-241 (1969)

CASTEL, M., ABRAHAM, M.: Effects of a dry diet on the antidiuretic hormone content of the neurohypophysis in spiny mice as compared to the albino rat and mouse. Gen. Comp. Endocrinol. 19 (1), 48-55 (1972)

CASTEL, M., HOCHMAN, Y.: Ultrastructural immunohistochemical localization of vasopressin in the hypothalamic-neurohypophysial system of three murids. Cell Tissue Res., 1976 (in press)

LECLERC, R., PELLETIER, G.: Electromicroscopic immunohistochemical localization of vasopressin in the hypothalamus and neurohypophysis of the normal and Brattleboro rat. Am. J. Anat. 140 (4), 583-588 (1974)

SILVERMAN, A.J., ZIMMERMAN, E.A.: Ultrastructural immunocytochemical localization of neurophysin and vasopressin in the median eminence and posterior pituitary of the guinea pig. Cell Tissue Res. 159, 291-301 (1975)

STERNBERGER, L.A.: Immunocytochemistry. Englewood Cliffs (N.J.): Prentice Hall 1974

THORN, N.A.: Mechanisms of release of neurohypophysial hormones. In: Aspects of Neuroendocrinology. BARGMANN, W., SCHARRER, B. (eds.). Berlin-Heidelberg-New York: Springer-Verlag 1970, pp. 140-152

Induced Spawning of *Clarias batrachus* (Linn) Using Clomid, and Observations on the Consequential Resulting Histochemical Changes Exhibited by the Nucleus lateralis tuberis (NLT), Pituitary Cyanophils, and Caudal Neurosecretory Neurons

K. CHANDRASEKHAR and C. VISWANATHA RAO
Surgical Research Laboratory, Institute of Medical Sciences, Varanasi, India

A. Introduction

Induced breeding of fish by hormones dates back to very early times, as has been extensively reviewed by PICKFORD and ATZ (1957), DODD (1960), and others. The disadvantages of hormones are obvious because of their species specificity, etc. In recent years, the chemical "Clomid" (clomiphene citrate) has been extensively administered to humans with positive results by GREENBLATT (1961), MELLINGER et al. (1970), COY et al. (1963), CROOK et al. (1969), SCHNEIDER et al. (1968), and others. Surprisingly, only PANDEY and HOAR (1972) have used Clomid to make gravid goldfish spawn in the laboratory. However, the goldfish is a laboratory animal, the experimentation was done only on gravid females, and the document does not throw light on the path of action of the drug. Therefore, we studied the effect of Clomid on a commercially important fish. This was done during its off-season because it was felt that it would help increase the production of protein-rich food. It was considered worthwhile recording the path of action of Clomid, as well as the reactions of the caudal neurosecretory neurons, as it would yield additional basic information in this area.

B. Materials and Methods

About 200 female *Clarias batrachus* weighing 65 ± 10 g were acclimated for 10 days, maintaining the photoperiod 10 LH/14 DH. They were then grouped into: (1) 0.5 ml distilled-water-injected controls, (2) 25 µg Clomid in 0.5 ml distilled-water-injected experimental-group I, (3) 50 µg Clomid in 0.5 ml distilled-water-injected experimental-group II. Intramuscular injections were given under MS 222 anesthesia, three times a week for 3 months - February through April, the off-season for this fish. Ten fishes from each group were sacrificed on days 15, 30, 45, 60, 75, and 90. Body and ovarian weights were recorded regularly. The brains with the pituitaries, the ovaries, and the caudal region of the spinal cord were fixed in Bouin's fluid. Transverse and sagittal sections of the brains (8-10 µm) were made for study of the NLT, pituitaries (4-5 µm) for cyanophils, caudal region of the spinal cord (8-10 µm) for neurosecretory neurons (CNSN), and ovaries (6-8 µm) were made and stained in (a) Masson's Trichrome, (b) PAS, (c) Mallory's Triple, (d) AF, (e) Acid Violet and (f) HE. The sizes of the neurons, cyanophils and their nuclei, and oocytes were measured by an ocular micrometer. Quantitative assessment of the granules in neurons and cyanophils were made by a five-grade arbitrary scale (CHANDRASEKHAR, 1970), and tables were made on mean values of 1000 cells gathered from ten fishes in a group. Statistical analysis was done using Student's 't' test.

C. Results

The ovarian responses to Clomid and the related changes exhibited by the neurons of the NLT, pituitary cyanophils, and the CNSN are collected in Tables 1, 2, 3, and 4. A few salient points are summarized here.

I. Ovary (Table 1)

In the 50 μg Clomid-administered fishes there was a steady increase in the size and percentage of oocytes leading to spawning in April, while in the controls, the ovaries at this time still contained only oogonia and type-I oocytes.

II. NLT, Pituitary Cyanophils and CNSN

In the experimental groups, the neurons of the pars medialis and pars ventrocaudalis (Table 2, types-I and -II cyanophils of the pituitary (Table 3), and type-I neurons of the CNSN (Table 4) enlarged and degranulated, consistent with the oocyte enlargement. Finally, when the fishes spawned, the neurons and the cyanophils reached their maximum size, but were depleted of their granules.

D. Discussion

This is, to our knowledge, the first report of a commercially important fish being made to spawn in the laboratory 4 months ahead of its normal schedule, using a chemical. The only other communication is that of PANDEY and HOAR (1972) who made the gravid goldfish spawn, but did not indicate the path of action of Clomid. The present article deals with the histochemical and morphologic changes exhibited by the neurons of the pars medialis and pars ventrocaudalis, the type-I and -II cyanophils, the type-I CNSN and the ovaries; it also points to the correlation existing between the two types of changes. The perceptible changes, although they took place during the off-season in response to the influence of the drug, apparently resulted from simulation of naturally occurring processes, thus indicating that the drug acts through the hypothalamogonadal-ovarian axis.

Acknowledgments. The authors are deeply indebted to Director K.N. Udupa, Institute of Medical Sciences for facilities and encouragement, and to Wm. S. Merrel Co., Australia, for a liberal supply of Clomid. The authors also wish to express thanks to Prof. M.S. Mitskevich, Institute of Developmental Biology, USSR Academy of Sciences, for help and encouragement.

Table 1. Changes in ovary after Clomid administration (mean ± SD)

	Ovarian weight mg/100 g body wt.			Percentage of mature oocytes			Diameter of mature oocytes (μm)		
	Control	Clomid 25 μg	Clomid 50 μg	Control	Clomid 25 μg	Clomid 50 μg	Control	Clomid 25 μg	Clomid 50 μg
15 days February	725 ±200	524[a] ±250	2200[b] ±300	7.2	16	27.5	205 ±25	382[a] ±45	305[b] ±29
30 days February	655 ±250	1945[a] ±600	3550[b] ±200	11	32.5	45	268 ±41	457[a] ±52	504[b] ±39
45 days March	1250 ±175	1645[a] ±300	3535[b] ±400	9	35	73.7	300 ±53	562[a] ±45	628[b] ±25
60 days March	1900 ±400	1555[a] ±175	5775[b] ±500	11.5	45.5	85	270 ±34	726[a] ±49	907[b] ±72
75 days April	2025 ±325	2625[a] ±700	6653[b] ±500	10	75	90	314 ±50	914[a] ±41	1168[b] ±85
90 days April	1450 ±250	2700[a] ±900	8350[b] ±1200	13.7	91	92.5	321 ±29	1019[a] ±80	1214[b] ±89

[a] $P < 0.05$ significant increase cf. corresponding controls

[b] $P < 0.05$ significant increase cf. corresponding controls and 25 μg Clomid administration

Table 2. Changes in the nucleus lateralis tuberis (NLT) after Clomid administration (mean ± SD)

	Pars rostralis Neuronal size (μm)			Pars medialis Neuronal size (μm)			Pars ventrocaudalis Neuronal size (μm)			Pars lateralis Neuronal size (μm)		
	Control	Clomid 25 μg	Clomid 50 μg	Control	Clomid 25 μg	Clomid 50 μg	Control	Clomid 25 μg	Clomid 50 μg	Control	Clomid 25 μg	Clomid 50 μg
15 days February	9.45 ±0.45	11.25 ±1.15	15.9 ±2.03	7.65 ±0.35	12.4 [a] ±1.01	17.8 [b] ±1.78	8.97 ±0.58	12.95 [a] ±0.95	16.2 [b] ±0.39	9.9 ±0.53	13.85 ±1.29	13.6 ±1.35
30 days February	10.02 ±0.10	11.90 ±1.34	16.70 ±2.41	8.40 ±0.76	13.25 [a] ±1.32	17.45 [b] ±1.08	9.59 ±0.47	13.60 [a] ±1.24	17.80 [b] ±1.39	10.6 ±0.98	14.8 ±1.42	15.6 ±1.98
45 days March	11.90 ±1.02	12.85 ±1.24	16.95 ±1.98	10.8 ±0.81	14.9 [a] ±1.21	19.79 [b] ±2.28	12.42 ±0.94	15.8 [a] ±1.32	20.85 [b] ±209	12.45 ±1.25	15.59 ±1.75	16.45 ±1.39
60 days March	15.25 ±1.52	14.3 ±1.50	16.8 ±1.65	12.6 ±1.41	17.95 [a] ±1.75	22.39 [b] ±2.34	13.82 ±1.35	18.95 [a] ±0.98	22.9 [b] ±0.74	12.90 ±1.29	17.45 ±1.86	19.6 ±1.28
75 days April	13.9 ±1.85	15.25 ±0.98	19.2 ±1.19	13.7 ±1.14	22.35 [a] ±1.89	24.9 [b] ±1.98	14.87 ±1.21	21.30 [a] ±1.53	25.85 [b] ±2.25	14.35 ±1.85	29.79 ±2.25	19.90 ±1.59
90 days April	14.8 ±1.23	16.28 ±0.94	18.6 ±1.76	15.7 ±1.53	24.85 [a] ±2.39	27.4 [b] ±2.75	14.45 ±1.35	19.80 [a] ±1.50	24.1 [b] ±2.09	15.2 ±1.25	23.2 ±1.39	17.8 ±2.01

[a] $P < 0.05$ significant increase cf. corresponding controls

[b] $P < 0.05$ significant increase cf. corresponding controls and 25 μg Clomid administered

Table 3. Changes in pituitary cyanophils after Clomid administration (mean ± SD)

	Cell diameter type-I (µm)			Nuclear diameter type-I (µm)			Cell diameter type-II (µm)			Nuclear diameter type-II (µm)		
	Control	Clomid 25 µg	Clomid 50 µg	Control	Clomid 25 µg	Clomid 50 µg	Control	Clomid 25 µg	Clomid 50 µg	Control	Clomid 25 µg	Clomid 50 µg
15 days February	5.9 ±0.34	6.3 ±0.39	6.1 ±0.54	2.75 ±0.19	3.29[a] ±0.21	3.5[a] ±0.27	7.2 ±0.35	6.85 ±0.75	7.5 ±0.39	3.79 ±0.31	4.65[a] ±0.29	3.95[a] ±0.19
30 days February	6.9 ±0.21	7.22 ±0.75	7.75[a] ±0.39	3.55 ±0.64	3.9 ±0.38	3.29 ±0.29	7.45 ±0.09	6.7 ±0.73	7.35 ±0.78	4.2 ±0.21	4.6 ±0.31	4.4 ±0.23
45 days March	6.3 ±0.35	7.5[a] ±0.67	8.25[a] ±0.97	3.8 ±0.33	4.85 ±0.46	3.97 ±0.91	7.05 ±0.68	7.25 ±0.15	7.8[a] ±0.21	4.49 ±0.23	5.2[a] ±0.19	5.6[a] ±0.25
60 days March	7.45 ±0.15	8.01[a] ±0.46	8.62[a] ±0.38	3.95 ±0.17	4.5[a] ±0.32	4.92[a] ±0.71	7.1 ±0.25	7.69[a] ±0.22	7.29 ±0.31	3.79 ±0.27	4.75[a] ±0.28	5.5[a] ±0.19
75 days April	7.1 ±0.51	9.1[a] ±0.37	9.3[a] ±0.41	4.35 ±0.41	4.87 ±0.45	4.6 ±0.29	7.05 ±0.43	7.75[a] ±0.25	8.29[a] ±0.31	3.95 ±0.19	5.95[a] ±0.25	6.32[a] ±0.12
90 days April	7.39 ±0.28	7.05[a] ±0.87	7.85[a] ±0.69	3.9 ±0.22	4.22[b] ±0.30	3.73[b] ±0.37	7.6 ±0.12	8.9[a] ±0.28	9.15[a] ±0.17	4.42 ±0.29	5.62[a] ±0.41	5.22[a] ±0.27

^{a} $P < 0.05$ significant increase cf. corresponding controls
^{b} $P > 0.1$ insignificant change cf. corresponding controls

Table 4. Changes in caudal neurosecretory neurons after Clomid administration (mean ± SD)

	Neuronal size type-I (µm)			Neuronal size type-II (µm)			Nuclear size type-I (µm)			Nuclear size type-II (µm)		
	Control	Clomid 25 µg	Clomid 50 µg	Control	Clomid 25 µg	Clomid 50 µg	Control	Clomid 25 µg	Clomid 50 µg	Control	Clomid 25 µg	Clomid 50 µg
15 days	34.9	40.2[a]	37.9[a]	9.8	27.5[a]	24.6[a]	12.9	14.8	14.3	9.50	10.50	10.20
February	±3.32	±3.05	±4.05	±1.21	±2.93	±3.41	±1.25	±2.15	±1.89	±1.05	±1.25	±1.20
30 days	32.5	42.5[a]	45.2[a]	12.5	27.25[a]	30.20[a]	14.05	15.9	16.60	7.30	9.20	10.10
February	±3.75	±2.99	±3.78	±1.09	±3.04	±3.39	±1.35	±1.15	±1.78	±0.75	±1.25	±0.69
45 days	30.1	47.5[a]	55.3[b]	14.95	30.6[a]	34.8[a]	15.04	16.07[a]	18.40[a]	9.90	11.30	11.09
March	±2.75	±3.91	±3.33	±1.59	±2.25	±4.01	±1.64	±2.09	±1.57	±1.34	±1.37	±1.49
60 days	37.5	52.5[a]	59.6[a]	10.4	35.4[a]	32.9[a]	15.90	18.80[a]	18.30[a]	8.51	13.7	10.90
March	±2.95	±3.38	±4.05	±0.98	±2.32	±3.35	±1.83	±3.40	±2.58	±0.76	±1.42	±1.39
75 days	40.9	55.12[a]	60.25[a]	14.95	35.29[a]	40.4[a]	12.9	17.6[a]	16.90[a]	8.90	14.3	13.83
April	±3.19	±4.42	±3.45	±1.25	±2.51	±3.38	±1.27	±1.65	±1.18	±1.09	±01.39	±1.48
90 days	39.5	53.3[a]	45.8[a]	15.6	32.5[a]	35.3[a]	14.9	19.3[a]	15.6[a]	9.80	16.25	14.12
April	±2.75	±3.91	±2.98	±1.75	±2.96	±3.19	±1.14	±1.31	±1.51	±1.14	±2.01	±1.98

[a] $P < 0.05$ significant increase cf. corresponding controls

[b] $P < 0.05$ significant increase cf. corresponding controls and 25 µg Clomid administered

References

CHANDRASEKHAR, K.: Retarded differentiation of the hypothalamic neurosecretory system in thiouracil treated chick embryos. Ind. J. Exp. Biol. 8, 84-88 (1970)

CROOKE, A.C., MEHROO, D.H., BERTRAND, P.V.: Joint action of clomiphene citrate and human pituitary gonadotrophins. Lancet 1969/I, p. 587-588

DODD, J.M.: Gonadal and gonadotrophic hormones in lower vertebrates. In: Marshall's Physiology of Reproduction, p. 417. PARKES, A.S. (ed.). New York: Longman's, Green 1960

GREENBLATT, R.B.: Chemical induction of ovulation. Fertil. Steril. 12, 402-420 (1961)

MELLINGES, R.C., THOMPSON, R.J., MANSOUR, J.A., SMITH, R.W.: Abstract in Programme of the 45th Meeting of the Endocrine Society, St. Louis, Missouri, June 13-15, 1970

PANDEY, S., HOAR, W.S.: Induction of ovulation in gold-fish by clomiphene citrate. Gen. J. Zool. 50, 1679-1680 (1972)

PICKFORD, G.E., ATZ, J.W.: The Physiology of the Pituitary Gland of Fishes. New York: Zool. Soc. 1957

ROY, S., GREENBLATT, R.B., MAHESH, V.B., JUNGCK, E.C.: Clomiphene citrate; further observations on its use in induction of ovulation in the human and its mode of action. Fertil. Steril. 14, 575-595 (1963)

SCHNEIDER, H.P.G., STAEMMLER, H.J., STRACHLER-POLL, K., SACHS, L.: Clomiphene and hypothalamic LH releasing function. Acta Endocrinol. 58, 347-351 (1968)

Role of the Preoptic Recess Ependyma in the Formation and Physiologic Regeneration of the Nucleus praeopticus in Amphibians

V.K. CHETVERUKHIN
Laboratory of Neuroendocrinology, Sechenov Institute of Evolutionary Physiology and Biochemistry of the Academy of Sciences of the USSR, Leningrad, USSR

It is well known that neurosecretory cells (NSC) in the nucleus praeopticus (NPO) of Teleostei and Amphibia are heteromorphous. In these species, large NSC occupy the dorsal part of the NPO and small NSC occupy the ventral part. Degeneration, especially during spawning and as a result of aging, was demonstrated in some large highly differentiated NSC in lower poikilothermic vertebrates (POLENOV, 1974; POLENOV et al., 1972).

It has been suggested that permanent growth and differentiation of NSC in the NPO, and their final natural degeneration occur in adult fish and amphibians. The ependyma of the preoptic recess is probably a source from which the population of NSC can be renewed (POLENOV, 1954, 1974; POLENOV et al., 1972).

Embryos, tadpoles, metamorphosed frogs, and adult individuals of *Rana temporaria* collected in their natural habitat were studied. The developmental age of animals was determined from their external form according to the stages established by TAYLOR and KOLLROS (1946) for *R. pipiens*. Paraldehyde-fuchsin (PAF) staining and a light-microscopic tritiated -thymidine autoradiographic method described previously (CHETVERUKHIN, 1971, 1973; POLENOV et al., 1972) were used. For details of this method see SIDMAN (1970). Electron-microscopic autoradiography (LARRA and DROZ, 1970) was also employed. Six adult frogs were exposed to ^{3}H-thymidine (18 Ci/mmol, 20 µCi/g body wt., three injections during the first 24 h with 12 h intervals). Animals were sacrificed 1 h after the first injection and on day 8 of the experiment. Thin epon-embedded sections of the NPO region were prepared for electron-microscopic autoradiography after dipping in NIKFI-M emulsion. After exposure for 7 weeks, autoradiograms were developed with Amidol and examined in a JEM-7 electron microscope.

The dorsoventral gradients in the time of formation of the NPO have been revealed both by light-microscopic thymidine autoradiography and on sections stained with PAF. In metamorphosed frogs exposed to ^{3}H-thymidine on larval stage 1, only labeled NSC of the dorsal part of the NPO can be seen (Fig. 1). Hence the dorsal part of the NPO generally has its final cell divisions at larval stage 1. The more ventrally placed NSC are unlabeled and arise later. It should be pointed out that the ventral portion of the NPO is generated over a more prolonged period of ontogenesis than the dorsal portion. The autoradiographic evidence of a distinctive dorsoventral gradient in the time of origin of NSC in the NPO is consistent with similar results obtained in classic morphologic investigations of the NPO in ontogenetic development of Amphibia (VOITKEVICH, 1967; CHETVERUKHIN, 1971; NOTENBOOM, 1972),

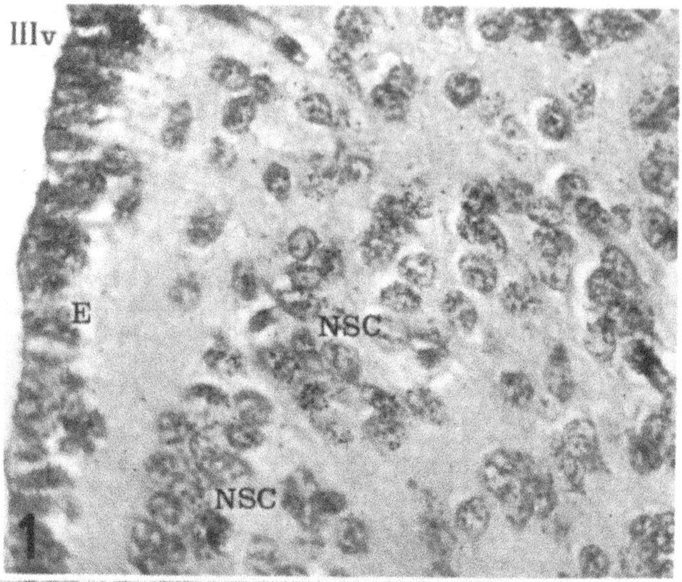
IIIv
E
NSC
NSC
1

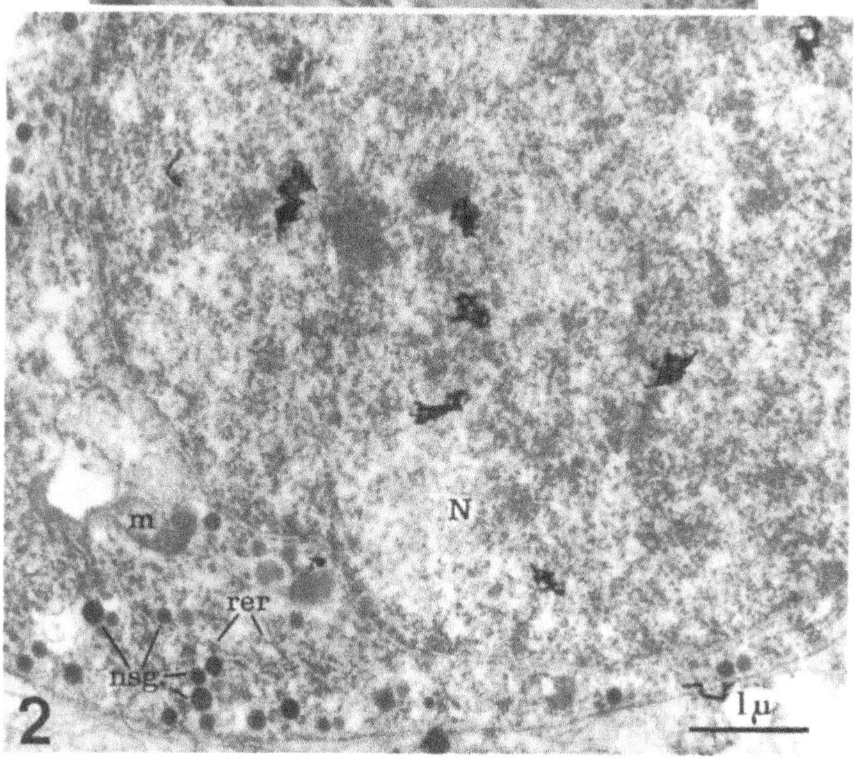
m
N
rer
nsg
1μ
2

Fig. 1. Photomicrograph of an autoradiograph of frontal section through dorsal part of NPO of metamorphosed frog injected with ^{3}H-thymidine at larval stage 1. Note a number of labeled *NSC* in dorsal part of NPO and absence of label over ventrally placed NSC. *IIIv* - third ventricle, *E* - definitive ependymal layer of third ventricle PAF + alum carmine stain. × 280
Fig. 2. Electron-microscopic autoradiograph of thin section through peptidergic NSC from 1-2 cellular position of preoptic recess-subependymal zone of adult frog sacrificed 8 days after exposure three times to ^{3}H-thymidine. Note presence of label over nucleus. *N* - nucleus, *m* - mitochondria, *rer* - rough endoplasmic reticulum, *nsg* - neurosecretory granules. × 16,000

Acipenseridae (JAKOVLEVA, 1964; JAKOVLEVA et al., 1974), and Teleostei (KOBAYASHI et al., 1959). It can thus be suggested that heterochronicity in formation of the NPO results in polar location of NSC in the NPO in adult animals - large cells in the dorsal area and small cells in the ventral one.

Proliferative activity of the ependymal cells in the ventral thalamic and dorsal hypothalamic areas as well as in the preoptic-recess area decreases in frogs after larval stage 4 (Fig. 3). The most dramatic decrease of the S-phase index and mitotic index can be observed in the ependymal zone of the dorsal hypothalamic region. This zone is situated above the magnocellular part of the NPO and in a short time becomes definitive in structure. It consists of a single compact uniform layer of ependymal perikarya and, in the metamorphosed frogs, practically ceases proliferative activity. Moreover, the proportion of postmitotic labeled cells that migrate laterally from the ependymal zone of the dorsal hypothalamus also decreases to a great extent at that time (Fig. 4). In contrast, proliferation in the ependyma of the preoptic-recess area, where the ventral portion of the NPO in adult individuals is localized, decreases negligibly (Fig. 3); until the end of metamorphosis, the number of labeled cells in this ependymal zone remains at a relatively high level. This level of proliferation apparently guarantees a high proportion of the postmitotic cells filling in the subependymal zone of the preoptic-recess area (Fig. 4). Some of these cells (so-called undifferentiated cells, UC) are small in size and poor in cytoplasm, which usually forms a narrow rim around the oval nucleus. Thus, preservation of the cambial-ependymal (matrix) cells can be revealed in the preoptic-recess area. Of particular interest in this connection is the observation that the proliferative cellular pool remains in the preoptic recess-ependymal zone in adult frogs. Similar but usually less pronounced proliferation of the ependymal cells occurs in the ventral portion of lateral ventricles in these animals. Comparing the pattern of migration in these two brain regions, it can be concluded that the migration of postmitotic cells into the preoptic-recess area is significantly more intensive. In fact, by day 25 of the experiment on adult frogs, the majority of labeled cells that left the cell cycle had migrated up to the 7th-8th cellular position of the preoptic recess-subependymal zone, i.e., to the area where the small NSC are localized (Fig. 5). The preliminary results of our electron-microscopic autoradiographic investigations on adult frogs demonstrate that by 8 days after ^{3}H-thymidine injections, some NSC of the ventral

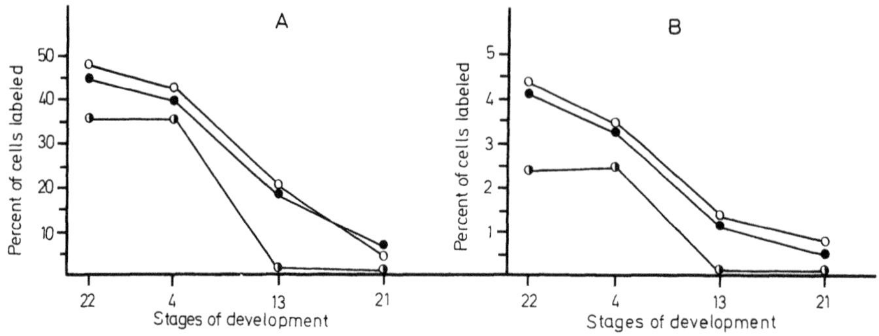

Fig. 3. S-phase index (A) and mitotic index (B) in ependymal zones of frog diencephalon as a function of age of animals. Animals of each stage of development were sacrificed 1 h after ^{3}H-thymidine injection. ● - ependymal zone of ventral thalamic region, ◑ - ependymal zone of dorsal hypothalamic region, o - preoptic recess-ependymal zone

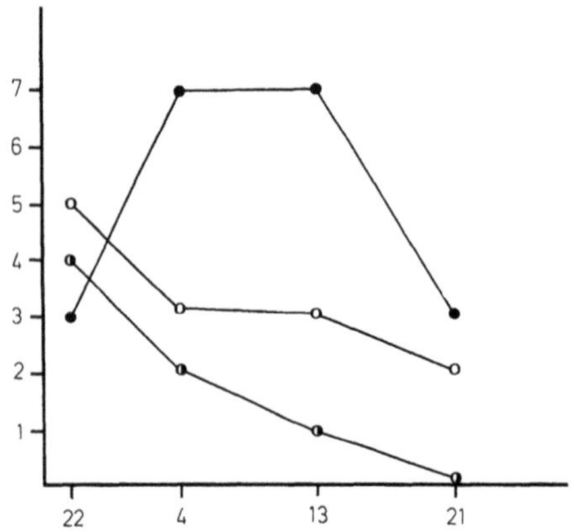

Fig. 4. Rate of migration of cells labeled with ^{3}H-thymidine from ependymal zones of frog diencephalon. *Abscissa* - stages of development, *ordinate* - number of cellular positions of subependymal zones filled by labeled cells within 48 h after single isotope injection. Symbols of ependymal zones are same as in Fig. 3

portion of the NPO with labeled nuclei are found in the 1-2nd cellular position of the preoptic recess-subependymal zone (Fig. 2). At present, however, the significance of these pictures is not yet clear.

Thus, in the first postembryonic stages, NSC originate only from the matrix layer of the third ventricle. Furthermore, in young frogs and in mature animals they seem to arise mainly from the preoptic-recess ependyma. Even in adults, this ependyma remains poorly differentiated. It retains a multiserial structure and a relatively high level of proliferation.

The ependymal matrix zones of the preoptic area have been observed in adult Cyclostomata, Fishes, Amphibia, and Reptilia (CROSBY and WOODBURNE, 1940; POLENOV, 1954, 1974; POLENOV et al., 1972; FLEISCHHAUER, 1957; PAUL, 1967; KIRSCHE, 1967; KRANZ and RICHTER, 1970). The UC accumulating subependymally in this region during ontogenesis seem to represent the "reserve" for the population of NSC. It may be assumed that at least some of the newly formed NSC are derived from a pool of these UC, originat-

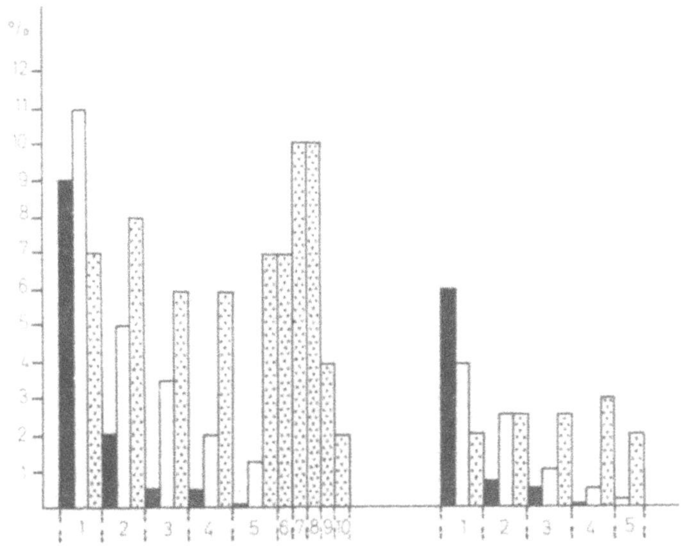

Fig. 5. Histogram demonstrating changes in labeling indexes in subependymal zones of recessus praeopticus (A) and of lateral ventricles (B) in adult frogs exposed to repeated ^{3}H-thymidine injections (daily for a week). This histogram reflects migratory process of labeled cells from ependyma on days 4, 8, and 25 of experiment. *Horizontal line* - ordinal number of subependymally located cell positions beginning with ependyma; *vertical line* - percentage of labeled cells. Each bar represents one cell position: *black* - on day 4, *white* - on day 8, and *dot* - on day 25

ing during a prolonged period of late ontogenesis. "Inhibition" in the utilization of matrix-ependymal zones of the ventral hypothalamus, as compared with those of the dorsal hypothalamus during development of some amphibian species has also been observed (KIRSCHE, 1967). RICHTER and HEINRICH (1969) and KRANZ and RICHTER (1970) have reported similar results based on ^{3}H-thymidine-autoradiography analysis of proliferation of ependymal matrix zones in the diencephalon of Teleostei. We believe that UC in adult individuals of lower vertebrates can be expected to differentiate either into macroglial elements or NSC and possibly into conventional neurons as well (POLENOV et al., 1972). A number of morphologic (see KIRSCHE, 1967), autoradiographic (see ALTMAN, 1970), and electron-microscopic (LEONHARDT, 1972; POLENOV, 1974; JAKOVLEVA et al., 1974) experiments have provided evidence regarding the formation *de novo* of neurons and/or glial cells from the reduced matrix zones and/or UC in some brain regions of different postnatal vertebrate species. The present investigation on adult frogs shows that UC in the hypothalamus originate from the preoptic-recess ependyma. The availability of transitional forms between UC and the small NSC indicates that the latter develop from the UC. As far as we know, no evidence has yet been presented for a possible division of both NSC and UC. One can assume that the nuclei of highly differentiated conspicuous NSC in Teleostei, and to a lesser degree in Anura, are divided only amitotically (POLENOV et al., 1972). Thus, the preoptic-recess ependyma is considered to be the matrix layer - "cambium" for the NPO. The existence of such a cambium appears to be necessary to restore the quantity of NSC, and the function of the NPO as well, because physiologic degeneration of NSC occurs constantly and is very intensive during certain periods (spawning, hibernation) of the animals' life.

References

ALTMANN, J.: Postnatal neurogenesis and the problem of neural plasticity. In: Developmental Neurobiology. HIMWICH, W.A. (ed.). Springfield, Ill.: Thomas 1970, pp. 283-321

CHETVERUKHIN, V.K.: The hypothalamo-hypophysial neurosecretory system of the frog *Rana temporaria* in early ontogenesis. J. Evol. Biochem. Physiol. (Leningrad) 7, 366-374 (1971)

CHETVERUKHIN, V.K.: Radiographic study of histogenesis of preoptic nucleus in *Rana temporaria* (in Russian). Arch. Anat. Histol. Embryol. Norm. Exp. 65, 60-69 (1973)

CROSBY, E., WOODBURNE, R.: The hypothalamus and central levels of autonomic function. III. The comparative anatomy of the preoptic area and the hypothalamus. Recent Publ. Assoc. Nerv. Ment. Dis. (New York) 20, 51-169 (1940)

FLEISCHHAUER, K.: Untersuchungen am Ependym des Zwischen- und Mittelhirns der Landschildkröte *(Testudo graeca)*. Z. Zellforsch. 46, 729-767 (1957)

JAKOVLEVA, I.V.: The hypothalamo-hypophysial neurosecretory system at some stages of early ontogenesis of Volga sturgeons. In: Development of Endocrine Functions During Ontogenesis (in Russian). AVCIN, A.P. (ed.). Moscow: Nauka 1964, pp. 48-51

JAKOVLEVA, I.V., EFIMOVA, N.A., SENCHIK, Yu.I.: The characteristics of ultrastructure of neurosecretory cells at different stages of differentiation from the nucleus preoptions in sexually immature sterlet *(Acipenser ruthenus)*. Ontogenesis (Moscow) 5, 180-186 (1974)

KIRSCHE, W.: Über postembryonale Matrixzonen im Gehirn verschiedener Vertebraten und deren Beziehung zur Hirnbauplanlehre. Z. Mikrosk. Anat. Forsch. 77, 313-406 (1967)

KOBAYASHI, H., ISHII, S., GORBMAN, A.: The hypothalamic neurosecretory apparatus and pituitary gland of a teleost, *Lepidogobius*. Gunma J. Med. Sci. 8, 301-321 (1959)

KRANZ, D., RICHTER, W.: Autoradiographische Untersuchungen über die Lokalisation der Matrixzonen des Diencephalon von juvenilen und adulten *Lebistes reticulatus* (Teleostei). Z. Mikrosk. Anat. Forsch. 82, 42-66 (1970)

LARRA, F., DROZ, B.: Techniques radioautographiques et leur application à l'étude du renouvellement des constituants cellulaires. J. Microscopie 9, 845-880 (1970)

LEONHARDT, H.: Elektronenmikroskopische Untersuchung der postembryonalen Matrixzone des Kaninchengehirns. Z. Mikrosk. Anat. Forsch. 85, 161-175 (1972)

NOTENBOOM, C.: The reaction of the preoptic nucleus of *Xenopus laevis* tadpoles to osmotic stimulation. A fluorescence microscopical investigation. Z. Zellforsch. 134, 383-402 (1972)

PAUL, E.: Über die Typen der Ependymzellen und ihre regionale Verteilung bei *Rana temporaria* L. mit Bemerkungen über die Tanycytenglia. Z. Zellforsch. 80, 461-487 (1967)
POLENOV, A.L.: On the physiological degeneration and restoration of the neurosecretory cells of the nucleus preopticus in sazan and the mirror carp. Dokl. Acad. Nauk SSSR 99, 625-628 (1954)
POLENOV, A.L.: On the life way and the secretory cycle of hypothalamic neurosecretory cells (in Russian). Arch. Anat. Histol. Embryol. Norm. Exp. 67, 5-19 (1974)
POLENOV, A.L., CHETVERUKHIN, V.K., JAKOVLEVA, I.V.: The role of the ependyma of the recessus praeopticus in formation and the physiological regeneration of the nucleus praeopticus in lower vertebrates. Z. Mikrosk. Anat. Forsch. 85, 513-532 (1972)
RICHTER, W., HEINRICH, D.: Über die postnatale mitotische Aktivität der Matrixzonen des Diencephalons von *Lebistes reticulatus* (Teleostei). Abhängigkeit vom Lebensalter. Z. Mikrosk. Anat. Forsch. 80, 433-449 (1969)
SIDMAN, R.: Autoradiographic methods and principles for study of the nervous system with thymidine-H^3. In: Contemporary Research Methods in Neuroanatomy. EBBERSSON, S.O.E., NAUTA, W.J.H. (eds.). New York: Springer-Verlag 1970, pp. 252-274
TAYLOR, A., KOLLROS, J.: Stages in normal development of *Rana pipiens* larvae. Anat. Rec. 94, 7-24 (1946)
VOITKEVICH, A.A.: Neurosecretion. Leningrad: Medicina 1967

Adrenergic Mechanisms in the Hypothalamic Regulation of Pituitary Thyrotropic Function

S. I. CHUPRINOVA, G. I. KHARAG, V. V. MAMINA, and B. V. ALESHIN
Kharkov Research Institute of Endocrinology and Hormone Chemistry, Kharkov, USSR

Using the 3-oxyindole procedure developed by OSINSKAYA in experiments performed on male rabbits, we found a slight but constant increase in the concentration of norepinephrine in the hypothalamus alongside the potentiation of pituitary-thyrotropic function (after total or partial thyroidectomy, castration, and cervical sympathectomy). A more significant increase in the catecholamine content of the hypothalamus was found after stimulation of the cervical sympathetic ganglia, but in this case epinephrine, which is not normally detected in the rabbit brain, appears with the norepinephrine. In rats, of which the brain (unlike that of rabbits) normally contains epinephrine together with norepinephrine, the potentiation of thyrotropic function induced by thyroidectomy, the action of 6-methylthiouracil, and cervical sympathectomy were all accompanied by an increase in the total concentration of both catecholamines in the hypothalamus. The combined action of the cervical sympathectomy and administration of 6-methylthiouracil resulted in a significant reduction of pituitary-thyrotropic function and not in its potentiation. At the same time, both the total concentration of catecholamines and the norepinephrine level dropped in the hypothalamus. This parallelism between the intensity of pituitary-thyrotropic function and the norepinephrine level in the hypothalamus suggests that hypothalamic thyroliberin secretion is stimulated by norepinephrine.

Efferent Projections from the Preoptic Area in the Hypothalamus

S. DAIKOKU, H. MATSUMURA, and Y. SHINOHARA
Department of Anatomy, School of Medicine, Tokushima University, Tokushima, Japan

A. Introduction

There is considerable evidence that the medial preoptic nucleus of the hypothalamus plays an essential role in reproductive physiology (KAASJAGER et al., 1971). However, morphologic evidence on the efferent projection of this nucleus is still obscure (SZENTÁGOTHAI et al., 1972). The present study was designed to examine the efferent projection from the preoptic area to the hypophysiotropic area, especially to the median eminence, using an autoradiographic method (COWAN et al., 1972).

B. Materials and Methods

Male Sprague-Dawley rats ranging from 250 to 280 g in body wt. were used. A volume of 0.2 μl containing 0.2 μCi ^{3}H-leucine (s.a. 58 Ci/mmol) was injected into the preoptic area sterotaxically through a glass cannula. After 72 h, the animals were killed by cardiac perfusion of 10% formalin. Eight-micron serial paraffin sections of the brain were cut in the frontal plane, and each fifth section was processed for autoradiography. Electric coagulation of the preoptic area was carried out by a thin platinum needle at 10 mA DC for 1 s. The animals were killed 3 days later by cardiac perfusion of Karnovsky fixative. The preoptic area and the basal hypothalamus with the infundibular stem were individually dissected from the brain. The brain tissue, including the preoptic area, was embedded in paraffin and the coagulated region was located. The electron-microscopic examination of the median eminence was made on the animals in which the preoptic area was coagulated to a suitable extent. Several normal, adrenalectomized, and gonadectomized male rats were sacrificed as controls, and the median eminence was examined electron microscopically.

C. Results

The injection of ^{3}H-leucine or the electric coagulation was made in the basal-periventricular (group 1), basal-medial (group 2), medial (group 3), and lateral (group 4) parts of the preoptic area; each group consisted of from three to six animals. In group 1, the labeled cells appear in the ventral part of the periventricular area, immediately rostral to the suprachiasmatic nucleus. The silver grains are distributed over both sides of the periventricular area, but the majority appear ipsilaterally

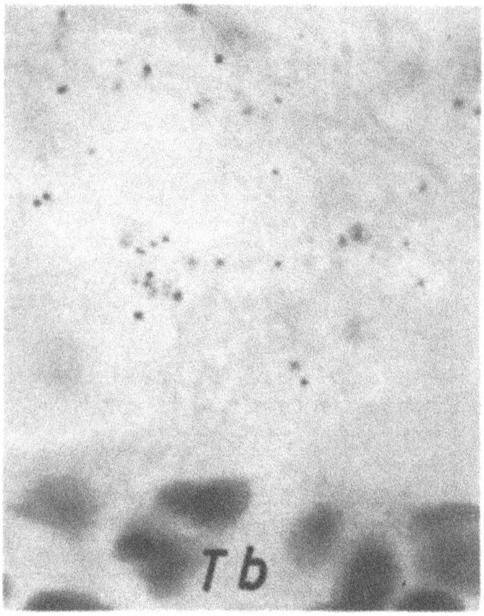

Fig. 1. Silver grains over external layer of median eminence of rat with ^{3}H-leucine injection in basal-periventricular part of preoptic area. *Tb* - pars tuberalis. × 1000

on the injected side. The labeled fibers are distributed throughout the periventricular area, and traced to the anterior, paraventricular, dorsomedial, and ventromedial nuclei, and posterior hypothalamic area. Some of the grains are associated with the suprachiasmatic and arcuate nuclei, and the median eminence. In the median eminence, the fibers appear ipsilaterally on the injected side and distribute in the external layer, but diminish in number caudally. Animals of group 2 had labeled cells on the ventral part of the medial preoptic area adjacent to the optic chiasm. On the injected side, silver grains are scattered ipsilaterally over the medial and periventricular preoptic areas. The labeled fibers are traced caudolaterally to the ventral zone of the lateral hypothalamus. Other fibers extend in a caudomedial direction scattering over the suprachiasmatic, anterior, paraventricular, dorsomedial, ventromedial and arcuate nuclei, and median eminence. In the median eminence, some fibers are revealed in the external layer. In group 3, labeled cells are found in the center of the medial preoptic area. On the injected side, the silver grains appear in the bed nucleus of the stria terminalis, periventricular area, and ventral zone of the lateral hypothalamus. More caudally, the labeled fibers are followed to the lateral, anterior, arcuate, ventromedial, dorsomedial, paraventricular and supraoptic nuclei. The median eminence contains silver grains, but relatively few are found in the external layer. In group 4, the labeled cells are located in the center of the lateral preoptic area. Silver grains are scattered mainly over the lateral preoptic area and the lateral part of the medial preoptic area. Labeled fibers are traced caudally to the supraoptic and lateral hypothalamic nuclei. In the periventricular, arcuate, ventromedial and dorsomedial nuclei, and the median eminence, labeled fibers are not detected.

The external layer of the median eminence consists of nerve terminals and glial or ependymal cell processes. Nerve terminals contain clear and cored vesicles (KOBAYASHI et al., 1970) in normal rats. In rats of groups 1 and 2, the median eminence contains many nerve terminals with dense lamellar or vesicular structures in various numbers; besides these, they occasionally contain intact small clear and cored vesicles of 80-100 nm diameter. These various structures seem to indicate lytic or degenerative processes within the terminals. Similar fibers are also encountered in normal or gonadectomized animals, but they are few in number. This is true in group 4 also.

D. Discussion

The present autoradiographic experiments show that the neurons situated in the medial and periventricular parts of the preoptic area have axons that project to the hypophysiotropic area of the hypothalamus, and that the neurons in the mediobasal preoptic area project to the external layer of the median eminence. The latter observation was substantiated by the results of the electric coagulation studies in groups 1 and 2. SWANSON (1976) indicated a similar projection from the preoptic area in rats, using the isotope-labeling method, but failed to show nerve fibers in the external layer of the median eminence. Recently immunohistochemical studies suggest that the LHRH-containing neurons are situated both in the preoptic and prechiasmatic areas, and more caudally in the arcuate nucleus, and that their axons terminate in the external layer of the median eminence in rats (NAIK, 1975; WHEATON et al., 1975). These findings suggest the dual origin of LHRH-containing axons in the median eminence. The labeled or degenerated fibers in the external layer of the median eminence shown here may indicate that the LHRH fibers originated in the mediobasal preoptic area. Electron-microscopic immunohistochemistry showed that LHRH-containing granules in the nerve terminals are 70-90 nm in diameter (PELLETIER et al., 1974; GOLDSMITH and GANONG, 1975). A similar size range was calculated for the dense-cored vesicles within the degenerated terminals in groups 1 and 2.

References

COWAN, W.M., GOTTLIEB, D.I., HENDRICKSON, A.E., PRICE, J.L., WOOLSEY, T.A.: The autoradiographic demonstration of axonal connections in the central nervous system. Brain Res. 37, 21-51 (1972)

GOLDSMITH, P.C., GANONG, W.F.: Ultrastructural localization of luteinizing hormone-releasing hormone in the median eminence of the rat. Brain Res. 97, 181-193 (1975)

KAASJAGER, W.A., WOODBURY, D.M., DIETEN, J.A.M.J. VAN, REES, G.P. VAN: The role played by the preoptic region and the hypothalamus in spontaneous ovulation and ovulation induced by progesterone. Neuroendocrinology 7, 54-64 (1971)

KOBAYASHI, H., MATSUI, T., ISHII, S.: Functional electron microscopy of the hypothalamic median eminence. Int. Rev. Cytol. 29, 281-381 (1970)
NAIK, D.V.: Immunoreactive LH-RH neurons in the hypothalamus identified by light and fluorescent microscopy. Cell Tissue Res. 157, 423-436 (1975)
PELLETIER, G., LABRIE, F., PUVIANI, R., ARIMURA, A., SCHALLY, A.V.: Immunohistochemical localization of luteinizing hormone-releasing hormone in the median eminence. Endocrinology 95, 314-317 (1974)
SWANSON, L.W.: An autoradiographic study of the efferent connections of the preoptic region in the rat. J. Comp. Neurol. 167, 227-256 (1976)
SZENTÁGOTHAI, J., FLERKÓ, B., MESS, B., HALÁSZ, B.: Hypothalamic control of the anterior pituitary. Buda-Pesth: Akadêmiai Kiadô 1972
WHEATON, J.E., KRULICH, L., MCCANN, S.M.: Localization of luteinizing hormone-releasing hormone in the preoptic area and hypothalamus of the rat using radioimmunoassay. Endocrinology 97, 30-38 (1975)

Classical ("Gomori-positive") Neurosecretory System in the Rat After Isolation of the Medial Basal Hypothalamus and Adrenalectomy

O. A. DANILOVA
Laboratory of Neuroendocrinology, Sechenov Institute of Evolutionary Physiology and Biochemistry, Academy of Sciences of the USSR, Leningrad, USSR

A. Introduction

The medial basal hypothalamus (MBH) is considered to be the site of releasing-factor production, parvicellular formations being the only source of hypophysiotropic factors (HALÁSZ, 1972). The role of the "Gomori-positive" neurosecretory (NS) system in the regulation of the anterior pituitary has been neglected or even rejected during past years. The appearance of Gomori-positive material in the external median eminence after adrenalectomy (AE) has been demonstrated repeatedly. This material is even termed "CRF-granules" (BOCK et al., 1976). It is still unknown whether it is synthesized in the MBH, where no cell perikarya with Gomori-positive granules have ever been seen, or in the Gomori-positive magnocellular formations outside the MBH. We prefer the latter suggestion. If this were so, no Gomori-positive material should be found in the external median eminence of MBH 2-3 weeks after AE when deafferentation (DA) was previously performed (DA + AE rats).

B. Materials and Methods

Male rats, of a Wistar-derived strain, ~ 150 g body wt., were operated on in early spring. DA of the MBH was performed according to HALÁSZ and PUPP (1965). AE, if performed simultaneously with DA, led to high mortality. It was therefore performed 6-11 days after DA. In this case survival of the animals was rather good, the rats receiving 1% saline with 5% glucose instead of drinking water. Brains of 15 were taken for histologic study from the rats decapitated 28-38 days after DA, and 15-27 days after AE respectively. The hypothalamic area and the hypophysis were fixed in Bouin's fluid; serial paraffin sections were stained with Gomori-Gabe's paraldehyde-fuchsin and counterstained with Heidenhain's azan.

C. Results

Out of the 15 brains studied, complete isolation of the MBH was found only in three brains. In one case the DA was perfect from one side and incomplete from another. The isolated area extended from behind the optic chiasm to the premamillary region and included the median eminence and the arcuate nuclei. In the other rats the isolated area was displaced laterally.

Fig. 1A and B. Knife cut *c* at the level of the median eminence in rat 25 days after DA of the MBH, and 15 days after AE. Note Gomori-positive fibers within isolated brain area near to knife cut (*open arrow*) and around vessel of brain sheath (*arrow*). Fig. 1A, × 360; Fig. 1B, × 900

Fig. 2A, B, and C. Median eminence of rat 25 days after DA and AE. 2A: Cut reaching base of brain *c* and incomplete separation *c*. Half of median eminence near side of complete isolation is folded and devoid of Gomori-positive material (for details see Fig. 2B). Some thin Gomori-positive NS fibers are found in external median eminence leading to portal capillaries (see Fig. 2C, *arrows*). Fig. 2A, × 360; Fig. 2B, C, × 900

Fig. 3. Median eminence of rat 3 weeks after incomplete DA and AE. Note Gomori-positive NS fibers and accumulation of Gomori-positive material in external zone. × 900

Fig. 4. The anterior commissural nucleus (*ACN*) in rat with DA 28 days before and AE 19 days before. Some Gomori-positive cells are seen lateral to the fornix (*Fx*) (*arrow*). × 360

Regeneration of the NS fibers and formation of new axovascular contacts as demonstrated in rats with DA (DANILOVA and MASLOVA, 1974; DANILOVA and POLENOV, 1977) were characteristic of the animals in this study. In the 3 rats with complete DA, the posterior lobes were absolutely depleted of NS material. The median eminence of these 3 rats was also devoid of NS fibers although some NS fibers entered the lateral part of the "isolated" area adjacent to the knife cut (Fig. 1). If the isolation was complete at one side only, the part of the median eminence close to the side with complete isolation was devoid of NS material (Fig. 2A and B). On the opposite side the median eminence showed a normal structure, and CRF-granules were visible near the portal capillaries (Fig. 2A, C). The same holds for all the other animals in which the median eminence was not isolated completely (Fig. 3). It is noteworthy that the DA + AE rats had more NS material in the NS fibers and in the NS cell perikarya as compared with DA or AE rats. The most striking finding was the abundance of NS material in the NS cells of the anterior commissural nucleus (PETERSON, 1966); 20-30 NS cells were sometimes seen in a single brain section in the DA + AE rats (Fig. 4), compared with 3-4 cells in sections of brains from intact rats.

D. Discussion

In spite of DA of the MBH, there is normal or even enhanced blood-corticoid level in the lesioned rats; only circadian rhythm is abolished (HALÁSZ and PUPP, 1965). Even ablation of the MBH does not lead to considerable lowering of the adrenal-cortical secretion (DUNN and CRITCHLOW, 1973). ALLEN et al. (1974) claimed that compensatory hypersecretion of ACTH was prevented by DA. Nevertheless, ACTH blood concentration was about 2.5 times higher in the DA + AE rats than in rats with only DA.

Recently it was shown that, within 3 weeks after DA of the MBH, Gomori-positive NS cells regenerate to form new active axovas-

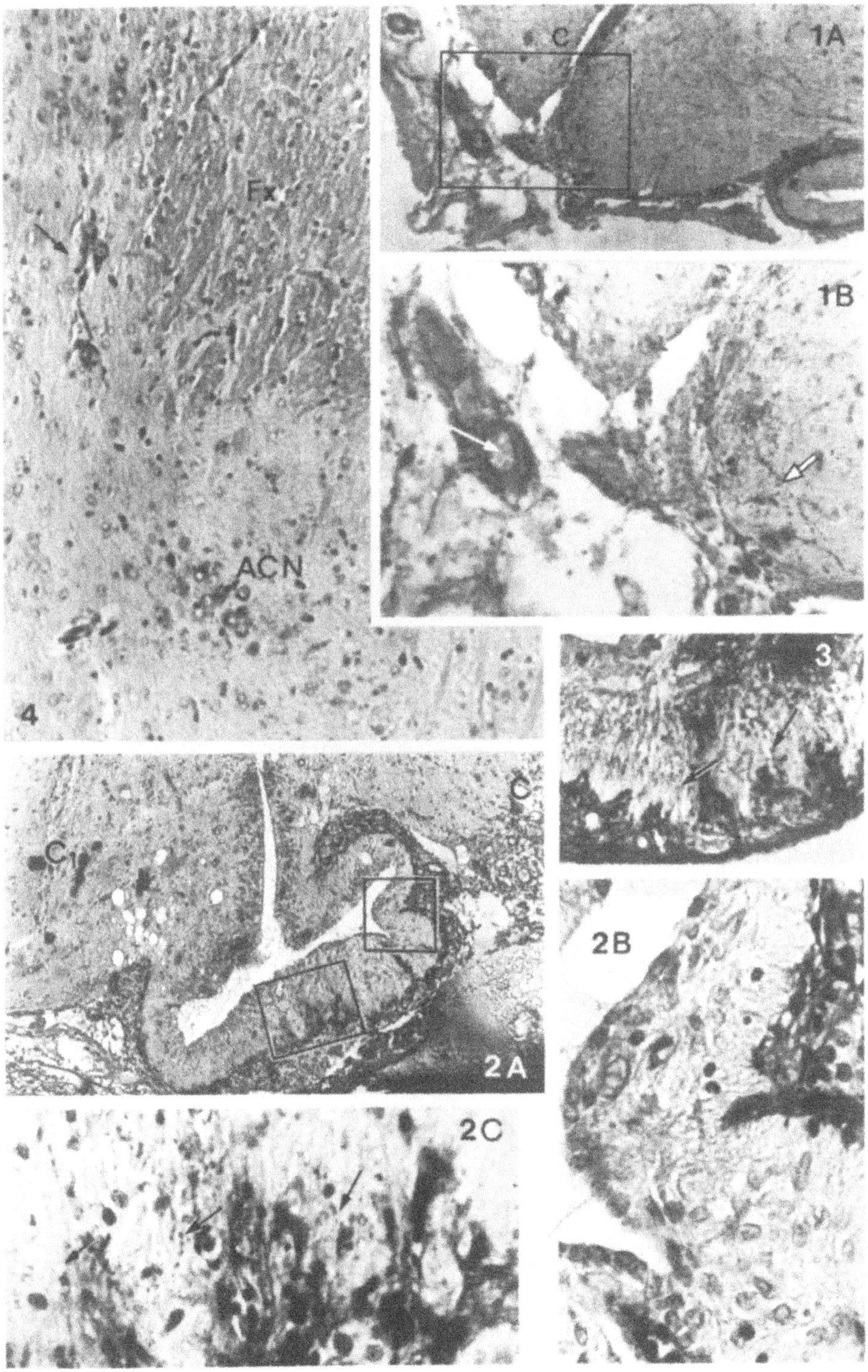
1A
C
1B
4
Fx
ACN
3
C
C1
2A
2B
2C

cular contacts (DANILOVA and MASLOVA, 1974; DANILOVA and POLENOV, 1977). One may suggest that in the DA rats CRF reaches the portal blood circulation and influences the anterior pituitary in spite of the hypothalamus lesion. This may account for a rather high level of adrenalcortical function in the rats with isolated or removed MBH. The possibility of regeneration of fibers carrying neurohormones after DA according to HALÁSZ was proposed by HARRIS as early as 1970.

Along with peptide releasing factor (CRF) the function of adrenals is influenced by monoamines (see GANONG, 1974). As proposed by DANILOVA and POLENOV (1977), monoamines do not enter the portal circulation in rats with DA. Absence of the monoamine component of the "dual control" (POLENOV, 1970) leads to the disappearance of circadian rhythm.

An increased amount of the Gomori-positive material is seen in the hypothalamus of the DA + AE rats, especially in the anterior commissural nucleus. We propose that this nucleus is the site of CRF synthesis. However, we must mention the possibility that the increase in the Gomori-positive material is due to the drinking of glucose solution, as was found in mice by POLENOV and YUSHKANTSEVA (1963).

E. Conclusion

DA of the MBH is followed by regeneration of Gomori-positive NS fibers and formation of new axovascular contacts. In the hypothalami of the DA + AE rats the amount of the Gomori-positive material is higher than in the hypothalami of rats with DA or only AE. Nevertheless, there are no CRF-granules in the external median eminence in the rats 2-3 weeks after AE, if complete isolation of the MBH is achieved. We suggest that Gomori-positive cells of the anterior commissural nucleus synthesize CRF.

Acknowledgments. Thanks are due to Dr. L.N. Maslova (Institute of Cytology and Genetic, Novosibirsk, USSR) for deafferentation of the rats.

References

ALLEN, C.F., ALLEN, J.P., GREER, M.A.: Anterolateral hypothalamic deafferentation prevents compensatory hypersecretion of ACTH following adrenalectomy in the rat. Proc. Soc. Exp. Biol. Med. 146, 840-843 (1974)

BOCK, R., SALLAND, Th., SCHWABEDAL, P.N., WATKINS, W.B.: Histochemical and immunohistochemical properties of the CRF-granules and other "Gomori-positive" substances of the rat. Histochemistry 46, 81-105 (1976)

DANILOVA, O.A., MASLOVA, L.N.: Distribution of "Gomori-positive" neurosecretory material in the rat hypothalamus and hypophysis with isolated medial basal hypothalamus. Dokl. Akad. Nauk SSSR 218, 986-987 (1974)

DANILOVA, O.A., POLENOV, A.L.: "Gomori-positive" neurosecretion in the rat after deafferentation of the medial basal hypothalamus. Cell Tissue Res. 176, 121-130 (1977)

DUNN, J., CRITCHLOW, V.: Pituitary-adrenal function following ablation of medial basal hypothalamus. Proc. Soc. Exp. Biol. Med. 142, 749-754 (1973)

GANONG, W.F.: Brain mechanisms regulating the secretion of the pituitary gland. The Neurosciences: Third Study Program. WORDEN, F. (ed.). Cambridge (Massachusetts): MIT Press 1974, pp. 549-563

HALÁSZ, B.: Hypothalamic mechanisms controlling pituitary function. In: Topics in Neuroendocrinology. KAPPERS, J.A., SCHADÉ, J.P. (eds.). Brain Res. 58, 57-122 (1972)

HALÁSZ, B., PUPP, L.: Hormone secretion of the anterior pituitary gland after physical interruption of all nervous pathways to the hypophysiotropic area. Endocrinology 77, 553-562 (1965)

HARRIS, G.W.: Some data to the paper By Knigge, M. and Scott, D.: Structure and function of the median eminence. Symposium "Brain-endocrine interactions". Am. J. Anat. 129, 245 (1970)

PETERSON, R.P.: Magnocellular neurosecretory centers in the rat hypothalamus. J. Comp. Neurol. 128, 181-185 (1966)

POLENOV, A.L.: Morpho-functional principles of neurosecretory (peptidergic) and adrenergic regulating mechanisms of the hypothalamus. In: Proceedings of the XIth All-Union Congr. of I.P. Pavlov Physiological Society. CHERNIGOVSKY, V.N. (ed.). Leningrad: Nauka 1970, Vol. I, pp. 311-315

POLENOV, A.L., YUSHKANTSEVA, S.I.: Morphology and localization of the accessory "Gomori-positive" neurosecretory elements in the hypothalamic area of the white mouse. Dokl. Akad. Nauk SSSR 148, 441-444 (1963)

Age- and Sex-Dependent Biotransformation of Androgens in the Pituitary, Pineal Gland, and Arcuate Nucleus of the Hypothalamus of Rats

W. G. DEGTIAR, S. A. PAVLINOV, L. A. LOSEVA, and W. A. ISACHENKOV
Central Scientific Research Laboratory of the Ministry of Health of the USSR, Moscow, USSR

Sex-steroid hormones are the principal mediators of feedback loops between reproductive and neuroendocrine organs. Hormone action on these structures may be accompanied by their biotransformation. Our present work is concerned with the investigation of androgen metabolism in the pituitary, pineal gland, and arcuate nucleus (AN) of the hypothalamus of rats. Isolated organs from male and female rats 5, 10, 15, 23, 30, 40, and 60 days old were incubated in 199 medium in the presence of ^{3}H-androgens (concentration ~ 10^{-8} *M*): 4-androstene-3,17-dione, testosterone, 5α-androstane-17β-ol-3-one, 5α-androstane-3α, 17β-, and 3β, 17β-diols. Steroid metabolites were separated by TLC and their quantity were determined by radiometry. In all organs, biotransformation was found to be carried out by two principal steps: reduction of the steroids by Δ^{4}-5α-steroid reductase, and reversible ketone-alcohol transformation by 3α- and 17β-hydroxysteroid oxido reductases. However, 5α-androstane-3β, 17β-diol was transformed only into polar-unidentified compound. The differences in androgen metabolism in the organs of both sexes were found to be only of a qualitative nature: the most intensive biotransformation of all androgens was observed in the pineal gland: the lowest was in the AN of the hypothalamus. The intensity of metabolism was strongly dependent on the age of the rat: in the pineal gland, androgen transformation (with the exception of testosterone) increases to a maximum on the 10th day of life (for testosterone - on the 15th day) and sharply decreases up to the 23rd day. In the AN of the hypothalamus and the pituitary, maximal activity has been observed on the 5th day of life; it drops sharply until the 23rd day, and reaches minimal values at day 60. Extreme differences in the steroidogenesis are of several orders of magnitude. This suggests the existence of "critical periods" for androgen biotransformation in the neuroendocrine structures of the brain, which are probably connected with age and sexual differentiation.

Experimental Studies of the Dynamics of Herring Bodies. Ultrastructure of Axon Dilatations Developing at the Site of Compression or Transection of Neurosecretory Axons in the Grass Frog *Rana pipiens*

H.-D. DELLMANN and J. R. CARITHERS
Department of Veterinary Anatomy, Pharmacology and Physiology, Iowa State University, Ames, Iowa, USA

A. Introduction

Herring bodies are dilatations of neurosecretory axons that have been well characterized ultrastructurally (for review see DELLMANN, 1973). Their formation and possible involution has been studied (PICKERING et al., 1975) and is more subject to hypothetical speculations. This study of the sequence of ultrastructural changes occurring during experimentally induced formation of axon dilatations, is the first step in elucidating dynamic changes in Herring bodies.

B. Materials and Methods

The ventral surface of the brain of 37 grass frogs was exposed through the roof of the pharynx, and neurosecretory axons were either compressed or transected in the ventral hypothalamus or the infundibulum. After periods ranging from 5 min to 2 days, the brain was fixed in 5% phosphate-buffered (0.1 *M*, pH 7.4) glutaraldehyde, postfixed in 2% osmium tetroxide and embedded in Epon-Araldite. Sections were stained with lead citrate and uranyl acetate.

C. Results and Discussion

The most striking ultrastructural changes occur during the first hour following partial or total arrest of the axoplasmic flow. Five minutes after transection there is evidence of leakage of axoplasm from the transected axons. Free cytoplasmic material is seen, and there is a concomitant increase in intercellular spaces (Fig. 1). There is a great number of axons that contain groups of irregular, seemingly empty vesicles 68-137 nm in diameter (Fig. 1). A few of these were discernable in controls, but 5 and 15 min after transection the majority of axon profiles contain at least a few of these vacuoles. In the 15-min group, terminal dilatations containing neurosecretory granulated vesicles (NGVs) are first observed (Fig. 3). Within 30 min, sealing of the axolemma and subsequent arrest of the axoplasmic flow causes even larger dilatations of the distal-most portions of axons. These, as well as many adjacent, undilated axons, contain accumulations of NGVs and in some cases anastomosing networks of tubular axoplasmic reticulum (AR). A slight increase in the number of microtubules is apparent. This has been shown to be associated with

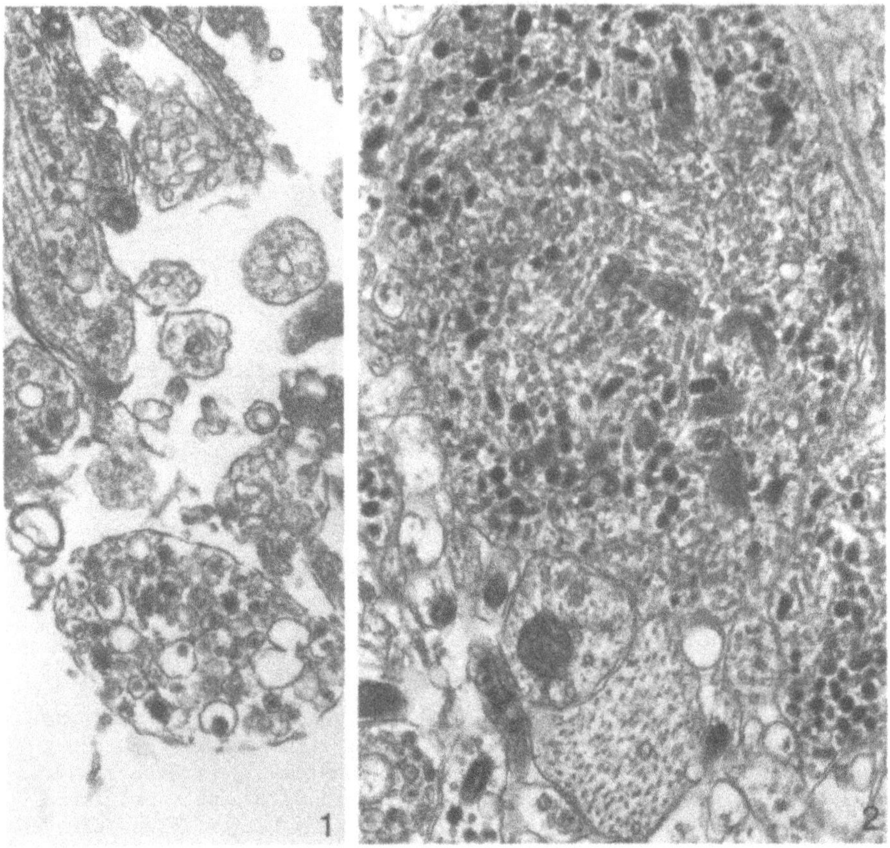

Fig. 1. Terminal axon dilatation 15' after transection, containing NGVs. Notice seemingly empty vesicles (axons). × 30,600
Fig. 2. Axon dilatation 6 h after compression with many NGVs and extensive tubular AR. × 21,600

increased transport activity (GRAINGER and SLOPER, 1974), in this case possibly as a response to injury of the neuron. There are still large numbers of seemingly empty vesicles and dilated intercellular spaces. At 1 h the responses first observed at 30 min are much more advanced (Fig. 3). There is a great hypertrohpy of the tubular AR, which now contains electron-dense material, sometimes in dilated areas resembling NGVs. The number of microtubules is strikingly increased. Terminal dilations are well developed, filled with AR and more NGVs, and there are similar dilations developing slightly proximal to the cut or compressed site. The number of seemingly empty vesicles is reduced and continues to decline throughout the two day observation period.

In the 2-, 3-, and 6-h groups the changes already described become progressively more pronounced. By 6 h, the contents of the dilatations often show segregation of NGVs from masses of AR

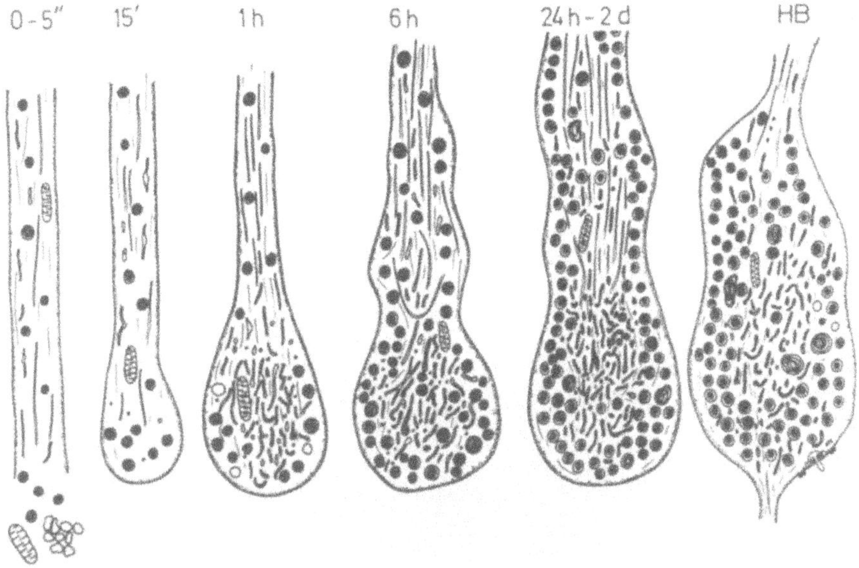

Fig. 3. Schematic drawing of morphologic changes in neurosecretory axons following transection or compression, as compared to Herring body (*HB*); for details see text

(Fig. 2). The NGVs most often are localized distally or peripherally in the enlargements. The simultaneous first appearance of accumulations of NGVs and AR, the presence of electron-dense material resembling neurosecretory granular content, the apparent continuity of the boundary membranes of some granules with membranes of AR, and the accumulation of NGVs in the environs of masses of AR all suggest that the smooth AR plays some role in the formation of neurosecretory granules. Dense bodies and dense lamellar bodies appear in the 6-h group, and increase in later groups. These structures are probably lysosomal, and their appearance indicates the onset of crinophagic activity.

The 12-, 24-, 36-, and 48-h groups continue to show quantitative increases in the amount of AR, number of NGVs, dense bodies, dense lamellar bodies and microtubules, and in size of the axonal dilations (Fig. 3). In each succeeding group there is an increase in the distance proximally from the transected or compressed site at which newly formed dilatations are seen. Also, axons in later groups contain occasional very large (maximum diameter of 440 nm) granulated vesicles amongst the normal NGVs.

Thus, partial or total arrest of the axoplasmic flow initiates a sequence of changes within neurosecretory axons that culminate within 6 h in axon dilatations with ultrastructural characteristics identical with those of naturally occurring Herring bodies. This confirms the previously hypothesized sequence of events DELLMANN and RODRÍGUEZ, 1970; POLENOV and GARLOV, 1971).

References

DELLMANN, H.-D.: Degeneration and regeneration of neurosecretory systems. Int. Rev. Cytol. 36, 215-315 (1973)

DELLMANN, H.-D., RODRÍGUEZ, E.M.: Herring bodies; an electron microcope study of local degeneration and regeneration of neurosecretory axons. Z. Zellforsch. 111, 293-315 (1970)

GRAINGER, F., SLOPER, J.C.: Correlation between microtubular number and transport activity of hypothalamo-neurohypophysial secretory neurons. Cell. Tissue Res. 153, 101-114 (1974)

PICKERING, B.T., JONES, C.W., BURFORD, G.D., McPHERSON, M., SWANN, R.W., HEAP, P.F., MORRIS, J.F.: The role of neurophysin proteins: suggestions from the study of their transport and turnover. Ann. N.Y. Acad. Sci. 248, 15-32 (1975)

POLENOV, A.L., GARLOV, P.E.: The hypothalamo hypophyseal system in acipenseridae. I. Ultrastructural organization of large neurosecretory terminals (Herring bodies) and axoventricular contacts. Z. Zellforsch. 116, 349-374 (1971)

Immunoenzyme Cytochemical Demonstration of Peptidergic Nerve Fibers in the Pars intermedia of the Amphibian Hypophysis

K. DIERICKX and F. VANDESANDE
Laboratorium voor Embryologie en Vergelijkende Histologie, Rijksuniversiteit, Godhuizenlaan, 4, B-9000 Gent, Belgium

A. Introduction

As in other vertebrates, the pars intermedia of the amphibian hypophysis contains peptidergic, catecholaminergic, and possibly cholinergic nerve fibers (see DIERICKX and VANDESANDE, 1976). The present paper reports the results of an immunoenzyme cytochemical study of the peptidergic nerve fibers of the amphibian pars intermedia.

B. Material and Methods

Four groups of adult animals were used. Three groups were normal animals: *Rana temporaria*, *R. esculenta*, and *Bufo bufo*. The fourth group consisted of nine *R. temporaria* from which, several months before being killed, the magnocellular hypothalamic neurosecretory preoptic nuclei had been removed. The details of the operative technique have been reported previously (DIERICKX, 1967). All animals were killed by decapitation. The brains, with the hypophysis attached, were fixed in Bouin-Hollande fluid with the addition of 10% saturated aqueous solution of sublimate. The fixed tissues were dehydrated in successive concentrations of ethanol, cleared in xylol, and then embedded in paraffin. Serial sections (5 µm) of the brain and hypophysis were made. The sections were stained using the technique of STERNBERGER et al. (1970) with unlabeled antibody peroxidase-antiperoxidase complex (PAP).

Two staining methods were used: (1) a single-staining method, and (2) a double-staining method. In the single-staining method, successive serial sections were stained, using alternately (1) rabbit antimesotocin serum (dilution 1:600), differentially adsorbed with Sepharose-4B-vasotocin, and (2) rabbit antivasotocin serum (dilution: 1:600), differentially adsorbed with Sepharose-4B-mesotocin.

With the double-staining method, described by VANDESANDE and DIERICKX (1976), mesotocinergic and vasotocinergic structures can be simultaneously identified in a single tissue section by their different color. In the present investigation this staining was performed as follows:

I. Localization of the First Antigen: Mesotocin

Successive incubations of the tissue sections in:

1. Normal goat serum (dilution 1:5), 10 min
2. Differentially adsorbed rabbit antimesotocin serum (dilution 1:600), 60 min

3. Goat antirabbit serum (dilution 1:20), 20 min
4. PAP complex (dilution 1:30), 20 min
5. 0.05 *M* Tris/HCl, pH 7.6, containing 0.003% H_2O_2 and 25 mg 3.3'-diaminobenzidine, ± 5 min

Result: selective brown staining of the mesotocinergic structures.

II. Localization of the Second Antigen: Vasotocin

Electrophoresis at 20 V/cm in 0.05 *M* glycine buffer pH 2.2 plus 30% dimethylformamide (60 min). Result: selective elution of the antibodies and the peroxidase used for the localization of mesotocin, without removing the brown reaction product-identifying mesotocin.

After electrophoresis, successive incubations of the tissue sections in:

1. Normal goat serum (dilution 1:5), 10 min
2. Differentially-adsorbed rabbit antivasotocin serum (dilution 1:600), 60 min
3. Goat antirabbit serum (dilution 1:20), 20 min
4. PAP complex (dilution 1:30), 20 min
5. 0.05 *M* Tris/HCl, pH 7.6, containing 0.01% H_2O_2 and 4-Cl-1-naphthol at saturation, ± 5 min

III. Results: Selective Blue Staining of the Vasotocinergic Structures

The rabbit antisera and the buffer solutions contained 1% goat serum. The antimesotocin serum and the antivasotocin serum were differentially adsorbed with Sepharose-4B-vasotocin and Sepharose-4B-mesotocin respectively. For the dilution of the antisera and the washing (2 × 5 min) of the sections before each incubation step, Tris/HCl buffered saline (pH 7.6) was used. The stained sections were mounted with chrome-glycerin jelly.

The tests for specificity of the method (including tests for selectivity and completeness of the elution of antibodies and of peroxidase from the tissue sections were done as described by VANDESANDE and DIERICKX (1976).

Finally, sections of the hypothalamus and hypophysis of the operated animals were also stained with standardized aldehyde-fuchsin (Gabe)-hemalum-orange G.

C. Results

I. The Tests for Specificity of the Histochemical Staining Methods

With the immunoenzyme histochemical stainings, it was always observed that background staining was almost eliminated. The tests for specificity of the method, done either by omitting one of the immune reagents, or by replacing the rabbit antisera by preimmune or antithyroglobulin rabbit serum, resulted only in a diffuse minimal staining of the tissue sections. The same negative staining result was obtained when antivasotocin serum exhausted with Sepharose-4B-vasotocin, and antimesotocin serum exhausted with Sepharose-4B-mesotocin were used.

In the double-staining method, the tests for selectivity and completeness of the elution of the antibodies and the peroxidase showed that the elution was selective and complete.

II. The Results in the Nonoperated Animals

The study of the single-stained and double-stained sections showed that in the three species:

1. The neural lobe contained two separate kinds of peptidergic nerve fibers: brown "mesotocinergic" fibers and blue "vasotocinergic" fibers.

2. The whole pars intermedia of the hypophysis contained an intercellular network of brown stained varicose "mesotocinergic" nerve fibers. It was observed that these nerve fibers were branches of axons leaving the pituitary stalk and the neural lobe.

3. In the pars intermedia of most of the animals, immunoreactive "vasotocinergic" fibers were totally absent. Only in a few animals, at the border with the neural lobe, the pars intermedia contained an occasional intercellular "vasotocinergic" dot or short thread, which might have been a part of a "vasotocinergic" nerve fiber.

III. The Results in the Operated Animals

The study of the serial sections of the whole hypothalamo-hypophyseal region, stained with the aldehyde-fuchsin method or with the immunoenzyme histochemical method showed that, in five of the nine operated animals, all the neurons of the hypothalamic magnocellular neurosecretory nuclei had been removed. In addition, the positively reacting nerve fibers of the preoptico-hypophyseal tract, of the median eminence, and of the neural lobe had completely disappeared. Moreover, in the pars intermedia, positively reacting nerve fibers were completely absent.

In the four other operated animals it was found that all the neurons of the ventral part of the hypothalamic magnocellular neurosecretory nuclei had been removed, but that the removal of their dorsal part was incomplete. In these animals, the pars intermedia contained a few immunoreactive mesotocinergic fibers.

D. Discussion

In contrast to normal animals, immunoreactive nerve fibers were totally absent from the pars intermedia of animals of which the hypothalamic magnocellular preoptic nuclei had been completely removed. This absence of immunoreactive nerve fibers in the pars intermedia was due to the complete removal of the magnocellular preoptic nuclei, as shown by the fact that in the pars intermedia of the animals of which these nuclei had been incompletely removed, positively-reacting nerve fibers were still present. Consequently, it may be concluded that the"mesotocinergic" nerve fibers of the amphibian pars intermedia are axons of neurosecretory perikarya located in the hypothalamic magnocellular preoptic nuclei.

On the other hand, VANDESANDE and DIERICKX (1976) have shown that the amphibian hypothalamic magnocellular neurosecretory nuclei contain separate mesotocinergic and vasotocinergic neurons. Taking account of this observation, and from the present results, it may be inferred that the "mesotocinergic" nerve fibers of the pars intermedia must contain mesotocin and/or parts of the mesotocin molecule. This inference has recently been confirmed by DIERICKX and VANDESANDE (1976).

As described, our light-microscopic immunocytochemical observations suggest that the amphibian pars intermedia contains no, or very few, vasotocinergic fibers. By contrast, according to our preliminary electron-microscopic studies, the amphibian pars intermedia would also contain separate vasotocinergic fibers, distributed throughout the whole gland. The reason for the discrepancy between our light- and electron-microscopic results is being investigated.

References

DIERICKX, K.: The function of the hypophysis without preoptic neurosecretory control. Z. Zellforsch. 78, 114-130 (1967)

DIERICKX, K., VANDESANDE, F.: Immuno-enzyme cytochemical demonstration of mesotocinergic nerve fibers in the pars intermedia of the amphibian hypophysis. Cell Tissue Res. (1976) (in press)

STERNBERGER, L.A., HARDY, P.H., Jr., CUCULIS, J.J., MEYER, H.G.: The unlabeled antibody enzyme method of immunohistochemistry. Preparation and properties of soluble antigen-antibody complex (horseradish peroxidase-antihorseradish peroxidase) and its use in identification of spirochetes. J. Histochem. Cytochem. 18, 315-333 (1970)

VANDESANDE, F., DIERICKX, K.: Immunocytochemical demonstration of separate vasotocinergic and mesotocinergic neurons in the amphibian hypothalamic magnocellular neurosecretory system. Cell Tissue Res. (1976) (in press)

Role of Biogenic Amines and M-Cholinergic Structures of the Rat Brain in the Hypothalamo-Hypophyseal Neurosecretory System (HHNS) Under Shock

V.N.ELSKY
Medical Institute, Health Protection Ministry of the Ukraine SSR, Donetsk, USSR

The functional state of the HHNS relating to the synthesis and secretion of CRF and ACTH was characterized in the different phases of shock. The level of norepinephrine decreased and the levels of epinephrine, serotonin, and histamine increased significantly in the short-duration phase. The synthesis of CRF and ACTH prevailed over their secretion. A tendency to decreased epinephrine and serotonin levels and to an increase of histamine and norepinephrine content was revealed in the second, longer-duration phase. CRF secretion exceeded its synthesis in this phase. In the third, longest-duration phase, the continued decrease of epinephrine and norepinephrine content, the increase of dopamine and additional increase of serotonin and histamine contents were accompanied by the steady decrease of CRF in the hypothalamus and a second wave of increase of ACTH synthesis and secretion. Both the pharmacologic decrease of the monoamine content of the brain and the blocking of adrenergic, serotoninergic, histamine sensitive, and M-cholinergic structures in the brain changed the initial excessive activation of HHNS on extreme influence. Production of CRF decreased, or its increase was late and was less evident; secretion lasted longer. The correlation between biogenic amines and CRF content was retained. Biogenic amines and acetylcholine are of great importance in the mechanism of HHNS activation.

Autoradiographic Studies on the Incorporation of Labeled Amino Acids in the Brain After Injection of Oxytocin

A. ERMISCH, B. AUERBACH, and H.-J. RÜHLE
Section of Biosciences, Karl Marx University, Leipzig, GDR

Considerable evidence suggests that oxytocin influences certain brain functions. The sites and mode of action of this and other peptide hormones are unknown. It was decided to study the influence of oxytocin on protein metabolism in different cell populations of the brain by autoradiography. Ten minutes after the intravenous injection of oxytocin (0.5 mU/g body wt.) the incorporation of ^{3}H-phenylalanine was significantly increased in the supraoptic nucleus and the cerebellar Purkinje cells of anesthetized rats. The ^{3}H-concentration was enhanced also in the paraventricular, arcuate and medial habenular nuclei, the pyramidal cells of the hippocampus and motor cortex, the choroid plexus, and the subcommissural organ. The ^{3}H-concentration in the subfornical organ, however, was significantly diminished. In conscious mice after a survival time of 15 min, an enhanced incorporation of ^{3}H-leucine was observed in eight of the above-mentioned cell populations. In contrast to our studies in the rat, an enhanced incorporation was also observed in the mouse subfornical organ. Increased amino-acid incorporation in cell populations of the brain may be specifically facilitated by oxytocin, as, by comparison, the incorporation of ^{3}H-phenylalanine in the pancreatic exocrine cells is significantly diminished by oxytocin.

Conclusions concerning the precise sites of action of oxytocin in the CNS cannot yet be made. Studies using other methods carried out in our laboratory support the hypothesis that the oxytocin action sites are located in the blood-brain barrier system, thereby influencing the amino-acid pool of the above-mentioned cell populations. The present results are of some interest in relation to the well-known effects of peptide hormones on such basic brain functions as learning and memory.

Comparative Account of the Hypothalamus of Amphibians; a Neuroanatomic Approach

A. FASOLO and M.F. FRANZONI
Institute of Comparative Anatomy, University of Turin, Turin, Italy

The hypothalamic organization in two representative amphibians (frog, newt) was studied by means of classic and experimental neuroanatomic methods.

Golgi-Method: Tufted, pear-shaped, or liquor-contacting neurons of relatively primitive type are encountered throughout the posterior hypothalamus of the newt. In the frog the overall pattern is more sophisticated; the CSF-contacting neurons seem more concentrated in some areas of the posterior hypothalamus, especially in the tuberal areas contiguous to the neurohypophysis. In the latter region, SF-contacting neurons send their axons to the median eminence. In the preoptic area, tufted and multipolar neurons of the isodendritic type are seen. A population of CSF-contacting cells is also prominent. Moreover, some large magnocellular elements also appear impregnated.

The HRP-Transport Method: After HRP injections or insertion of pellets in the neurointermediate complex, preoptic cells are observed, while after HRP applications into the median eminence, the posterior hypothalamus is largely labeled. Particularly in the frog, neurons are filled in areas corresponding to the so-called nucleus infundibularis dorsalis and nucleus infundibularis ventralis. In the posterior hypothalamus the HRP-positive cells of the tufted or pear-shaped type often appeared consistent with the Golgi results.

Conclusions: The present results stress the relations between the posterior hypothalamus and the median eminence in amphibians. Moreover, the application of HRP in the frog shows distinct tracts arising from discrete areas in the periventricular gray matter and directed towards the neurohypophysis. This confirms the efficacy of the neuroanatomic approach to the elucidation of the structural basis of neurosecretory mechanisms.

Functional Organization of the Hypothalamus in the Regulation of CRF-Producing Neurons

A. A. FILARETOV, M. I. MITYUSHOV, and L. V. VASSILEVSKAYA
Laboratory of Experimental Endocrinology, I. P. Pavlov Institute of Physiology, Academy of Sciences of the USSR, Leningrad, USSR

A. Introduction

The hypothalamus is the center of coordination of adrenocortical function. Its role consists of the inhibition or facilitation of one of its afferent inputs. The redistribution of the activity of hypothalamic nuclei results in the excitation or inhibition of CRF-producing neurons and can be revealed by recording hypothalamic electric activity. Such recordings suggest that the anterior and medial hypothalamus enter into antagonistic interaction in the regulation of the adrenocortical system (FILARETOV, 1976). The lateral hypothalamus seems to connect the medial hypothalamus and extrahypothalamic structures (SZENTÁGOTHAI et al., 1968; EAGER et al., 1971; MILLHOUSE, 1973).

The aim of the present study was to estimate changes in the activity of the anterior (AHA), medial (MHA), and lateral (LHA) hypothalamus during inhibition (following cortisol administration) and activation (immobilization stress) ofthe adrenocortical system.

B. Methods

Experiments were performed on intact unrestricted rabbits with permanent implanted semimicroelectrodes (for details see FILARETOV et al., 1976). Electrodes were implanted in AHA (retrochiasmatic area), MHA (areas of ventro- and dorsomedial nuclei), and LHA (at the level of ventrodorsomedial nuclei). The frequency of discharges of neuronal pools was compared before and after interference (Student's t-test). Inhibition of the adrenocortical system was investigated after administration of cortisol (1 mg/kg, i.v.) activation was investigated during immobilization stress. The rate of firing was followed during the 30 min preceding and for 60 min during immobilization or after cortisol administration. Excitation of the adrenocortical system was estimated by measurement of plasma corticosteroid levels (fluorometric method (VIES et al., 1960)). At the end of the experiments the electrode placements were verified histologically.

C. Results and Discussion

Administration of cortisol (1 mg/kg body wt., i.v.) resulted in the inhibition of the adrenocortical system. The initial plasma level of corticosteroids was 4.9 ± 0.4 μg%. It decreased to 3.9 ± 0.22 μg% ($p < 0.05$) by 120 min and to 3.7 ± 0.22 μg% ($p < 0.05$) by 180 min after injection of the hormone. Similar data were obtained by ZIMMERMAN and CRITCHLOW (1969) and DAFNY et al. (1973).

Cortisol administration caused variations in the firing frequency of multiunit activity of the AHA, MHA, and LHA. There was a decrease in firing rate in most pools in MHA. Out of 22, 12 decreased, three increased, five did not change their discharge rate, and two pools showed biphasic responses. Out of 26, 13 pools in the AHA responded to cortisol by a rise in the frequency of discharges. The rate of firing did not change in six, increased in six, two pools had biphasic responses. There was inhibition of firing in the LHA in eight out of 15 pools, three increased, four did not change their rate. Neurons that were excited following cortisol administration predominated in the AHA ($p < 0.001$, d-criterion), neurons that were inhibited predominated in the MHA ($p < 0.002$). It may be supposed that precisely such a pattern of neuronal activity is responsible for the suppression of CRF-producing neurons.

Activation of the pituitary-adrenocortical system resulted from immobilization. Immobilization stress caused an increase in plasma corticosteroid levels to from 9-19 μg%. The majority of the pools in the MHA responded by activation (17 out of 33 ($p < 0.002$, d-criterion)). Firing rate was reduced in ten pools, in five there was no change observed, one had a biphasic response. There was inhibition of firing rate in the AHA. Out of 30, 18 pools decreased ($p < 0.001$), seven increased their firing rate, three showed no change, one had a biphasic response. In the LHA the majority of neuronal pools (ten out of 17) were inhibited ($p < 0.05$), five were activated and one had a biphasic response. Excitation of the pituitary-adrenocortical system seems to result from the activation of the MHA and inhibition of the AHA.

It may be concluded that the AHA and MHA are the centers responsible for the control of CRF-producing neurons. The data suggest an antagonistic interaction between the AHA and MHA in the control of the function of the pituitary-adrenocortical system. The LHA seems to be less specific with respect to the regulation of pituitary-adrenocortical function than AHA and MHA. These data confirm our previous results obtained in experiments on single cells of the hypothalamus (FILARETOV, 1976).

References

DAFNY, N., PHILLIPS, M.I., TAYLOR, A.N., GILMAN, S.: Dose effects of cortisol on single unit activity in hypothalamus, reticular formation and hippocampus of freely behaving rats correlated with plasma steroid levels. Brain Res. 59, 257-272 (1973)

EAGER, R.P., CHI, C.C., WOLF, G.: Lateral hypothalamic projections to the hypothalamic ventromedial nucleus in the albino rat: demonstration by means of simplified ammoniacal silver degeneration method. Brain Res. 29, 128-132 (1971)

FILARETOV, A.A.: The afferent input and functional organization of the hypothalamus in reactions regulating pituitary-adrenocortical activity. Brain Res. 107, 39-54 (1976)

FILARETOV, A.A., ELISEEV, Yu.M., VASSILEVSKAYA, L.V.: Recording of hypothalamic multiunit activity with chronic implanted semi-microelectrodes. Sechenov Physiol. J. (USSR) 62, 475-476 (1976) (in Russian)

MILLHOUSE, O.E.: Certain ventromedial hypothalamic afferents. Brain Res. 55, 89-105 (1973)

SZENTÁGOTHAI, J., FLERKÓ, B., MESS, B., HALÁSZ, B.: Hypothalamic Control of the Anterior Pituitary. Budapest: Akadémiai Kiadó 1968

VIES, J. VAN DER, BAKKER, R.F.M., WIED, D. de: Correlated studies on plasma free corticosterone and on adrenal steroid formation rate in vitro. Acta Endocrinol. (Kbh). 34, 513-523 (1960)

ZIMMERMANN, E., CRITCHLOW, V.: Suppression of pituitary-adrenal function with pyhsiological plasma levels of corticosterone. Neuroendocrinology 5, 183-192 (1969)

Pituicytes: Their Reaction to Microtubule Poisons in vivo and in vitro

J. FLAMENT-DURAND, A. M. COUCK, J. P. HUBERT, and P. DUSTIN
Departments of Pathology and Electron Microscopy, Université Libre de Bruxelles, rue aux Laines 97, B-1000 Brussels, Belgium

A. Introduction

Pituicytes are peculiar glial cells found in the posterior lobe of the pituitary, in close proximity to axonal endings loaded with neurosecretory granules. They are easily recognizable, contain a large spheroid nucleus, a prominent Golgi apparatus, numerous free ribosomes, large lipid droplets, and an occasional centriole. Microtubules are present in the pituicyte cytoplasm and in their processes surrounding axonal neurosecretory endings. Since the first description of these cells by BUCY (1930), numerous studies of pituicytes have appeared (GERSH, 1939; ORTMANN, 1951; RENNELS and DRAGER, 1955; LEVEQUE and SMALL, 1959; LEVEQUE et al., 1966; WITTKOWSKI, 1968; STERBA and BRÜCKNER, 1969; DELLMANN and OWSLEY, 1969; BOUDIER et al., 1970; KRSULOVIC and BRÜCKNER, 1969; KRSULOVIC et al., 1970; HANSSON and NORSTRÖM, 1971; ERKOÇAK, 1973). In these publications, however, cilia have not been mentioned. The possible role of pituicytes in the control of the release of neurohormones has been suggested in relation to the mitotic figures observed after dehydration (SELVE and HALL, 1943; DESCLIN, 1947; ORTMANN, 1951; LEVEQUE and SMALL, 1959; KRSULOVIC and BRÜCKNER, 1969).

We report here a series of results obtained in pituicytes in various experimental conditions, in vivo and in vitro. Some of these results have already been presented (HUBERT et al., 1974; DUSTIN et al., 1975a,b; FLAMENT-DURAND et al., 1976).

B. Materials and Methods

The Sprague-Dawley strain of albino rats was used.

I. In vivo Experiments

1. Normal rats 7, 14, 21, and 30 days old, and adults 3 months old were studied as controls.

2. Five rats 3 months old were injected (i.p.) with 400 μg colchicine diluted in distilled water, and received three subsequent injections of 20 mg Lasix®

---

[1]This work was supported by a grant from the Belgian National Fund for Scientific Research and grant No. 3.4539.76 from the Belgian National Fund for Medical Research.

every second h, to reach a total dose of 60 mg Lasix® (Furosemid). The animals were killed 8 h after the colchicine injection, or 4 h after the last injection of Lasix®. Five rats received three injections of 20 mg Lasix®. They were killed 8 h later.

3. Five rats 3 months old were injected (i.p.) daily 5 days a week with 10 µg vincristine (VCR). The animals were killed after a total dose of 0.85 mg/kg body wt.

II. In vitro Experiments

The pituitaries of rats 13 days old were incubated at 37°C in Hanks' solution alone or with added 10^{-5} *M* colchicine or 10^{-5} *M* VCR (Oncovin Lilly)[2].

The posterior lobes were fixed by immersion in 4% glutaraldehyde in a phosphate buffer with added 0.50% sucrose at pH 7.4 for 90 min at room temperature. The specimens were then postfixed in 2% OsO_4 and prepared for electron microscopy.

C. Results

I. In vivo Experiments

1. Whereas in the pituicytes of adult rats, only occasional centrioles and no cilia have been reported in the literature, we have observed in the posterior lobe of adult rats and of young animals, 7, 14, and 21 days old, one or two cilia in spatial relation with a basal body. The cilia of the "9+0" or "9+2" type bud into a ciliary vesicle.

2. In rats treated with Furosemid and colchicine, numerous centrioles are seen in the pituicytes. They are either of the classic pattern, with parent and daughter centrioles in precise spatial relationship, or they are randomly distributed. A dense granular matrix of precursor material appears along with these newly formed centrioles. Numerous cilia at various stages of formation are seen. Occasional arrested metaphases are observed. In the five rats treated only with Furosemid, without microtubular poison, occasional centrioles of normal configuration are seen.

3. Repeated injections of VCR induce changes comparable to those described in I.2. All steps of formation of centrioles and cilia from a a dense matrix are visible. Some centrioles are incomplete and exhibit a "U" shape. Some cilia are abnormal (Fig. 1).

II. In vitro Experiments

After incubation in Hanks' solution for 1 h, one can see procentrioles as dense clusters of osmiophilic material ("deuterosomes")

---

[2]Oncovin was kindly supplied by Lilly and Co.

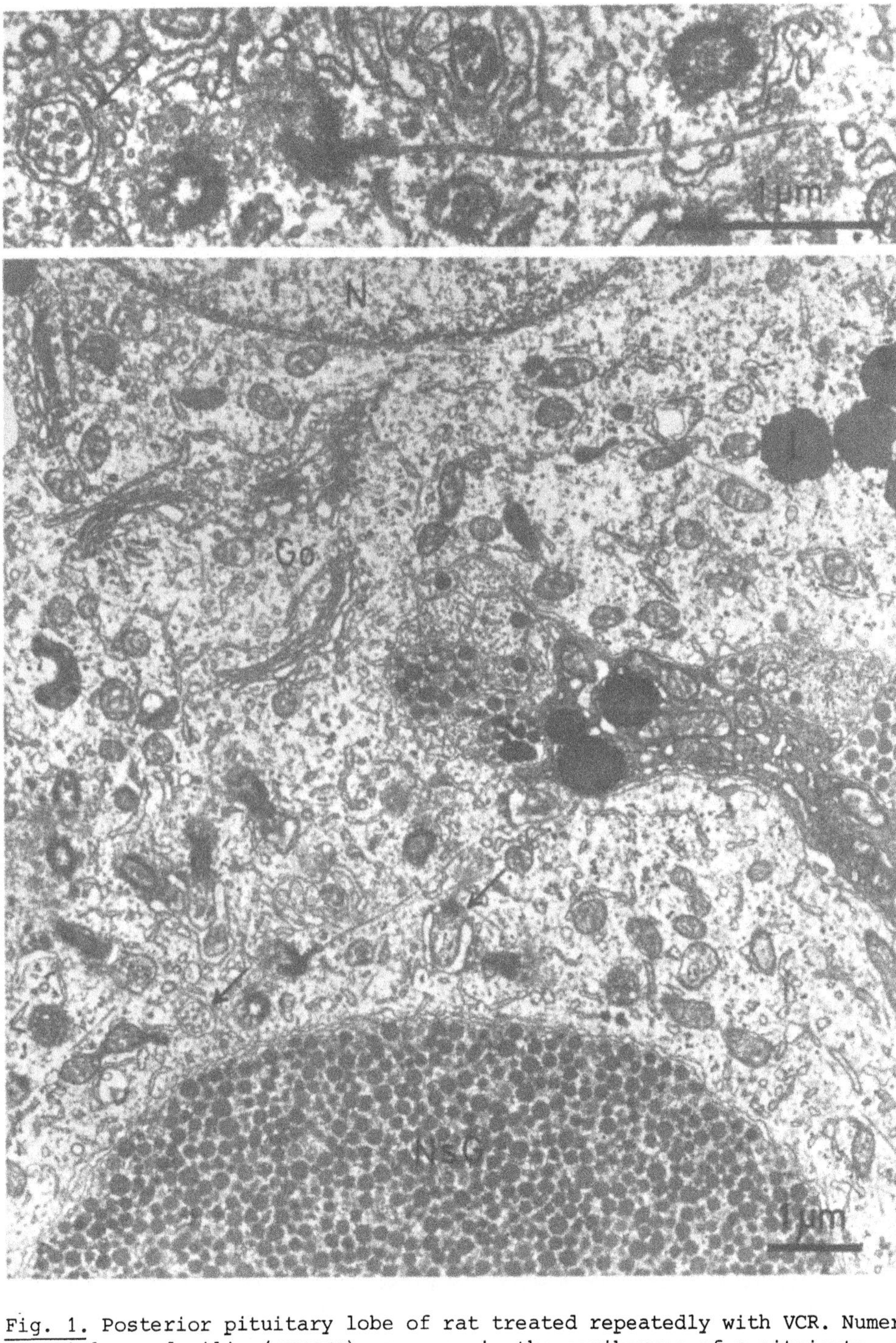

Fig. 1. Posterior pituitary lobe of rat treated repeatedly with VCR. Numerous centrioles and cilia (*arrows*) are seen in the perikaryon of a pituicyte, surrounding axonal swelling loaded with neurosecretory granules (*NsG*). *N* - nucleus, *L* - lipid droplets, *Go* - Golgi apparatus. Inset: higher magnification. Long microtubule attached to a rootlet and near a centriole and cilium

and centrioles at various stages of formation. When 10^{-5} *M* colchicine is added to the incubation medium, this centriologenesis still occurs, and numerous procentrioles, centrioles, and cilia are seen. When VCR is added to the incubation medium, numerous large paracrystals of tubulin are seen, as already described by RUFENER et al. (1972). In addition, centrioles and occasional cilia are observed. Peculiar macrotubules are frequently seen, mainly in the axonal endings but not in the pituicytes. They are in close proximity to normal microtubules and resemble the "decorated" microtubules described by BEHNKE and FORER (1972).

D. Discussion

Whereas in adult pituicytes only occasional centrioles have been reported, we have observed that in the posterior pituitary lobe of adult rats and of young animals, 7, 14, and 21 days old, one or two typical cilia of the 9+0 or 9+2 configuration extend into a ciliary vesicle and are seen in relation of the presence of cilia in such cells. It is not surprising, however, as pituicytes appear to be derived from ependymal cells (SHANKLIN, 1944; WINGSTRAND, 1966). An apparent multiplication of centrioles and cilia was observed in various conditions:

1. in vivo, after forced diuresis, produced by a potent diuretic (Furosemid), in the presence of colchicine;
2. in vivo, after habitual treatment with VCR (i.p.), without any stimulation of diuresis;
3. in vitro, in Hanks' solution alone, or with an added microtubular poison.

Cilia formation appears to be a normal function of pituicytes, as seen from studies of posterior lobes of all animals. It is influenced by conditions modifying the ionic environment of the posterior lobe, suggesting a possible role of pituicytes in the release of antidiuretic hormone (ADH). Cilia formation is not prevented by microtubular poisons. A similar formation of centrioles and cilia in the presence of microtubule poisons has been described by WUNDERLICH et al. (1974). The addition of colchicine to the incubation medium appears to enhance the centriologenesis. A similar paradoxical effect of colchicine in vitro was described by STUBBLEFIELD and BRINKLEY (1966) in hamster fibroblast cultures[3]. Treatment with VCR is known to produce an abnormal secretion of ADH in human patients (ROBERTSON et al., 1973). Our experimental data suggest that an abnormal release

[3]Addendum (May 1977). Since this work was presented, additional data have been obtained from normal rats of various ages, ranging from newborn to adults. Cilia and centrioles were regularly observed in their pituicytes. However, a precise quantitative estimation of their frequency appears difficult. The significance of the apparent multiplication of centrioles and cilia we have observed in various conditions deserves further study.

of ADH, instead of abnormal secretion, may occur. Pituicytes might thus be involved in the control of the release of neurohormones through ionic modifications. Further experiments are needed to confirm this hypothesis. As concluded by VOLLRATH (1974) during the last meeting on neurosecretion (London, 1973), "pituicytes require special attention." They appear to have an activity quite different from that of supporting cells (LIVINGSTON, 1976).

References

BEHNKE, O., FORER, A.: Vinblastine as a cause of direct transformation of some microtubules into helical structures. Exp. Cell Res. 73, 506-508 (1972)

BOUDIER, J.L., BOUDIER, J.A., PICARD, D.: Ultrastructure du lobe postérieur de l'hypophyse du rat et ses modifications au cours de l'excrétion de vasopressine. Z. Zellforsch. 108, 357-379 (1970)

BUCY, P.C.: The pars nervosa of the bovine hypophysis. J. Comp. Neurol. 50, 505-511 (1930)

DELLMANN, H.D., OWSLEY, P.A.: Investigations in the hypothalamo-neurosecretory system of the gree frog (*Rana pipiens*) after transection of the proximal neurohypophysis. II. Light and electronmicroscopic findings in the disconnected neurohypophysis with special emphasis on the pituicytes. Z. Zellforsch. 94, 325-336 (1969)

DESCLIN, L.: A propos des réactions morphologiques du lobe postérieur de l'hypophyse au cours des états de déshydratation chez le rat blanc. C. R. Soc. Biol. (Paris) 141, 438-439 (1947)

DUSTIN, P., HUBERT, J.P., FLAMENT-DURAND, J.: Centrioles and cilia formation in rat pituicytes after treatment with colchicine and vincristine. Studies in vivo and in vitro. In: Microtubules and Microtubule Inhibitors. BORGERS, M., BARBANDER, M. de (eds.). Amsterdam: North-Holland 1975a, pp. 289-296

DUSTIN, P., HUBERT, J.P., FLAMENT-DURAND, J.: Action of colchicine on axonal flow and pituicytes in the hypothalamopituitary system of the rat. Ann. N.Y. Acad. Sci. 253, 670-684 (1975b)

ERKOÇAK, A.: Etude au microscope électronique de la neurohypophyse du rat normal, ou après surrénalectomie bilatérale. Recherches sur les pituicytes et sur le mode de libération du neurosécrétat. Acta Anat. (Basel) 84, 178-201 (1973)

FLAMENT-DURAND, J., HUBERT, J.P., DUSTIN, P.: Centriolo- and ciliogenesis in the rat's pituicytes under the influence of microtubule poisons in vitro. Exp. Cell Res. 99, 435-438 (1976)

GERSH, L.: Structure and function of parenchymatous glandular cells in neurohypophysis of the rat. Am. J. Anat. 64, 407-443 (1939)

HANSSON, H.A., NORSTRÖM, A.: Glial reactions induced by colchicine treatment of the hypothalamic-neurohypophyseal system. Z. Zellforsch. 113, 294-310 (1971)

HUBERT, J.P., FLAMENT-DURAND, J., DUSTIN, P.: Centrioles and cilia multiplication in the pituitary of the rat after furosemid and colchicine treatment. Cell Tissue Res. 149, 349-361 (1974)

KRSULOVIC, J., BRÜCKNER, G.: Morphological characteristics of pituicytes in different functional stages. Z. Zellforsch. 99, 210-220 (1969)

KRSULOVIC, J., ERMISCH, A., STERBA, G.: Electron microscopic and autoradiographic study on the neurosecretory system of albino rats with special considerations of the pituicyte problem. In: Aspects of Neuroendocrinology. BARGMANN, W., SCHARRER, B. (eds.). Berlin-Heidelberg-New York: Springer-Verlag 1970, pp. 166-172

LEVEQUE, T.F., SMALL, M.: The relationship of the pituicyte to the posterior lobe hormones. Endocrinology 65, 909-915 (1959)

LEVEUQE, T.F., STUTINSKY, F., PORTE, A., STOECKEL, M.E.: Morphologie fine d'une différenciation glandulaire du récessus infundibulaire chez le rat. Z. Zellforsch. 69, 381-394 (1966)

LIVINGSTON, A.: Pituicytes in normal and jimpy mice. Cell Tissue Res. 167, 111-116 (1976)

ORTMANN, R.: Über experimentelle Veränderungen der Morphologie der Hypophysen-Zwischenhirnsysteme und die Beziehung der sog. "Gomorisubstanz" zum Adiuretin. Z. Zellforsch. 36, 92-140 (1951)

RENNELS, E.G., DRAGER, G.A.: The relationship of pituicytes to neurosecretion. Anat. Rec. 122, 193-200 (1955)

ROBERTSON, G.L., BHOOPHALAM, N., ZELKOWITZ, L.J.: Vincristine neurotoxicity and abnormal secretion of antidiuretic hormone. Arch. Intern. Med. 132, 717-722 (1973)

RUFENER, C., ROUILLER, C., ORCI, L.: Effect of vincristine on the ultrastructure of rat neurohypophysis. Experientia 29, 837-838 (1972)

SELYE, H., HALL, C.E.: Further studies concerning the action of sodium chloride on the pituitary. Anat. Rec. 86, 579-583 (1943)

SHANKLIN, W.N.: Histogenesis of the pig neurohypophysis. Am. J. Anat. 74, 327-353 (1944)

STERBA, G., BRÜCKNER, G.: Elektronmikroskopische Untersuchungen über die Reaktion der Pituizyten nach Hypophysenstieldurchtrennung bei *Rana esculenta*. Z. Zellforsch. 93, 74-83 (1969)

STUBBLEFIELD, E., BRINKLEY, B.R.: Cilia formation in Chinese hamsters fibroblasts in vitro as a response to colcemid treatment. J. Cell Biol. 30, 645-652 (1966)

VOLLRATH, L.: New trends in vertebrate neurosecretion. In: Neurosecretion - The Final Neuroendocrine Pathway. KNOWLES, F., VOLLRATH, L. (eds.). Berlin-Heidelberg-New York: Springer-Verlag 1974, pp. 276-284

WINGSTRAND, K.G.: Comparative anatomy and evolution of the hypophysis. In: The Pituitary Gland. HARRIS, G.W., DONOVAN, B.T. (eds.). London: Butterworths 1966, Vol. I, pp. 58-126

WITTKOWSKI, W.: Zur funktionellen Morphologie ependymaler und extraependymaler Glia im Rahmen der Neurosekretion. Z. Zellforsch. 86, 111-128 (1968)

WUNDERLICH, F., HEUMANN, H.G.: In vivo reassembly of microtubules in the presence of intracellular colchicine. Cytobiologie 10, 140-151 (1974)

Hypothalamo-Hypophyseal System in *Calamoichthys calabaricus smithi* (Polypteriformes)

M. F. FRANZONI, A. FASOLO, and V. MAZZI
Institute of Comparative Anatomy, University of Turin, Turin, Italy

A. Introduction

Polypteriformes are a singularly primitive group of African freshwater bony fishes, regarded as paleoniscid relicts, which are the extinct ancestors of the entire actinopterygian stock (MOY-THOMAS, 1939; ROMER, 1946). The hypothalamo-hypophyseal complex of Polypteriformes was studied from a general point of view by DODD and KERR (1963) and WINGSTRAND (1966). LAGIOS (1968) and KERR (1968) independently supplied important observations on the median eminence, the portal system, and the hypophyseal vascularization of *Calamoichthys calabaricus* , at both light- and electron-microscopic levels.

B. Neurohypophysis

The neurohypophysis of *Calamoichthys calabaricus* can be subdivided into a pars nervosa and a median eminence. The saccus vasculosus is seen dorsal to the pars nervosa. The pars nervosa consists of complicated digitations projecting deeply into the pars intermedia. They are made up of aldehyde-thionine-positive nerve fibers containing elementary neurosecretory granules 1000-1500 Å in diameter, and sometimes larger neurosecretory granules 1800-2000 Å in diameter. Some pituicytes scattered among neurosecretory nerve fibers, and ependymal cells lining the infundibular lumen are present. The median eminence is typically stratified; it shows three different types of nerve fibers and terminals containing: (1) granular vesicles 600-800 Å in diameter and clear vesicles of 300-450 Å; (2) granular vesicles of 900-1200 Å, polymorphous dense granules of 1300-1600 Å, and clear vesicles of 300-450 Å; (3) dense granules of 1600-1800 Å and clear vesicles of 300-450 Å.

In *Calamoichthys*, the organization and vascularization of the median eminence (LAGIOS, 1968), along with the lack of direct innervation of the adenohypophyseal pars distalis, probably reflects the primitive situation among bony fishes. On the other hand, the organization of the hypothalamo-hypophyseal system resembles that of dipnoans and of some primitive tetrapods like the urodeles. Significant in this context is the occurrence of synaptoid contacts between nerve fibers of different types and ependymal-glial cells, active points between nerve fibers and the perivascular space, and typical synapses between nerve fibers.

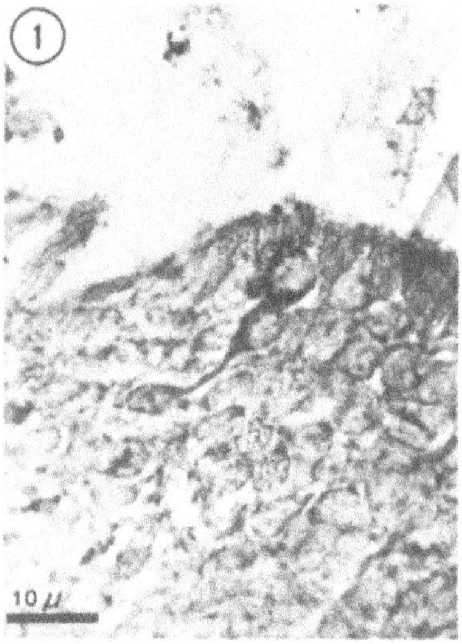

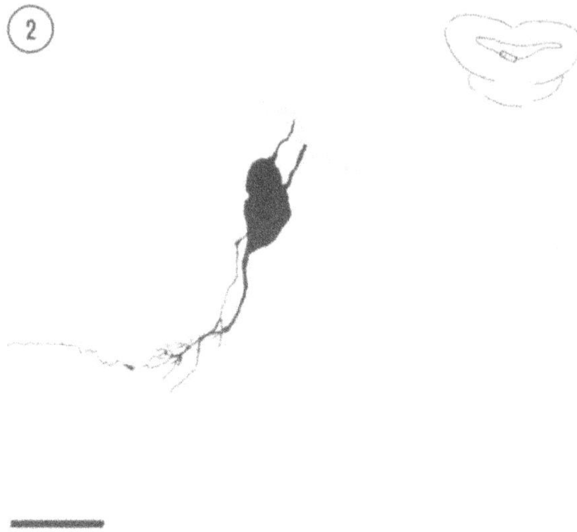

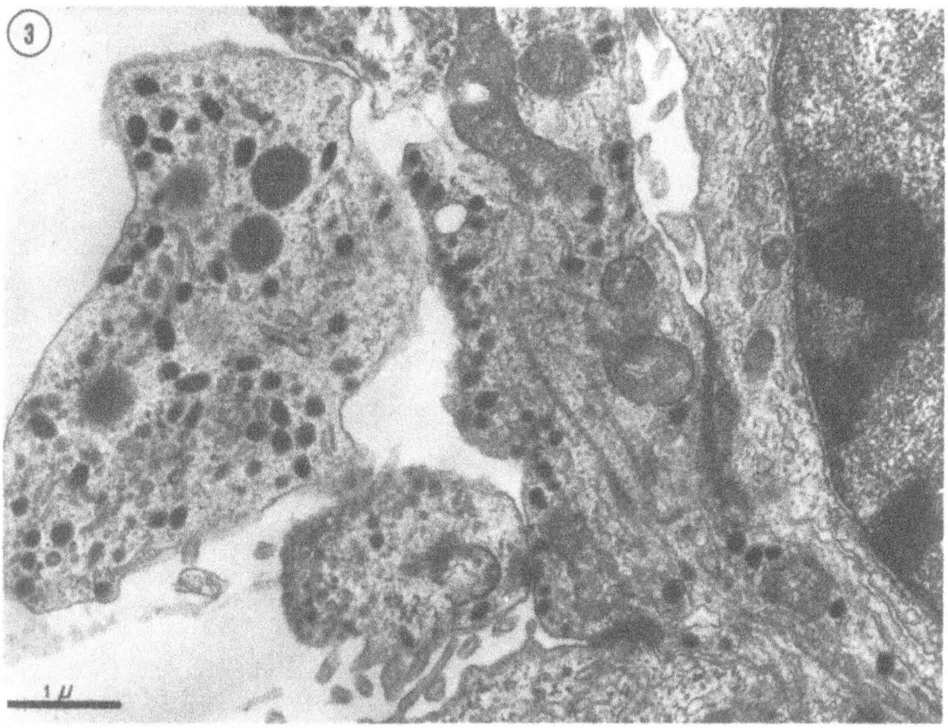

Fig. 1. Aldehyde-thionine-positive bipolar cells in posterior hypothalamus
Fig. 2. Drawing of Golgi preparation of same region
Fig. 3. Electron micrograph of CSF-contacting processes in posterior hypothalamus

C. Neurosecretory Systems

At the light microscopic level, an aldehyde-thionine-positive, extensive preoptic nucleus can be observed. Moreover, in the perinfundibular grey of the caudal hypothalamus, close to the median eminence, some aldehyde-thionine-positive bipolar cells with CSF-contacting processes are present (Fig. 1, 2). At the ultrastructural level, this region shows CSF-contacting cells of different types. In particular, a number of cells containing elementary neurosecretory granules 1600-2000 Å in diameter, or containing dense granules of 1100-1800 Å, granular vesicles of 750-1000 Å and multivesicular bodies are encountered (Fig. 3).

At least some of the afferent fibers to the median eminence are likely to be supplied by the region that passes almost indistinctly into the median eminence, where some neurosecretory neurons are still found. This characteristic emphasizes the ill-defined demarcation between the hypothalamus proper and the neurohemal areas.

References

DODD, J.M., KERR, T.: Comparative morphology and histology of the hypothalamo-neurohypophysial system. Symp. Zool. Soc. (Lond.) 9, 5-27 (1963)

KERR, T.: The pituitary in polypterines and its relationship to other fish pituitaries. J. Morphol. 124, 23-36 (1968)

LAGIOS, M.D.: Tetrapod-like organization of the pituitary gland of the polypteriformid fishes, *Calamoichthys calabaricus* and *Polypterus palmas*. Gen. Comp. Endocrinol. 11, 300-315 (1968)

MOY-THOMAS, J.A.: Paleozoic Fishes. London: Methuen 1939, p. 149

ROMER, A.S.: The early evolution of fishes. Q. Rev. Biol. 21, 31-69 (1946)

WINGSTRAND, K.G.: Comparative anatomy and evolution of the hypophysis. In: The Pituitary Gland. HARRIS, G.W., DONOVAN, B.T. (eds.). London: Butterworths 1966, Vol. I, p. 58-126

Vasotocin Immunoreactive Neurons in the Hypothalamus of Some Nonmammalian Vertebrates

J. GABRION[1], B. KERDELHUE[2], G. ALONSO[3], O. BOSLER[3], I. ASSENMACHER[3], and A. CALAS[3]
[1]Laboratoire d'Histologie et Embryologie, Faculté de Médecine, Université de Montpellier I, F-34000 Montpellier, France, [2]Laboratoire des Hormones Polypeptidiques du CNRS, F-91190 Gif-sur-Yvette, France, [3]Laboratoire de Physiologie Animale, Université des Sciences et Techniques du Languedoc, F-34060 Montpellier, France

A. Introduction

Vasotocin has been demonstrated to be a posthypophyseal antidiuretic factor in amphibians, reptiles, and birds (ACHER et al., 1969; BENTLEY, 1971). Using specific antibodies directed against this peptide, we have tried to explore, using immunocytochemistry, the vasotocin-producing system in the hypothalamus of some nonmammalian vertebrates that are commonly used as neuroendocrine models.

B. Material and Methods

Animals studied were *Triturus helveticus*, *Pleurodeles Waltlii*, *Rana esculenta*, and *Bufo bufo* (Amphibia); *Natrix viperinus* and *Malpolon monspessulanus* (Reptilia); *Anas platyrhynchos*, *Columba columba*, and *Coturnix coturnix* (Aves). These animals were either collected in the field or kept in the laboratory under natural conditions. Their brains were fixed by immersion or aortic perfusion with 4% paraformaldehyde in phosphate buffer, or with a modified Bouin-Hollande fixative.

Cryostat or paraffin sections (7 µm thick) of formaldehyde and Bouin-Hollande-fixed brains were incubated 1 h with specific antisera (AS), diluted 1:40 in 0.005 *M* veronal-buffered saline. These AS were obtained in rabbits injected with synthetic vasotocin (Hoffmann-Laroche) coupled with guinea pig γ-globulins. After washing, sections were incubated with another anti-rabbit-γ-globulin fluorescein-coupled AS (Pasteur Institute) for 45 min. They were counterstained with 1:10,000 Evans blue in veronal-buffered saline, then observed with a Leitz fluorescence microscope.

For ultrastructural investigation, thick sections (50 µm) of formaldehyde-fixed brains were incubated with the first specific AS, then with an anti-rabbit-γ-globulin-peroxidase-coupled AS. After disclosure of peroxidase, the pieces were processed for electron microscopy (NAKANE, 1970).

C. Results and Discussion

I. In amphibians (Figs. 1-3), fluorescent reactions were observed in the preoptic area (POA), ventral hypothalamus (VHT), median eminence (ME), and neural lobe (NL). In each species studied, the localization of the immunoreactive material was similar: immunofluorescent cell bodies were observed only in the POA. Their fluorescence was greatly increased after hypophysectomy in *Triturus* and was less intense in *Bufo* than in other species studied. Numerous immunofluorescent axons occurred in the anterior hypothalamus. They ran towards the optic chiasm and formed, behind it, a rather dense network in the ventromedial hypothalamus. This bundle of fluorescent fibers reached the ventral surface of the diencephalon and the rostral ME, in the vicinity of the rostral adenohypophysis, where corticotropic cells are located. In the caudal ME, immunoreactive axons and Herring bodies were more restricted to the inner zone, while an intense reaction affected the whole NL. On the other hand, in *Triturus* and *Rana*, we noticed a peculiar localization of a few reactive axons, which were directed rostrally to the posterior limit of the telencephalon.

II. In reptiles (Figs. 4 and 5), numerous dispersed reactive perikarya were observed in the perichiasmatic area of the hypothalamus. Some fluorescent neurons were aggregated in front of the optic chiasm. These reactions were more evident in *N. viperinus* than in *M. monspessulanus*. As in amphibians, immunofluorescent axons were localized in the superficial ventromedial hypothalamus. In the rostral ME, which is well developed in reptiles (and in anurans), two clusters of reactive axons were recognized. The external bundle reached the surface of the ME, while the most internal one extended into the caudal ME to the NL, which exhibited very strong fluorescence.

III. In birds (Figs. 6-9), the localization of the fluorescent reaction in the anterior hypothalamic area, the ME, and NL was similar in the three species studied. Numerous fluorescent cell bodies were observed in the anterior hypothalamus, specifically in the supraoptic and paraventricular regions. Bundles of fluorescent axons occurred in the fiber layer of the rostral and caudal ME, while the whole NL appeared intensely fluorescent. Moreover, fluorescent fibers were observed in the palisade layer of the rostral ME.

In the duck, at the ultrastructural level (Figs. 10 and 11), immunoreactive ME axons contained granular inclusions of different sizes (120-160 nm in diameter), which were responsible for the immunoreactivity. Some reactive fibers, also containing clear vesicles (40-60 nm in diameter) reached the external basal lamina.

In all these cases, no fluorescent reactions of the type described above were observed after incubation with a first AS against the carrier protein (guinea pig γ-globulins). When the specific vasotocin AS had been saturated with synthetic vasotocin, no reaction was observed in the amphibian brains. In the avian hypothalamus it was strongly decreased but not abolished. Thus, we may conclude that the major part of the fluorescent reaction is due to vasotocin. This conclusion is corroborated by the results obtained in our laboratory after treatment with an anti-LHRH AS (unpublished results). The localization of the vasotocin-contain-

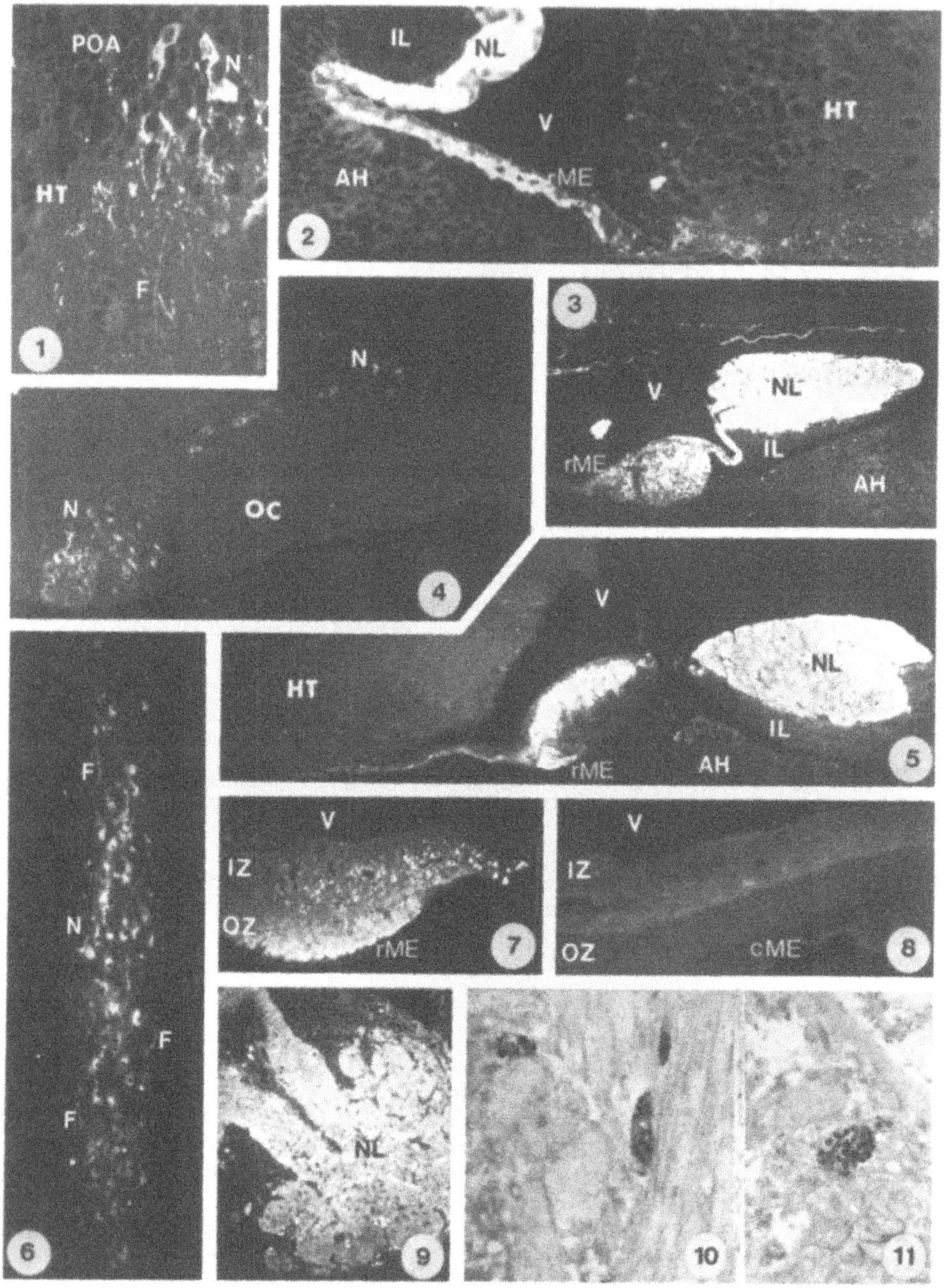
POA
N
HT
F
1
IL
NL
V
HT
AH
rME
2
3
V
NL
rME
IL
AH
N
N
OC
4
V
HT
NL
IL
rME
AH
5
F
N
F
F
6
V
IZ
OZ
rME
7
V
IZ
OZ
cME
8
NL
9
10
11

Figs. 1-11. Sagittal sections of brains treated first with vasotocin-AS, then with fluorescein- or peroxidase-coupled rabbit-γ-globulin AS.
Fig. 1. *T. helveticus*. Immunoreactive neurons are located in *POA*. Fluorescent fibers (*F*) are directed towards suprachiasmatic area of hypothalamus (*HT*)
Fig. 2. *T. helveticus*. Fluorescent fibers are localized in ventral hypothalamus, rostral median eminence (*rME*), caudal median eminence, and *NL*. *AH* - anterior lobe of adenohypophysis, *IL* - intermediate lobe, *V* - ventricle
Fig. 3. *B. bufo*. Immunoreactivity is intense in rostral and caudal median eminence and in neural lobe
Fig. 4. *N. viperinus*. Immunoreactive neurons are located in front of and above optic chiasm (*OC*)
Fig. 5. *N. viperinus*. Fluorescent fibers occur in ventral hypothalamus, rostral median eminence (where they constitute two bundles), and neural lobe
Figs. 6-11. *A. platyrhynchos*
Fig. 6. Immunoreactive cell bodies and proximal parts of axons are localized in anterior hypothalamus
Fig. 7. Rostral median eminence. Two groups of fluorescent fibers are clearly distinguished: one bundle is localized in outer zone (*OZ*) while another group of fibers and Herring bodies is located in inner zone (*IZ*)
Fig. 8. Caudal median eminence. Immunoreactivity is restricted to fibers of inner zone while outer layer is devoid of fluorescence
Fig. 9. Neural lobe. Immunoreactivity is intense in whole organ
Fig. 10. Inner zone of rostral median eminence (peroxidase-coupled AS). Immunoreactive fibers contain granular inclusions 120-160 nm in diameter
Fig. 11. Outer zone of rostral median eminence. Immunocytochemical reaction appears to be related to 120-160 nm granular inclusions

ing elements in all species examined was distinctly different from that of LHRH-reactive structures (CALAS et al., 1973; DOERR-SCHOTT and DUBOIS, 1974). Furthermore, in the rostral ME of all species studied, it appeared that the vasotocin immunoreactivity corresponded to the aldehyde-fuchsin stainability. So, the presence of vasotocin-containing axons in the external layer of the rostral ME provides morphologic support for the hypothesis that vasotocin is not only a posthypophyseal antidiuretic hormone but also functions as an adenohypophysiotropic principle at the rostral level of the hypothalamus. An experimental study is now in progress in order to clarify this adenohypophysiotropic role.

References

ACHER, R., CHAUVET, J., CHAUVET, M.T.: Evolution of the neurohypophysial hormones with reference to amphibians. Nature 221, 759-760 (1969)

BENTLEY, P.J.: Endocrines and Osmoregulation. Berlin-Heidelberg-New York: Springer-Verlag 1971

CALAS, A., KERDELHUE, B., ASSENMACHER, I., JUTISZ, M.: Les axones à LHRH de l'éminence médiane. Mise en évidence chez le Canard par une technique immunocytochimique. C. R. Acad. Sci. (Paris) (D) 277, 2765-2768 (1973)

New Protein Complexes in the Gomori-Positive Neurosecretion of the Hypothalamo-Neurohypophyseal System

A. A. GALOYAN, R. M. SRAPIONIAN, and F. M. SAHAKIAN
Institute of Biochemistry, Academy of Sciences of the Armenian SSR, Yerevan, USSR

It is now more than fifteen years since we postulated that the hypothalamus produces not only releasing hormones that regulate the function of the adenohypophysis, but also a family of new hormones that regulate cardiac activity and its coronary circulation. These peptide hormones, discovered by GALOYAN, act without the hypophysis in an organotropic mode (GALOYAN, 1962, 1965, 1975).

Three coronary-dilatator neurohormones were isolated from the hypothalamo-neurohypophyseal system of animals. We refer to these as K-, C-, and G-substances. In amounts of 0.1-0.5 µg/kg they induce a significant increase of about 200-300% in the volume of venous blood flowing out of the heart. This effect lasts for 2-3 h or more and has been shown to be due to an increase in the diameter of small capillaries and in the functions of the reserve vessels of the heart.

Thus, a family of neurohormones is produced in the hypothalamus for the regulation of cardiac activity and its coronary circulation. We have been able to show that neurohormones K and C are produced in the magnocellular areas of the hypothalamus, where vasopressin and oxytocin are produced. Substances K and C have been isolated from neurosecretory granules of the hypothalamus and neurohypophysis by the method of LaBELLA (1968).

We have made an electron microscopic investigation of the granules isolated from the neurohypophysis and hypothalamus. The largest granules have a diameter of 1200-1800 Å, and are characterized by a granular matrix of medium electron density. The other granules are smaller, 700-1100 Å. Among them we encountered separate granules with an electron-dense core described in the literature as containing the biologically active amines noradrenalin and serotonin. The other granules, the majority, have a rather high electron density and a homogeneous inner structure. They are surrounded by a membrane, and vary little in their size. It is interesting that, in the fraction isolated from the hypothalamus, granules of larger size predominate, and in the fraction isolated from the neurohypophysis, small granules are more often found.

Such an investigation was made on the fractions containing neurosecretory granules in which the coronary-dilatator substances are found. By paper chromatography some ninhydrin-positive compounds were revealed in the composition of the neurosecretory granules. Biologic testing revealed a definite coronary-dilatory effect of two fractions, by RF coinciding with the neurohormones

K and C (0.35 and 0.15). In 1964 GALOYAN discovered a specific protein from the hypothalamus that produced very pronounced coronary dilatation. This protein was located in the hypothalamus, was water soluble, and had a molecular weight of ca. 40-50,000. The presence of neurophysin in the neurosecretory cells and in the neurosecretory granules of the hypothalamus has been demonstrated (PLIŠKA and MEYER-GRASS, 1975; ZIMMERMAN et al., 1975).

Our experiments showed that protein isolated from the hypothalamus was different from neurophysin in both its biologic and physicochemical properties. Our calculations show that these protein carriers represent ca. 0.003% of the soluble proteins of the hypothalamus. It was necessary to show the presence of protein carriers in the neurosecretory granules. We have worked out a method for the isolation of water-soluble protein carriers from the neurosecretory granules. Table 1 shows the scheme of isolation of neurosecretory granules and protein carriers. In a density gradient of sucrose (1.21-1.31) neurosecretory granules are distributed in layers III, V, and VII. Coronary-dilatatory neurohormones are also found in those layers.

We were able to isolate water-soluble proteins from the neurosecretory granules by ammonium-sulfate precipitation. One of the proteins isolated from layer III is identified by its physicochemical properties with protein carriers isolated from the hypothalamus. This protein possesses coronary-dilatatory properties. However, proteins isolated from layers V and VII do not influence the coronary circulation. A protein from layer VII was isolated with the properties of vasopressin.

The data obtained show that the neurosecretory granules contain not only Van-Dyke protein but also new protein-peptide complexes, which possess cardiotropic activities. Protein-peptide components, C-AMP-dependent protein kinase, Van-Dyke protein and hexosamine together with other unidentified membrane proteins of neurosecretory granules are part of a special chemical system that is changed by nervous activity. In 1961, GALOYAN postulated that there is a functional-biochemical interrelationship between neurosecretory hormone formation and transmitters of nervous activity within the same neurons of the hypothalamus.

Phosphorylation of the neurosecretory granules plays an important role in their release and probably also in the formation of biologically active peptides (McKELVY, 1975). A spontaneous phosphorylation of neurosecretory granules by endogenous protein kinases also occurs. Thus, neurosecretory granules can be phosphorylated by both exogenous and endogenous protein kinases of the brain.

What are the substrates that are phosphorylated in the neurosecretory granules? GALOYAN has shown (unpublished work) that bovine neurophysin cannot be phosphorylated by C-AMP-dependent protein kinases of the brain. The same result was obtained by McKELVY (1975), who also indicated that neurophysin does not possess protein-kinase activity. Our experiments, however, (GALOYAN et al., 1976, unpublished work) indicated that neuro-

Table 1. Isolation of neurosecretory granules and hormones (K and C) from the hypothalamus-hypophyseal system

HOMOGENIZATION
0.25 *M* sucrose
0.02% heparin
↓
CENTRIFUGATION
(775 *g*, 15 min)

← SUPERNATANT
mitochondria,
microsomes,
granules
↓
CENTRIFUGATION
(6780 *g*, 15 min)

→ SEDIMENT
(nuclei and debris)

SEDIMENT

SUPERNATANT
microsomes,
granules,
light mitochondria
↓
CENTRIFUGATION
(20,000 *g*, 15 min)

← SEDIMENT
(light mitochondria)

→ SUPERNATANT
(microsomes + granules)

CENTRIFUGATION
(39,000 *g*, 4-5 h)

← SEDIMENT
microsomes and large numbers of neurosecretory granules
↓
ULTRACENTRIFUGATION
in 0.25 *M* sucrose and
0.02% heparin (1.12-1.13)
150,000 *g*, 1.5 h
↓
DIALYSIS
(against water 2-4°C)
↓
HOMOGENIZATION
↓
PRECIPITATION
$(NH_4)_2SO_4$
↓
DIALYSIS
↓
LYOPHYLIZATION
↓
BIOLOGIC ACTIVITY

secretory granules contain not only C-AMP-dependent protein kinase, but also the regulators of activity of C-AMP-dependent protein kinase. Neurohormones K, C, and G possess those properties. We have already begun the investigations of these substances, using as a substrate a specific protein of the hypothalamus, isolated from the neurosecretory granules. We expect that coronary-dilatatory neurohormones in the neurosecretory granules can play an important role in the phosphorylation of protein precursors of neurohormones.

References

GALOYAN, A.A.: Changes in Neurosecretion During Various Effects on the Central Nervous System. Pathalogie et Biologie, Paris, 9, 5-6, 682, 1961

GALOYAN, A.A.: Two Hypothalamic Hormones Affecting Coronary Circulation. Dokl. Akad. Nauk Arm. SSR, 34, 109, 1962

GALOYAN, A.A.: The Presence of the Specific Protein with Coronarodilatatory Properties in the Hypothalamus. Dokl. Akad. Nauk Arm. SSR, 38, 305, 1964

GALOYAN, A.A.: Some Problems of the Biochemistry of Hypothalamic Regulation. Erevan, Haiastan, 1965 (monograph)

GALOYAN, A.A.: Neuropeptides and Proteins. Proc. IVth American Peptide Symposium. WALTER, R., MEINHOFFER, J. (eds.), 651, 1975

LaBELLA, F.S.: Storage and Secretion of Neurohypophyseal Hormones. Canad. J. Physiol. Pharmacol. 46, 33, 1968

McKELVY, J.F.: Neurophysins: Carriers of Peptide Hormones, Annals of the New York Acad. Sci. 248, 80, 1975

PLIŠKA, V., MEYER-GRASS, M.: Neurophysins: Carriers of Peptide Hormones, Annals of the New York Acad. Sci. 248, 80, 1975

Morphofunctional Characteristics of Hypothalamo-Hypophyseal Structures Following Adrenalectomy

V. M. GORDIENKO, Yu. N. ZURNADJI, V. G. KOZYRITSKI, and I. I. DROZDOVICH
Institute of Endocrinology and Metabolism, Kiev, USSR

The supraoptic (SON), paraventricular (PVN), and arcuate (AN) hypothalamic nuclei and the adenohypophysis were examined at the light- and electron-microscopic levels in healthy dogs, rats, and guinea pigs at different periods after adrenalectomy.

Bilateral adrenalectomy causes changes connected with corticosteroid deficiency. At early periods following adrenalectomy, the ultrastructure of the SON is characterized by the presence of three main types of neurosecretory cells. The first type is a light neurocyte rich in organelles, with abundant neuroplasm, a euchromatin-rich nucleus with a large nucleolus, and abundant granular content. The second type is a large cell with a widened and degranulated ergastoplasm, a heterochromatin-rich nucleus, and an accumulation of neurosecretion in its axoplasm. The third type is a degenerating, inactive cell with electron-dense neuroplasm, swollen mitochondria, individual granules of neurosecretion, and a markedly pyknotic nucleus. At later periods following adrenalectomy, these ultrastructural characteristics of all three types of neurons are preserved; the first or the second type of neuron continues to be functionally active. While in the early periods there seems to be a characteristic increase in the release of neurosecretion, in later periods an increase in synthesis predominates. Accordingly, in the caudal neurohypophysis there is observed an increase or decrease in the content of empty vesicles in neuron terminals. In the supraoptic nuclei, active neurons adjoin the perivascular spaces of capillaries and are separated from their basal lamina by neuroglial cells. These latter cells penetrate closely, by their perikarya and processes, through the structures of the basal layers, and also contact neuropil, synapses, oligodendroglia, dendrites, and neurosecretory cell bodies. With decreasing corticosteroid levels in the blood, there is observed in neuroglial-cell cytoplasm a widening of hydrolized hyaloplasm, fibrillation of gliofibrils, change of mitochondrial size, and a change of glycogen and ribosome contents. These observations suggest that the neuroglial components of the supraoptic nuclei play a significant role in the mechanisms of osmo- and volume reception and that these components may be able to induce specific synthesis in neurosecretory cells.

Adrenalectomy increases the adrenocorticotropic function of the hypophysis. This function is mainly influenced by a regulatory effect of the parvicellular nuclei of the posterior hypothalamus. Our studies have shown that in adrenalectomized guinea pigs the most pronounced changes are observed in the ultrastructure of the AN. Depending on the degree of hypocorticoid condition, changes are detected in neuronal nuclei, which swell and have deep invaginations. In cytoplasm, the endoplasmic reticulum tubules are wide and their number increases, and large cisterns appear. The Golgi apparatus is more developed than in untreated animals and occupies a considerable part of the perinuclear zone. Golgi elements also appear in proximal parts of axons, and the number of microvesicles increases against the background of the tubular structures. Corresponding to an increase in the number of secretory granules, there is an increase in the number of lysosomelike bodies. Sometimes they are situated among the structures of the Golgi apparatus. Their number is especially large in the axonal part of the cytoplasm and the proximal parts of some axons. In some neurons, changes in cytoplasmic ultrastructure are insignificant or even absent. It is possible that these neurons do not take part in the regulation of adrenocorticotropic function.

Against the background of the described changes, which also occur in the AN in adrenocortical-hormone deficiency, there are changes observed in the ultrastructure of almost all cell types in the adenohypophysis of adrenalectomized animals. However, the most pronounced changes occur in the corticotrophs and folliculostellate cells. Deep degranulation and corticotroph-cell hypertrophy are observed as early as 2 h after adrenalectomy. By their size and ultrastructure these cells resemble adrenal cells. However, accumulations of intact and fragmentized secretory granules that are characteristic for corticotrophs are often detected on the vascular pole of these cells. The number of adrenal cells increases sharply within 5 h following the operation. In 14 h, the adrenal cells are very numerous, and folliculostellate cells appear to transform into corticotrophs. The analysis of sequential changes in corticotrophs, as the deficit of adrenocortical hormones increases, reveals a three-phase development. At early periods after adrenalectomy (in 2 h) a sharp degranulation is observed. In 5 h the number of secretory granules increases, and at 14 h a repeated pronounced degranulation with increased transformation of folliculostellate cells into corticotrophs is observed. Studies of blood-plasma-hydrocortisone levels at the same periods have shown that, in spite of adrenalectomy, the hormone levels decrease sharply at first, then increase, and decrease again. Hence, the three-phase response of the corticotrophs correlates with changes in the peripheral blood hydrocortisone levels.

Our studies show that the mechanisms of hypothalamic regulation of disturbed homeostasis as a result of adrenalectomy incorporates participation of both magnocellular and parvicellular nuclei. But if the participation of parvicellular neurons in corticosteroid deficiency is mainly connected with the regulation of adrenocorticotropic function of the hypophysis, then the influence of supraoptic nuclei is significally larger. These influences include first, maintenance of the water-salt balance and blood-pressure level, which undergo pronounced changes in the absence of adrenocortical hormones. The participation of these nuclei in the regulation of adenohypophyseal hormonopoiesis is also possible, and is confirmed by the synchronism of changes in neuronal ultrastructure in the SON and changes in the adenohypophysis. Evidently, however, these changes have no causal dependence on the SON.

Role of the Pineal Gland in the Hypothalamic Regulation of Adenohypophyseal Functions

I. I. GRACHEV, and R. I. USANOVA
A. A. Zhdanov State University, Leningrad, USSR

Extrahypothalamic influences of both a neural and an endocrine nature play an important role in the regulation of adenohypophyseal functions. In this connection the pineal gland, producing a few hormones of various chemical compositions, has attacted the particular attention of investigators. Studies that were carried out in our laboratory show that pineal factors of polypeptide origin play a significant role in the regulation of hypophyseal functions (GRACHEV et al., 1972, 1973). Shortly after the administration of pineal extract and some of its fractions to rats, we observed changes in the production of somatotrophic, luteinizing (LH), and follicle stimulating (FSH) hormones by the adenohypophysis. A few examples of the changes in the functional state of the hypothalamic nuclei in conditions of pineal hypo- and hyperfunction suggest the existence of pinealhypothalamic connections (REITER, 1973; BARANOV et al., 1974; CHAZOV and ISATCHENKOV, 1974). It seems that the influence of pineal hormones on the hypothalamic production of releasing and inhibiting factors, which respectively stimulate or inhibit hypophyseal hormonal secretion, is one of the mechanisms by which the pineal influences the adenohypophysis.

To verify this hypothesis we studied the effect of pineal extract on the secretion of gonadotrophin-releasing factors (GRF) in the hypothalamus of rats by in vivo and in vitro experiments. We used extracts of cattle pineal glands (produced by use of our method, GRACHEV et al., 1972) containing mainly polypeptides. The levels of gonadotrophin-releasing activity (GRA) in the hypothalamus and levels of gonadotrophic hormones in the hypophysis and blood plasma were determined by biologic assay. We observed that 1 h after the single intraperitoneal injection of the pineal extract (5 mg/100 g body wt.) the level of LH- and FSH-releasing activity in the anterior mediobasal hypothalamus of rats was considerably increased and the hypophyseal and plasma levels of gonadotrophic hormones were reduced (Fig. 1). This indicates that the administration of the pineal extracts to rats is followed by the suppression of release of GRF from the hypothalamus into the portal system. To study the possibility of direct action of pineal hormones on the hypothalamus we studied changes of GRF secretion in the tissue of the anterior mediobasal hypothalamus, incubating it in the presence of the pineal extract (150 mg/1 mg tissue). Pineal substances in vitro proved to suppress the release of GRF without changing the LH- and FSH-releasing activity in the incubated hypothalamic fragments. The increment of GRA in the hypothalamus observed in vivo is much less obvious in the in vitro experiments, i.e., the mechanisms of action of pineal substances in the whole body and those in isolated tissue are considerably different. In general, the results obtained in vivo and

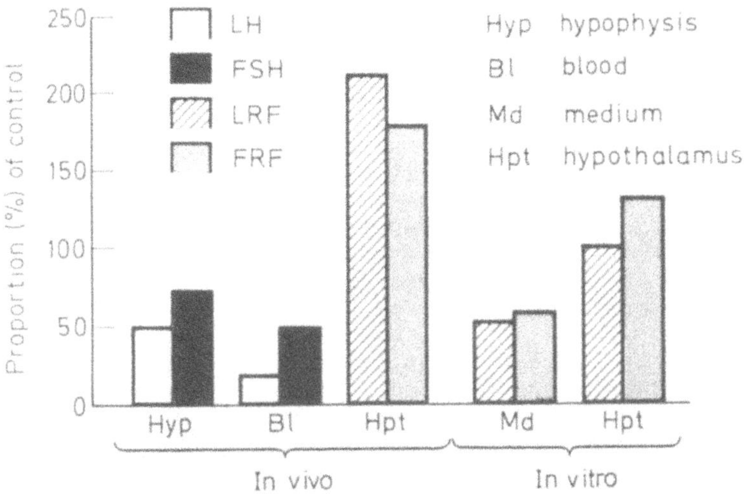

Fig. 1. Effect of pineal extract on secretion of hypothalamic GRF in vivo and in vitro

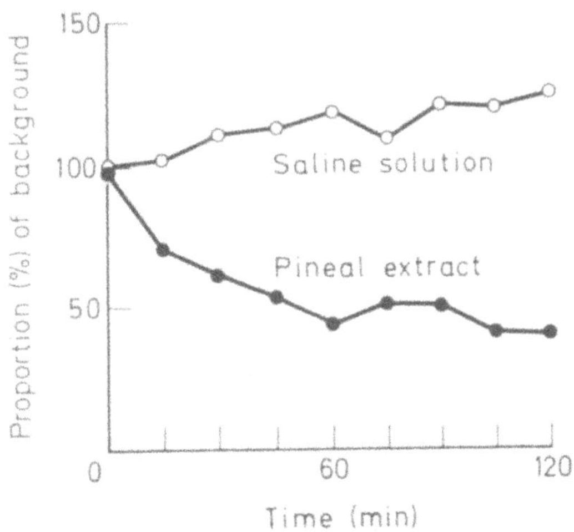

Fig. 2. Dynamics of changes in amplitude of EP in preoptic hypothalamus of rat in response to stimulation of hippocampus after injection of saline and pineal extract

in vitro suggest that pineal hormones have a direct effect on the hypothalamic centers responsible for the production of GRF. The changes of the functional state of the hypothalamic nuclei are reflected in bioelectric activity at different stages of reproduction (SAWYER, 1970). In this connection, we have studied the effect of pineal extract on the bioelectric activity of the preoptic hypothalamus, which is a neural center that triggers ovulation through the production and release of the LH-releasing factor in response to afferent impulses. We have studied the dynamics of amplitude changes of evoked potentials (EP) in the preoptic hypothalamus of the rat, when the hippocampus was stimulated after the i.p. injection of the pineal extracts. In every group of animals it was found that pineal substances considerably influenced EP of the preoptic hypothalamus, reducing the amplitude of both positive and negative phases of EP (Fig. 2). The first statistically significant changes of the amplitude of EP caused by the pineal extract were observed 15-30 min after the injection, and these changes gradually increased. The dynamics of amplitude changes in all the phases of EP was different from that of control animals, in which we were unable to observe an amplitude decrease. The same tendency in the changes of all the phases indicates that the observed effect is a consequence of functional activity changes in preoptic hypothalamic cells rather than of changes in multisensory pathways to the hypothalamus. It is of interest to note that the effect of pineal extract was more obvious in pinealectomized than in sham-operated animals. It is known that the production of releasing and inhibiting factors in the hypothalamus is regulated by feedback mechanisms and depends on the level of gland-target hormones in the blood. It was found that the combined daily administration of diethylstilbestrol (4 μg) and the pineal extract (2 mg/100 g body wt.) for 7 days, beginning from the day of operation, reduced the inhibitory influence of estrogen on the development of compensatory ovary hypertrophy.

Thus, one of the mechanisms by which pineal hormones control the release of GRF, secretion of hypophyseal gonadotrophins, and gonadal activity, is a decrease of sensitivity to the inhibiting influences of estrogen. This electrophysiologic and endocrinologic evidence supports the hypothesis of an indirect action of pineal substances on gonadotrophic hypophyseal function via the hypothalamus.

References

BARANOV, V.G., GRACHEV, I.I., PROPP, M.V., SAVCHENKO, O.N., SELIVERSTOV, Y.A., STEPANOV, G.S., USANOVA, R.I.: The influence of the epiphysis on the function of the hypothalamus, the hypophysis and the sex glands in rats prior to sexual maturation. Physiol. J. USSR 60, 1352-1359 (1974)

CHAZOV, E.I., ISCHENKOV, V.A.: In: The Pineal Gland: Site and Role in Neuroendocrine Regulatory System. Moscow: Science 1974, pp. 109-155

GRACHEV, I.I., SELIVERSTOV, Y.A., USANOVA, R.I., SABANIN, V.N.: The influence of epiphysis on the hypophyseal follicle stimulating function. Physiol. J. USSR 59, 647-651 (1973)

GRACHEV, I.I., USANOVA, R.I., SELIVERSTOV, Y.A.: The influence of the pineal extract on the growth activity of the rat pituitary gland. Physiol. J. USSR 58, 272-275 (1972)

REITER, R.I.: Comparative physiology of the pineal gland. Ann. Rev. Physiol. 35, 305-328 (1973)

SAWYER, C.H.: Some endocrine applications of electrophysiology. In: The Hypothalamus. MARTINI, L., MOTTA, M., FRASCHINI, F. (eds.). New York: Acad. Press 1970, pp. 83-101

Role of the Amygdaloid Complex in the Secretion of Antidiuretic Hormone and Oxytocin

Y. GUERNE and F. STUTINSKY
Laboratoire de Physiologie générale, ERA 178 du CNRS, Université Louis Pasteur, F-67000 Strasbourg, France

In previous studies we have shown that electric stimulation as well as microinjections of neurotransmitters (NA and ACh) into the paraventricular (NPV) and supraoptic (NSO) nuclei produce simultaneous secretion of oxytocin (OT) and antidiuretic hormone (ADH) (STUTINSKY, 1974; STUTINSKY and GUERNE, 1972). The stimulation of many other cell groups of the CNS produces the same results. This can easily be observed by stimulating different nuclei of the amygdaloid complex (GUERNE and STUTINSKY, 1975).

A. Material and Methods

Wistar rats weighing 230-380 g, anesthetized with Nembutal or urethane, were placed in a stereotaxic instrument following preparation for pressure recording of antidiuresis (62 rats, ♂), arterial (248 rats, ♂), intramammary (55 rats, ♀), and intrauterine (58 rats, ♀).

Electric stimulation was produced with concentric bipolar electrodes during 10-15 s, with a frequency of 60/s, a duration of 0.5 ms, and an intensity of 4 V (2 V for antidiuresis). The microinjections of neurotransmitters or other substances were done with a Hamilton syringe (0.5-4 µg in 1 µl NA or ACh); the inhibitors were injected into the NPV, the NSO, or the third ventricle (50 µg in 5 µl).

B. Results

Injections of NA into the nucleus reticularis, the inferior part of the putamen, and the n. amygdalae medialis, lateralis, corticalis, and centralis induce antidiuresis. Positive results were also obtained with injections into or in the vicinity of the n. amygdalae intercalatus and the n. amygdalae lateralis basalis. If a different test, such as blood pressure recording, is used, the location of the sites producing positive results is generally the same, but nevertheless, in some cases, the positive spots seem less numerous (Fig. 1). These positive reactions (antidiuresis or increase in blood pressure) can be inhibited by prior injection of alpha- or beta-blocking agents into the third ventricle or the neurosecretory nuclei themselves.

Electric stimulations produce similar results as NA- or ACh-injections. However, an increase in blood pressure is only observed

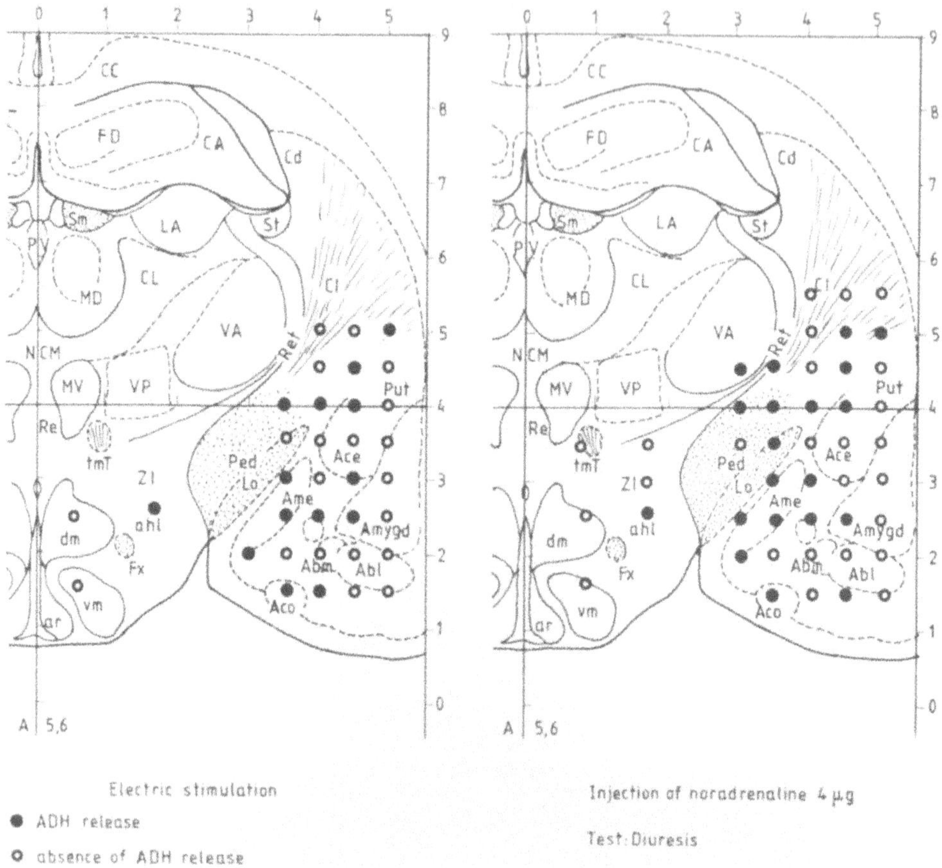

Fig. 1

in two locations: n. amygdalae corticalis and n. amygdalae lateralis basalis. Here also alpha- and beta-blocking agents inhibit the reation.

If other tests are applied, e.g., intramammary pressure recording, in order to detect oxytocin release, and the same stimulation parameters are used, negative results are obtained with the application of NA, ACh, or electric stimulation (Fig. 2).

C. Discussion

Our results show that pathways originating in the amygdala project not only to the ventromedial (NVM) and dorsomedial (NDM) nuclei and the preoptic region, as noted in the monkey (ADEY and MEYER, 1952; NAUTA, 1961, 1962) and in the cat (HALL, 1963; JOHNSON, 1965), but also directly or indirectly to the NPV and the NSO.

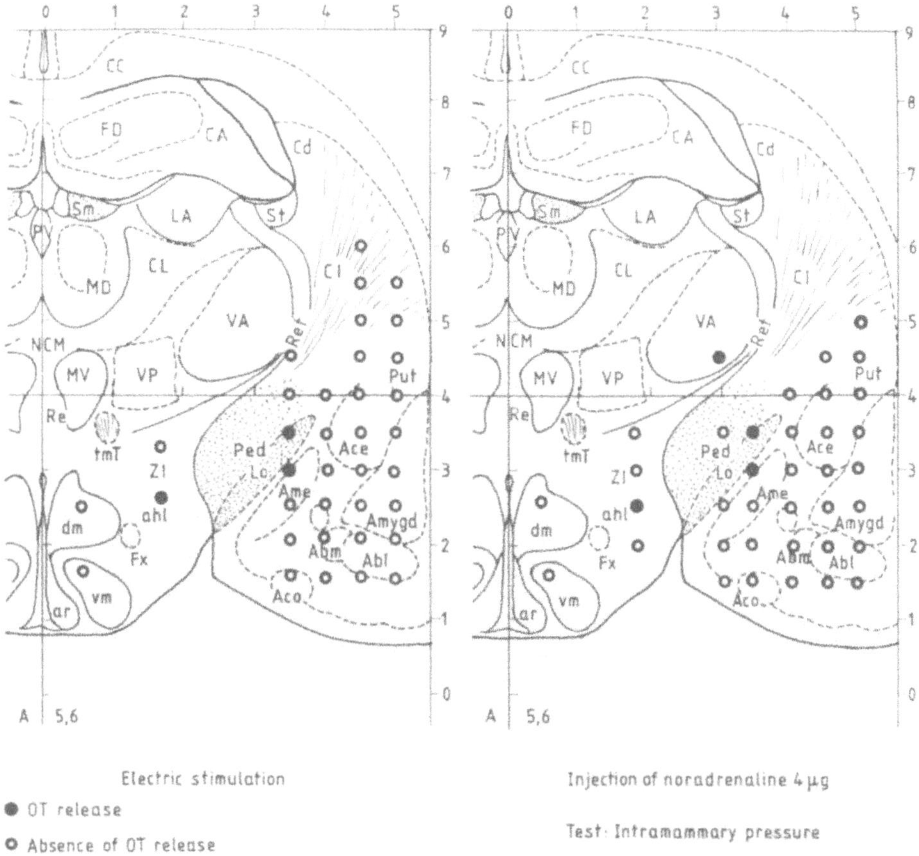

Fig. 2

This observation agrees with earlier histologic studies in the cat, where a connection between the amygdala and the NPV has been described (FOX, 1943). Nevertheless, our study indicates that all amygdalofugal fibers have no relays in the NVM before projecting to the NPV or NSO, since direct stimulation of the NVM (electric or humoral) does not induce ADH or oxytocin release.

Electrophysiologic evidence for a connection between the amygdala and some hypothalamic nuclei has been given by EGGER (1967), DREIFUSS et al. (1968), MURPHY et al. (1968), and recently by RENAUD (1976). In spite of a clear decrease in the activity of the neurosecretory cells after bilateral destruction of the amygdaloid complex (AZZALI et al., 1966), and despite the difficulties the pups have in getting milk if similar destruction has taken place in the mother during the second half of gestation (STUTINSKY and GUERNE, 1972), TINDAL et al. (1967), and RICHARD (1970) have clearly shown that there are no amygdalofugal pathways projecting to the neurosecretory cells. Such projections are, however, observed to the NVM (RENAUD, 1976).

These negative results contrast with our positive reactions after electric or humoral stimulation in the anterior and lateral hypothalamic areas and the medial preoptic area, all of which are connected with the amygdaloid complex through the stria terminalis (LEONHARD and SCOTT, 1971).

On the other hand, it is well known that the limbic system plays an important role in ADH secretion. Electric stimulation of the prepyriform area and the anterior cingulate area increases ADH in the jugular blood in the dog (YOSHIDA et al., 1965). In the monkey, electric stimulation of the n. amygdalae medialis lateralis, and the medial and lateral portions of the n. amygdalae basalis, induces antidiuresis (HAYWARD and SMITH, 1963). In the rat, differences seem to arise depending on whether the stimulation is applied to the anterior, medial, or posterior parts of the basal amygdala. Electric stimulation increases thirst if applied to the anterior region and decreases thirst if applied to the posterior part (GROSSMAN and GROSSMAN, 1963). This last observation suggests an increased ADH secretion. Other results, such as release of ADH by stimulation of the anterior cingulate area, or the hippocampus (TOMAS et al., 1973), or the role of the amygdaloid complex in the uptake of water and salt, underline the importance of the limbic system in modulating neurohypophyseal secretion.

Our results are in agreement with these data; however, some points need to be clarified. The observation that fewer sites give positive results when assessing ADH secretion with the blood-pressure test instead of the antidiuresis test may well be due to the lower sensitivity of the former. This explanation probably also accounts for the absence of variation in all experiments measuring intramammary pressure. This interpretation is corroborated by the very recent detection of minute quantities of OT, revealed by radioimmunoassay. This low OT concentration may well explain the failure of the intramammary pressure test.

Several questions remain unanswered. What is the physiologic significance of such a low hormonal secretion? What physiologic meaning has this result, and on which system can these low secretions act?

The inhibition of ADH and OT secretions after prior injection of alpha- and beta-blocking agents (into third ventricle and NSO and NPV) suggests that the nerve terminals ending on the neurosecretory cells belong to the alpha- and beta-types. In situ injection is more effective than intraventricular injection. The injection into the third ventricle induces an inhibition that lasts for only 10-25 min, whereas the effect of the in situ injections definitely lasts throughout the experiment.

References

ADEY, W.R., MEYER, M.: Hippocampal and hypothalamic connections of the temporal lobe in the monkey. Brain 75, 358-384 (1952)

AZZALI, G., MACCHI, G., CARRERAS, M., DALLA ROSA, V., LECHI, A.: Rhinencéphale et fonction neuroendocrine: aspects structuraux de l'hypothalamus neurosécrétoire et du complexe endocrine après lésions rhinencéphaliques. Acta Anat. 64, 10-47 (1966)

DREIFUSS, J.J., MURPHY, J.T., GLOOR, P.: Contrasting effects of two identified amygdaloid efferents pathways on single hypothalamic neurons. J. Neurophysiol. 31, 237-248 (1968)

EGGER, D.: Responses of hypothalamus neurons to electrical stimulation in the amygdala and the hypothalamus. Electroencephalogr. Clin. Neurophysiol. 23, 6-15 (1967)

FOX, C.A.: The stria terminalis longitudinal association bundle and precommissural fornix fibers in the cat. J. Comp. Neurol. 79, 277-295 (1943)

GROSSMAN, S.P, GROSSMAN, L.: Food and water intake following lesions or electrical stimulation of the amygdala. Am. J. Physiol. 205, 761-765 (1963)

GUERNE, Y., STUTINSKY, F.: Intervention du complexe amygdalien dans l'excrétion de vasopressine. J. Physiol. 71, 135A (1975)

HALL, E.A.: Efferent connexions of the basal and lateral nuclei of the amygdala in the cat. Am. J. Anat. 113, 139-151 (1963)

HAYWARD, J.N., SMITH, W.K.: Influence of limbic system on neurohypophysis. Arch. Neurol. 9, 171-177 (1963)

JOHNSON, T.N.: An experimental study of the fornix and hypothalamo-segmental tracts in the cat. J. Comp. Neurol. 125, 29-40 (1965)

LEONHARD, C.M., SCOTT, J.W.: Origin and distribution of the amygdalofugal pathways in the rat: an experimental neuroanatomical study. J. Comp. Neurol. 141, 313-330 (1971)

MURPHY, J.T., DREIFUSS, J.J., GLOOR, P.: Topographical differences in the responses of single hypothalamic neurons to limbic stimulation. Am. J. Physiol. 214, 1443-1453 (1968)

NAUTA, W.H.J.: Fibre degeneration following lesions in the amygdaloid complex in the monkey. J. Anat. 95, 515-531 (1961)

NAUTA, W.H.J.: Neural associations of the amygdaloid complex in the monkey. Brain 85, 505-520 (1962)

RENAUD, L.P.: An electrophysiological study of amygdalo-hypothalamic projections to the ventromedial nucleus of the rat. Brain Res. 105, 45-58 (1976)

RICHARD, Ph.: An electrophysiological study in the ewe of the tracts which transmit impulses from the mammary glands to the pituitary stalk. J. Endocrinol. 47, 37-44 (1970)

STUTINSKY, F.: Morphological and physiological reactions of the supraoptic and paraventricular nuclei. In: VI Int. Symp. on Neurosecretion. Neuro-Secretion, The Final Neuroendocrine Pathway. KNOWLES, F., VOLLRATH, L. (eds.). Berlin-Heidelberg-New York: Springer-Verlag 1974, pp. 15-23

STUTINSKY, F., GUERNE, Y.: Rôle des catécholamines dans la libération des hormones post-hypophysaires. C. R. Acad. Sci. (Paris) 275, 573-576 (1972)

STUTINSKY, F., TERMINN, Y.: Effets des lésions du complexe amygdalien sur le réflexe d'éjection de lait chez la ratte. J. Physiol. 57, 249-250 (1965)

TINDAL, J.S., KNAGGS, G.S., TURVEY, A.: Studies on the ascending path of the milk-ejection reflex in the brain of the guinea pig. J. Endocrinol. 37, xli (1967)

TOMAS, T., TRACZYK, W.Z., GUREK, J.W.: ADH release from cut pituitary stalk and intact pituitary gland during hippocampal stimulation of various frequencies in the rat. Neuroendocrinology 11, 257-267 (1973)
YOSHIDA, S., BAYASHI, H.I., MURAKAWA, S., NAKAO, K.: Cerebral control of secretion of antidiuretic hormone: effect of electrical stimulation of the prepyriform area on the neurohypophysis in the dog. Endocrinology 77, 597-601 (1965)

Hypothalamic Nuclei of Rats Treated with Corticosteroids

M. HRISTIĆ and V. PANTIĆ
Institute for Biological Research "Siniša Stanković", Belgrade, Yugoslavia

A. Introduction

Autoradiographic examinations have shown that radioactive cortisone is incorporated into the hypothalamus, and radioactive substances were found to be selectively concentrated in neurons in the ventral part of the nucleus arcuatus (NAR) and in the infundibular region (WARENBOURG, 1975). The aim of these investigations was to establish whether a high dose of hydrocortisone (Hy) given at the age of 5, 15, or 30 days has any effect on the selective and specific binding of ^{3}H-hydrocortisone (^{3}H-Hy) to the cells of the nuclei of the anterior and medial hypothalamus, and whether there are any changes in the structural characteristics of the nuclei examined.

B. Material and Methods

Rats at the age of 5, 15, or 30 days were injected with a single dose of Hy (10 mg/10 g body wt.) and sacrificed at the age of 3 months. The ^{3}H-Hy (100 µCi/100 g body wt.) was administered 1 h before sacrifice. The hypothalamus, with the pituitary, was fixed in Bouin's solution and stained with Gabe-Azan and hematoxylin-eosin methods. Ilford L_4 emulsion was used and the period of exposure was 3 months. The results were statistically analyzed according to SNEDECOR (1965).

C. Results

Upon examining the neurosecretory cells of the nucleus supraopticus (NSO) of animals treated with Hy at the age of 5 days, the following results were obtained: an increased incorporation of ^{3}H-Hy of 140%, and in glia cells of 360%, compared to the controls (Fig. 1a). Neurosecretory cells were significantly hypertrophied up to 15% and their nuclei up to 11%, and the amount of neurosecretory substance was decreased (Fig. 2a). Cell degeneration was seen only at the periphery of the nucleus (Fig. 2b).

The NSO of rats treated at the age of 15 days with a single dose of Hy also showed intense binding of ^{3}H-Hy, to neurosecretory cells of the NSO of 100% and to glia cells of 130% more than in controls. In most of the animals the amount of neurosecretory material was the same as in animals treated on day 5. Cells and

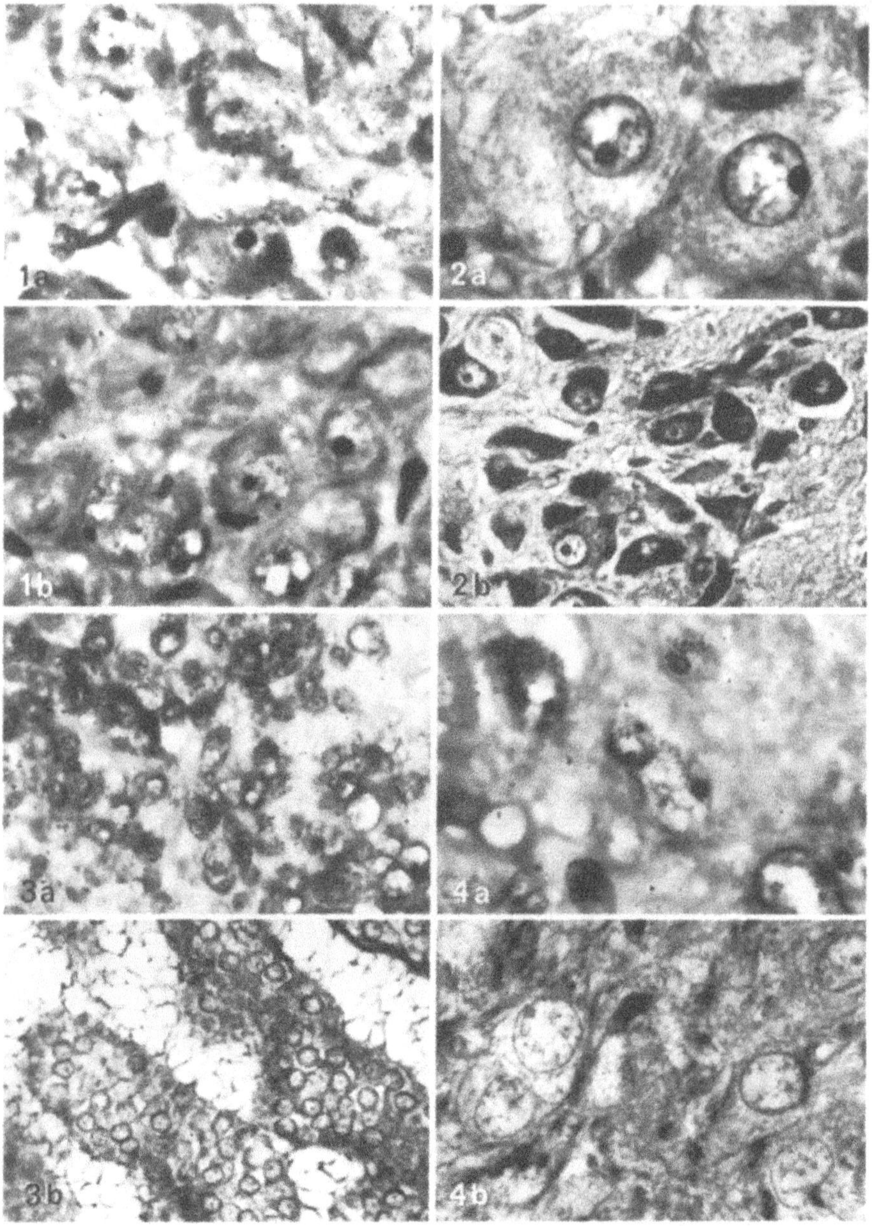
1a
2a
1b
2b
3a
4a
3b
4b

Fig. 1. NSO (a) and NPV (b) of rats treated with Hy at age of 5 days labeled with ^{3}H-Hy 1 h before sacrifice. (a) and (b) - × 1750
Fig. 2. Neurosecretory cells of NSO of rats treated with Hy at age of 5 days: (a) hypertrophy - × 2240, and (b) degeneration - × 900
Fig. 3a and b. Ependymal cells of rats treated with Hy at age of 15 days, with some ^{3}H-Hy-labeled cells (a) × 1750, (b) × 900
Fig. 4. ^{3}H-Hy-labeled glia cells in NAR (a) and accumulation of Gabe-positive substances in nerve terminals (b) between neurons. (a) and (b) - × 2240

nuclei of NSO were not significantly hypertrophied. In animals injected with Hy at the age of 30 days the binding of ^{3}H-Hy was intensive only in the glia cells of the NSO, reaching up to 246% of control values. No significant changes in the diameter of the cells were noticed and the amount of neurosecretory material was smaller than in the controls. There were no differences in the amount of ^{3}H-Hy incorporation nor in the amount of neurosecretory material in the nucleus paraventricularis (NPV) nor any changes in cell and nuclei diameter of experimental and control animals (Fig. 1b).

In treated animals, ependymal cells were increased in number and some of them were labeled with ^{3}H-Hy (Fig. 3a). The population of ependymal cells was greatest in animals treated with Hy at the age of 15 days (Fig. 3b). In the region of the NAR of all animals treated, a considerable amount of incorporated ^{3}H-Hy was noticed (Fig. 4a). Accumulation of Gabe- and Gomori-positive substance was noticed in animals with marked hyperplasia of ependymal cells in the NAR (Fig. 4b).

In the nucleus ventromedialis (NVM), as in the NPV, there were no significant changes in the incorporation of ^{3}H-Hy. Silver granules in glia cells of the hypothalamopituitary system were located mainly in the nucleus and primarily around the nucleolus (Fig. 4a).

D. Discussion

The presence of receptors for corticosteroids in the hypothalamus and pituitary has been suggested (BOHUS and STRASHIMIROV, 1970). The incorporation of labeled Hy has also been reported (STUMPF, 1971). Consideration of our results suggests that Hy injected into neonatal rats chiefly stimulates the activity of the central part of the NSO and partially stimulates the NAR.

E. Summary

The incorporation of ^{3}H-hydrocortisone (^{3}H-Hy) in the anterior and medial hypothalamus and the differences in the amount of neurosecretory material and diameter of the cells were examined in rats treated with a single dose of hydrocortisone (Hy) at the age of 5, 15, or 30 days and the following results were obtained: Intense incorporation of ^{3}H-Hy in NSO, enlargement of cells and their nuclei, and a decreased amount of neurosecretory material; in the medial hypothalamus, intense binding of ^{3}H-Hy in the region of the NAR; proliferation of ependymal cells; no significant changes were noticed in the NPV and NVM.

References

BOHUS, B., STRASHIMIROV, D.: Localization and specifity feedback receptors at the hypothalamo-hypophyseal level: comparative effects of various steroids implanted in the median eminence on the anterior pituitary of the rat. Neuroendocrinol. 6, 197-210 (1970)

SNEDECOR, G.W.: Statistical Methods. 5th ed. Ames: Iowa State College Press 1965, p. 534

STUMPF, W.E.: Autoradiographic techniques and the localization of estrogen, androgen and glucocorticoid in pituitary and brain. Am. Zool. 11, 725-739 (1971)

WARENBOURG, M.: Radioautographic study of the rat brain and pituitary after injection of ^{3}H-dexametasone. Cell Tissue Res. 161, 183-191 (1975)

Neurosecretory System of Dogfish, *Scylliorhinus caniculus*, Under Normal Conditions and After Osmotic Loading

J. C. VAN DE KAMER
Zoologic Laboratory, University of Utrecht, Utrecht, The Netherlands

The present paper deals with an old problem: the morphology of the hypothalamo-hypophyseal system of dogfish (*S. caniculus*) and its functional significance. SCHARRER (1952) and BARGMANN (1953) stressed the point that in these fishes a neurointermediate lobe is present, which complicates the analysis of the fiber endings of the hypothalamo-hypophyseal tract. KNOWLES (1965) demonstrated that neurosecretory fibers make intimate contact with the peripheral cells of the neurointermediate lobe, but did not obtain clear evidence for the termination of neurosecretory fibers on the walls of blood vessels in the lobe. MELLINGER (1963), however, studying *Scyliorhinus* demonstrated fiber endings also on the blood vessels, although their number was restricted. Since in dogfish the hypothalamo-hypophyseal system is extremely well developed, the question arises whether all fibers of this system fulfill only the function of a transmitter in stimulating the peripheral intermediate cells, or whether the system also releases hormones into the blood vessels and plays a role in osmoregulation, as is the case in the other vertebrate groups.

To study this problem, sections of the neurointermediate lobe were examined electron-microscopically, with the result that the presence of fibers, filled with granules about 1700 Å in diameter and ending on blood vessels, was established beyond doubt. According to MAETZ and LAHLOU (1974): "practically nothing is known about the possible action of neurohypophyseal hormones on salt and water balance in fishes other than teleosts." As early as several years ago the author discussed these matters with Francis KNOWLES and Manfred GABE. The discussion gave the impetus for a series of experiments in which dogfish taken from 3.5% seawater were placed in seawater to which so much NaCl was added that final salt concentrations of 5% and 10% were reached. Other animals were placed back into normal seawater after the salt-load period, while a reverse experiment in which the animals were placed in seawater diluted to 50% with distilled water was also performed. If the system were related to osmoregulation, one could expect release of material into the vascular system after the saltload, or accumulation of material in the system in the reverse experiment. This view seems justified, as exocytosis of the carrier-hormone complex appears to have been established beyond doubt (VOLLRATH, 1974), and therefore the quantity of AF-stainable material may be related to the hormonal content. The results of the experiments are presented in graphs, in which the quantity of neurosecretion, indicated in arbitrary units ranging from 0-7, is plotted against time (Plate 1, Fig. A). During osmotic loading, using 5% salt solution, the quantity of neurosecretion in the preoptic nucleus diminished gradually (Figs. 1 and 2). If one compares the nuclear area with the region of the

Scylliorhinus caniculus

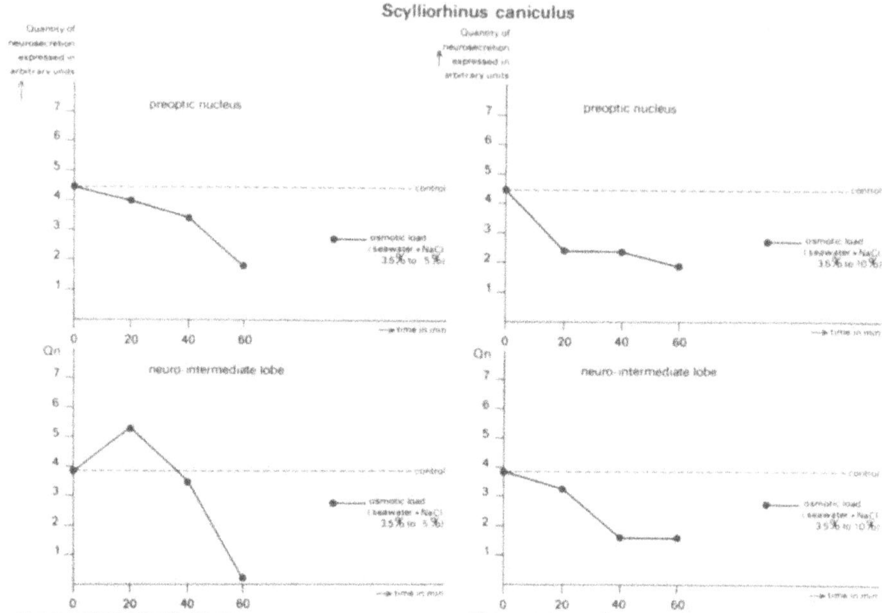

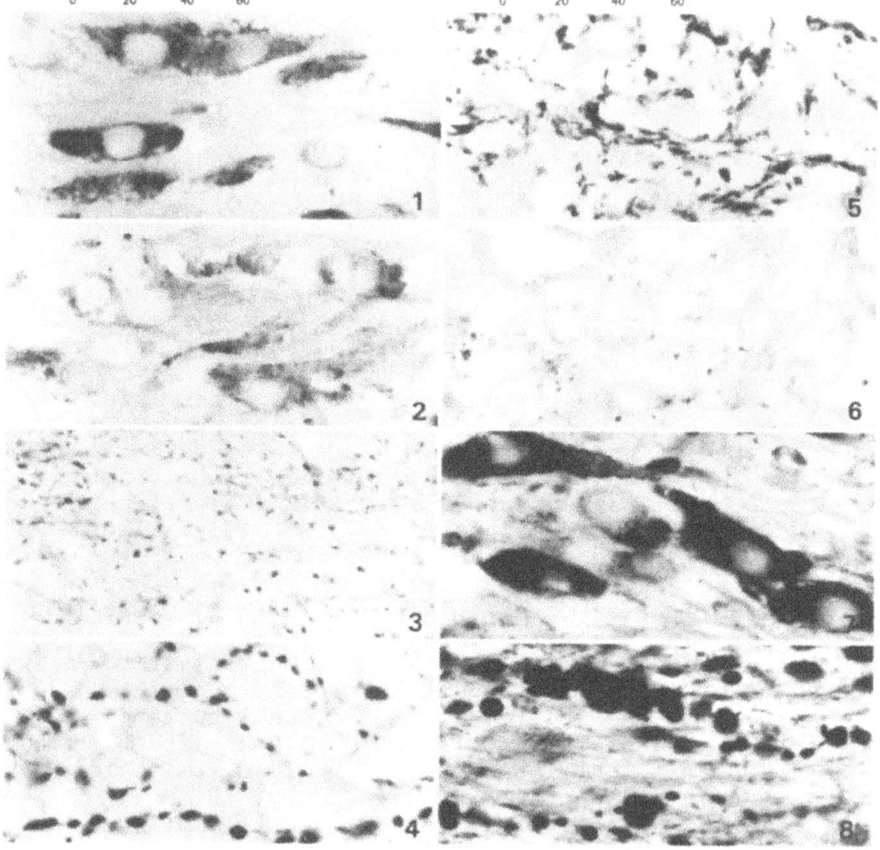

Plate 1 (*above*). Graphs showing effect of osmotic load upon quantity of AF-positive material in preoptic nucleus and neurointermediate lobe of *Scylliorhinus caniculus*. Ordinate: quantity of neurosecretion expressed in arbitrary units. Abscissa: time in minutes
Fig. 1. Preoptic nucleus. Control
Fig. 2. Preoptic nucleus. Degranulation after 60 min of saltload (5% solution)
Fig. 3. Hypothalamohypophyseal tract. Control
Fig. 4. Hypothalamohypophyseal tract after 40 min of saltload (5% solution)
Fig. 5. Fiber endings in neurointermediate lobe. Control
Fig. 6. Fiber endings in neurointermediate lobe after 60 min of saltload (5% solution)
Fig. 7. Preoptic nucleus after 40 min of saltload (5% solution) followed by a stay of 20 min in seawater
Fig. 8. Hypothalamohypophyseal tract of animal kept for 2.5 h in 50:50 mixture of seawater and distilled water.
All photographs × 560

fiber endings in the neurointermediate lobe, one observes in the latter an accumulation of the secretion in the beginning of the experiments (after 20 min), and a very clear and marked release leading to a nearly empty stage after 60 min (Figs. 5 and 6). This means that if the transport also occurs gradually, the tract must show a marked accumulation after about 40 min. This is exactly what was observed (Figs. 3 and 4). During osmotic loading, using a 10% salt solution, the quantity of neurosecretion in the preoptic nucleus decreased much faster than in the foregoing experiments. The fiber endings were - after only 40 min - practically devoid of selectively stainable material. In conclusion, these results indicate that an acceleration of the transport occurs during a stronger osmotic load. Remarkable was the fact that animals, replaced after the salt-load period into normal seawater, showed a marked accumulation of the secretion in the cells of the preoptic nucleus (Fig. 7). These results were reproducible. The explanation of these observations, however, is difficult and full of uncertainties. Comparable experiments are only available for teleosts. The results of ARVY and GABE (1954), obtained with the sea fishes *Callionymus lyra* and *Ammodytes lanceolatus*, strongly resemble our observations in *Scylliorhinus*. Although the results can be related to osmoregulation, the possibility remains that the reactions observed are the result of stress. Several authors share this view. At first sight this explanation seems acceptable. However, in general, stress produces a shock of short duration. In contrast to this, the present results cover a longer period and are gradual in time; a stronger load produces a correspondingly greater effect. Furthermore, placing the animals immediately after saltload into normal seawater has a marked effect on the accumulation of the secretion in the cells of the preoptic nucleus, which suggests that the synthesis of material in the preoptic cells had been stimulated by the foregoing experiment. Moreover, the reverse of the salt-load situation, in which the animals are placed in diluted seawater, might also have a "stress" effect; it shows, however, the opposite reaction - an accumulation of material in the system (Fig. 8). All these facts speak in favor of an adaptation process. It is known from the work of ACHER (1974) that in spiny dogfish (*Squalus acanthias*) two oxytocinlike substances, valitocin and aspargtocin, are present, as well as arginine vasotocin. Hormones with an antidiuretic effect are thus very probably also present in *Scylliorhinus*. In this connection it is interesting to note that HELLER, as early as 1941, demonstrated the presence in *Scylliorhinus* of an antidiuretic principle, although in small quantities. He stressed the fact that in mammals the antidiuretic principle exerts two functions: (1) it regulates the excretion of water, (2) it increases the excretion of certain ions. Furthermore, he remarked: "it seems significant that the antidiuretic principle influences the chloride excretion of frogs in very small doses. The question arises therefore whether the action of the postpituitary antidiuretic hormone on the mineral metabolism is not developmentally the older one." In discussing the present results with MAETZ, he suggested that neurohypophyseal hormones are released to increase chloride excretion by the gills. Although real proof is not available and will not be possible before the purified hormones of *Scylliorhinus* are available in sufficient quantity, the present results suggest that in the dogfish - a representative of the ancient group of cartilaginous fishes - the hypothalamo-hypophyseal system is already involved in ionic regulation. Since our laboratory will not continue this line of research at this time, it seems important to introduce this problem to the present audience, hoping that some colleagues will continue to use dogfish in further research of the hypothalamo-hypophyseal system.

Acknowledgments. Thanks are due to Dr. J. Peute for his support, to Ina J.C. Wilschut, Mrs. R.W. Schenk-Bijleveld, and M. Zandbergen for their technical assistance, and to the members of the staff of the photographic department for making the illustrations.

References

ACHER, R.: Chemistry of the neurohypophysial hormones: an example of molecular evolution. In: Handbook of Physiology, 1974, Sect. 7, Vol. I, Chapt. 6, pp. 119-130

ARVY, L., GABE, M.: Modifications du système hypothalamo-hypophysaire chez *Callionymus lyra* L. et *lanceolatus* Les. au cours des variations de l'équilibre osmotique. C. R. Assoc. Anat. 41, 843-849 (1954)

BARGMANN, W.: Über das Zwischenhirn-Hypophysensystem von Fischen. Z. Zellforsch. 38, 275-298 (1953)

HELLER, H.: The distribution of the pituitary antidiuretic hormone throughout the vertebrate series. J. Physiol. (London) 99, 246-256 (1941)

KNOWLES, F.: Evidence for a dual control by neurosecretion of hormone synthesis and hormone release in the pituitary of the dogfish *Scylliorhinus stellaris*. Philos. Trans. R. Soc. Lond. (Biol.) 249, 435-455 (1965)

LEATHERLAND, J.F., DODD, J.M.: Activity of the hypothalamo-neurohypophysial complex of the european eel (*Anguilla anguilla* L.) assessed by the use of an in situ staining technique and by autoradiography. Gen. Comp. Endocrinol. 13, 45-59 (1969)

MAETZ, J., LAHLOU, B.: Actions of neurohypophysial hormones in fishes. In: Handbook of Physiology, 1974, Sect. 4, Vol. I, Chapt. 19, pp. 521-544

MELLINGER, J.: Les relations neuro-vasculo-glandulaires dans l'appareil hypophysaire de la Roussette, *Scylliorhinus caniculus* L. Thesis, Université de Strassbourg - 238 E, 1963, pp. 1-211

SCHARRER, E.: Das Hypophysen-Zwischenhirnsystem von *Scyllium stellare*. Z. Zellforsch. 37, 196-204 (1952)

VOLLRATH, L.: New trends in vertebrate neurosecretion. In: Neurosecretion - The Final Neuroendocrine Pathway. VI Int. Symp. on Neurosecretion, London, 1973. Berlin-Heidelberg-New York: Springer-Verlag 1974, pp. 276-284

Fluorescence and Electron-Microscopic Study of the Meta-Adenohypophysis of the Carp, *Cyprinus carpio* L.

M. S. KONSTANTINOVA and G. G. KORNIENKO
Sechenov Institute of Evolutionary Physiology and Biochemistry of the Academy of Sciences of the USSR, Leningrad, USSR

There are varying opinions concerning the demonstration (using the Falck-Hillarp technique) of monoaminergic (MA) structures in the teleost hypophysis. Some authors have failed to detect any specific fluorescence, or the fluorescence of the fibers was very weak. The hypophysis of the adult carp, *Cyprinus carpio* L. was studied 2 h after injection of nialamid (300 mg/kg body wt.). Nialamid, an inhibitor of monoamine oxidase, causes an accumulation of monoamines, and it can make easier the detection of aminergic fibers. After pretreatment with nialamid, very thin MA fibers with yellowish-green fluorescence were distinguished in the carp neurohypophysis (NH). The fibers are more numerous in the parts of the NH adjacent to the metaadenohypophysis (MAH). The fine thin fluorescent fibers were found between the endocrine cells of the MAH. The MA fluorescence in the MAH of the carp is unsteady, low in intensity, and varied significantly in different specimens. The electron-microscopic study revealed that after treatment with nialmid, in the MAH of the carp, the dense-core vesicles in the neurosecretory fibers and terminals of type B, making mostly synaptoid contacts with endocrine cells of the MAH, became more numerous. The number of synaptic vesicles was slightly decreased, and some swollen mitochondria were found. The combined use of fluorescence- and electron microscopy establish the MA innervation of the endocrine cells in the MAH of the carp.

Effects of Temperature on the Preopticohypophyseal Neurosecretory System of Carp, *Cyprinus carpio* L.

G. G. KORNIENKO and N. S. POGREBNYAKOVA
Sechenov Institute of Evolutionary Physiology and Biochemistry of the Academy of Sciences of the USSR, Leningrad, USSR

Effects of low (+4 to +10°C) and high (+34 to +40°C) temperatures (T) on the preoptico-hypophyseal neurosecretory system (PHNS) of carp were studied. All the animals, including controls, were kept in a tank at 20-27°C before the experiments. A tendency to a decrease in size of the perikarya and nucleoli of the neurosecretory cells (NSC) of the nucleus praeopticus (NP) is noted in fish exposed to T 4-10°C for 1-2 h. The size of the nuclei is not changed, but they become denser. The amount of the neurosecretory material (NSM) in the cells of NP increases up to 4-4.5 units (3-4 units in controls). The NSM is intensely stained and looks homogeneous. The amount of NSM in the proximal and distal parts of the neurohypophysis (Nh) increases up to 4-5 units (3-4 units in controls). Capillaries in the NP (in comparison to the controls) are not very pronounced; the hyperemia of the Nh increases up to 2.5 units (2 units in controls). A decrease in size of the perikarya, nuclei, and nucleoli is seen in the NP of fish exposed to a gradual fall of T to 4-10°C for 6 h, and after keeping them at this T for 2-2.5 h. The amount of NSM decreases to 1-2 units. In the proximal parts of Nh 2.5 units of NSM are contained; no change is found in the NSM content in the distal parts of Nh. NSM is loosely arranged, finely granulated, and palely stained. The capillaries are not pronounced in the PHNS. An increase in size of the perikarya, nuclei, and nucleoli is found in NP under the influence of high T, which has a lethal effect. Basophilia of the cytoplasm is lowered. NSM is poorly stained. Its amount is increased up to 4 units. NSM is displaced from the proximal into the distal parts of Nh, where its amount exceeds 5 units. NP and Nh are strongly hyperemic. Thus, under the influence of T changes, inhibition of discharge of the neurohormones takes place. At low T, inhibition of synthesis of NSM, and at high T an activation of synthesis of NSM occurs in the NP. Under the gradual influence of low T, an activation of release of neurohormones into the blood circulation is observed against the background of inhibition of the synthesis of NSM in NP.

Ecologic-Histophysiologic Analysis of Neuroglial and Blood Elements in the Neurohypophysis of Sturgeon, *Acipenser güldenstädti* Brandt

E. D. KORYAKINA
Sechenov Institute of Evolutionary Physiology and Biochemistry of the Academy of Sciences of the USSR, Leningrad, USSR

Activation of the neurosecretory elements and tanycytes in the neurohypophysis (Nh) of female sturgeons soon after spawning has been well established. Sixty-three animals caught in the Volga were divided into three groups according to the stage of gonadal maturity (sgm): group I - before spawning (III-IV sgm), group II - soon after spawning (VI sgm), and group III - 1-1.5 months after spawning (VI-II sgm). A great amount of NSM ($\leq$ 4 U) is found in the Nh of groups I and III. Tanycytes chiefly have elongated nuclei (width = 3.5 ± 0.2 µm). Dark pituicytes (nuclear diameter 6-10 µm) are few. A smaller amount of NSM ($\leq$ 2 U) is contained in the Nh of group II. The nuclei of tanycytes are 4.5 ± 0.17 µm ($p < 0.001$) in width. The length of tanycyte nuclei in all groups of fish is practically constant. Pictures of "migration" of some tanycytes and loosening of the ependymal layer are observed. The number of (mainly light) pituicytes having nuclei 8-13 µm in diameter increases up to 3-7 and more in the field of vision. The infiltration of the Nh by leucocytes is most marked in group II. Medium-sized (nuclear diameter 5-7 µm) and small (nuclear diameter 3 µm) lymphocytes are most numerous in the Nh of groups I and III. Up to 30% of the fish of group II contain pituicytes and blood cells with PAF-positive inclusions (up to 10% in groups I and III). Mitotic division of the pituicytes occurs rarely in the Nh of all groups of fish (more frequently in group II). Increased functional activity of glial cells and increased phagocytic activity of the pituicytes and blood cells, as well as infiltration of the Nh by a greater number of leucocytes are all considered to be indirect signs of the increased functional activity of the hypothalamo-hypophyseal neurosecretory system most noticeable in fish soon after spawning.

Neurosecretory Supply to Extrahypothalamic Structures: Choroid Plexus, Circumventricular Organs, and Limbic System

G. P. KOZLOWSKI, M. S. BROWNFIELD, and G. HOSTETTER
Department of Anatomy, Colorado State University, Fort Collins, Colorado, USA

A. Introduction

> "We must not however forget that because we have chosen to give the name neurosecretion to those peptidergic neurones which form the final common pathways between nervous and endocrine systems, this should not bind us to the fact that it has been claimed that peptidergic neurones may be widely distributed in nervous tissue and could act as specific modulators of neuronal activity. The neurosecretion that we neuroendocrinologists study may be but one specialized form of a more widespread activity."
>
> (Sir Francis KNOWLES - Sixth International Symposium on Neurosecretion, London, 1973).

These prescient words expressed by the late Sir Francis KNOWLES in his introduction to the last International Symposium on Neurosecretion both remind and foretell that the concept of neurosecretory neurons as predominantly residing within the hypothalamohypophyseal pathway should be expanded to include an extensive system of neurosecretory fibers involved in numerous brain functions.

This ideatum of Sir Francis KNOWLES provides the theme for this report, which will describe extrahypothalamic neurosecretory projections to a variety of brain structures other than the median eminence and pars nervosa of the neurohypophysis. The extensive contribution of neurosecretory input as an integrative system of fibers to choroid plexus, limbic system structures, and circumventricular organs has received sporadic consideration; they have been studied only by indirect means, such as staining methods for neurosecretory material, ultrastructural characteristics of peptidergic terminals, and size measurements of their granules. These methods have been viewed *cum grano salis* in the previous symposium. We now are able to report a summary of our findings of the last few years, whereby we attempted to locate all brain areas having neurophysins as a distinguishing feature of magnocellular neurosecretory neuronal input. We examined serially sectioned brains of rat, mouse, and kangaroo rat, using immunocytochemistry in order to render neurosecretory projections visible, thus providing direct evidence for their existence and distribution.

B. Materials and Methods

The brains of Wistar rats, kangaroo rats, and Swiss Webster mice were fixed via intracardiac perfusion with Bouin's fluid and processed as described previously (KOZLOWSKI et al., 1974). Deparaffinized sections were immunoreacted with rabbit antibovine neurophysin I, which cross-reacts with all possible neurophysins. Whole brains were sectioned serially in either the transverse or sagittal planes. Every tenth section was immunostained for neurophysin, and adjacent sections were stained with luxol-fast blue and cresyl-echt violet for confirmation of the location, seen with identifiable regions described in various brain atlases. In some instances, cresyl-echt violet was applied to immunoreacted sections to improve delineation of cytoplasmic boundaries.

C. Topographic Distribution of Major Neurosecretory Fields

Immunocytochemistry of neurophysin applied to sections of the anterior hypothalamus of the rat reveal major areas of concentration of neurosecretory neuronal fields (Fig. 1). A paraventricular nuclear field gives rise to fibers that mainly course ventrolaterad towards a supraoptic nuclear field. Scattered along this tract are numerous isolated neurosecretory neurons, which at places form aggregates termed by some authors as the nucleus intermedius. Sections as far rostral as the anterior commissure reveal aggegates of such nuclear groups as rostral accessory nuclei. The paraventricular nuclear field also gives rise to an easily discernable tract of fibers directed dorsad towards the stria terminalis. As before, neurosecretory neurons can occur either in aggregates or singly along this tract. Paraventricular neurons (Fig. 1B, C) are largely bipolar, with their projections giving rise to other branches (Fig. 1C).

D. Choroid Plexus

Extracts of choroid plexuses of toad (RODRÍGUEZ and HELLER, 1970) and sheep (HELLER and ZAIDI, 1974) have antidiuretic activity, which may be abolished by thioglycolate, suggesting the presence of vasopressin in the choroid plexus. DAVSON and SEGAL (1970) demonstrated that infusion of 3 mU/min of vasopressin (Petressin, Parke-Davis) in rabbits causes a 50% reduction in the rate of secretion of cerebrospinal fluid (CSF). We reviewed other studies implicating a functional relationship between vasopressin and the choroid plexus, and further described vasopressin-induced ultrastructural modifications of the choroid plexus induced by dehydration and administration of Pitressin-tannate (KOZLOWSKI et al., 1976). These modifications included intracellular vacuolization and expansion of the lateral and basal intercellular spaces (Fig. 2A), and paralleled those described for vasopressin-sensitive epithelial tissues, such as the renal collecting

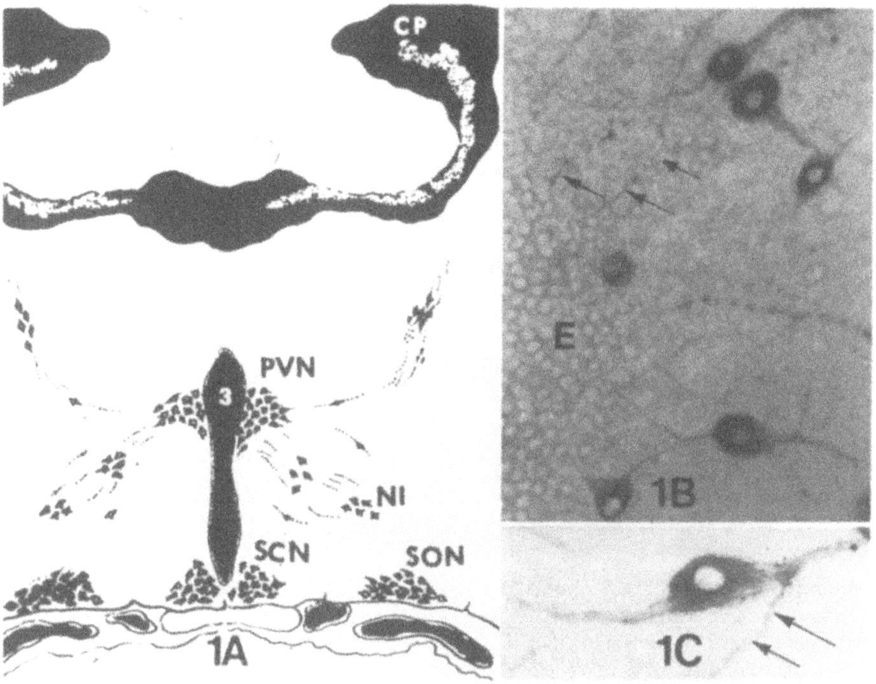

Fig. 1. (A) Distribution of major neurosecretory groups in rat anterior hypothalamus. *PVN* - paraventricular nucleus, *NI* - nucleus intermedius, *SON* - supraoptic nucleus, *SCN* - suprachiasmatic nucleus, *3* - third ventricle, *CP* - choroid plexus. (B) Region of rat paraventricular nucleus. Neurophysin is seen in cytoplasm of neurons and fibrous processes, some of which enter ependymal (*E*) layer (*arrows*). × 100. (C) Rat paraventricular nucleus neuron is typically bipolar. Here, a collateral branch is observed (*arrows*). Fibrous processes proximal to the perikaryon have an even distribution of neurophysin in distinction to the beaded nature of distal portions of the fiber, as in Fig. 1B

tubule and toad urinary bladder, during periods of bulk fluid reabsorption. Since the choroid plexus represents one of the anatomic substrates of the blood-CSF barrier, we proposed that the choroid plexus reabsorbs CSF under the influence of vasopressin. In this respect, we are encouraged by our recent finding that ^{125}I-arginine vasopressin binds to rat choroid plexus and that the binding kinetics observed mimic the binding kinetics for the kidney under similar conditions.

Immunocytochemistry for neurophysin demonstrated at least two easily observable projections of extrahypothalamic neurosecretory fibers that can be traced to the sites of origin of the choroid plexus of both horns of the lateral ventricles (KOZLOWSKI et al., 1976). Neurophysin-containing axons originating from the paraventricular and intermediate nuclei course dorsolaterad to enter the choroidal fissure of the dorsal horn (Fig. 2B, C). A caudally directed group of fibers, with fibrous contributions from the supraoptic nucleus, course ventrolaterad towards the choroidal

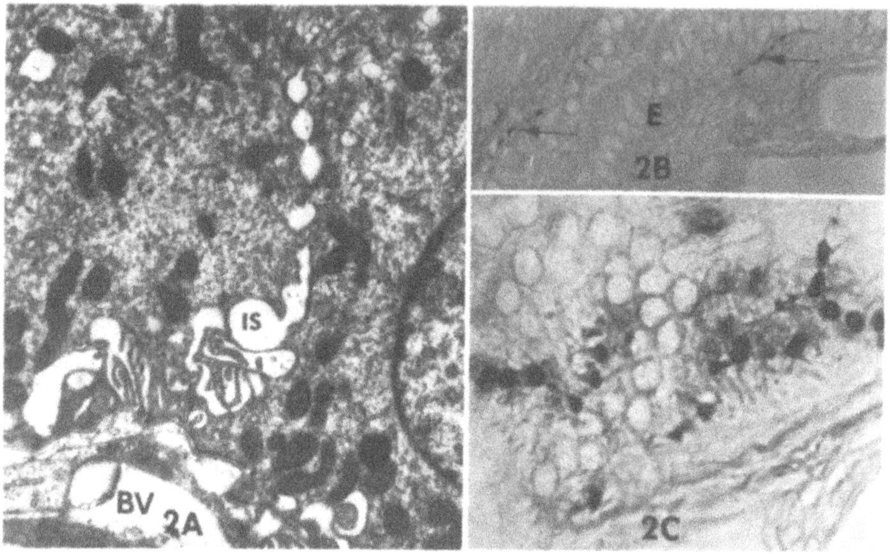

Fig. 2. (A) Ependymal cells from choroid plexus of rat deprived of water for 48 h prior to sacrifice. Intercellular space (*IS*) and basal infoldings proximal to blood vessels (*BV*) are dilated in comparison to control animals. × 7500. (B) Rat choroidal fissures of lateral ventricle. Neurophysin fibers are seen in close association to ependymal (*E*) cells. × 400. (C) High magnification of neurophysin in ependymal layer of rat choroidal fissure. × 600

fissure of the ventral horn. Scattered neurosecretory neurons are found in association with both pathways, usually in contact with blood vessels supplying the choroid plexus. The mode of termination of neurosecretory endings on choroidal tissue is yet unknown. However, both fibers (Fig. 2B) and Herring bodies (Fig. 2C) can be observed within the choroid plexus at its site of attachment. This situation at least allows us to propose that the extrahypothalamic system of neurosecretory fibers may directly influence the vasopressin-induced reabsorption of CSF by the choroid plexus.

E. Circumventricular Organs

Stainable neurosecretory material and peptidergic neurosecretory terminals have been reported for the pineal gland, neurohypohysis, median eminence, organum vasculosum laminae terminalis, subfornical organ, subcommissural organ, and area postrema (for review see STERBA, 1969). Of these, we have located neurophysin in the OVLT (Fig. 3A), SFO (Fig. 3B), median eminence, neurohypophysis, and AP. Neurophysin is also seen in sites adjacent to some of these organs such as in the epithalamic area associated with the epithalamoepiphyseal complex of the SCO and pineal, and in the tractus solitarius and dorsal vagal nucleus associated with the AP.

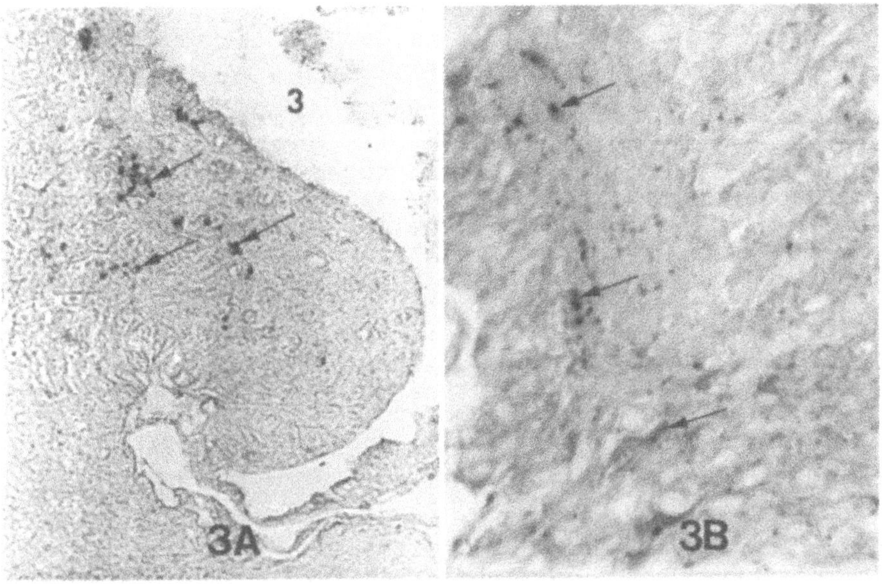

Fig. 3. (A) Sagittal section of subfornical organ of kangaroo rat, seen protruding into third (*3*) ventricle. *Arrows* indicate distribution of neurophysin fibers. × 250. (B) Neurophysin fibers (*arrows*) are most numerous in basal region of rat OVLT. × 250

F. Limbic System

Historically, the neurosecretory neuron was regarded as distinguishable from other neurons in that they possessed terminals that ended on the perivascular space of blood vessels, there forming a neurohemal organ. However, SCHARRER (1974) and KNOWLES (1974) at the last Neurosecretion Symposium reviewed the changing attitude throughout the years, in which the concept developed that neurosecretory neurons could form synaptoid contact with, for example, cells of the pars intermedia, salivary gland, corpus allatum, and other neurons. At that same symposium, CROSS (1974) showed peptidergic collateral axons from neurosecretory cells forming synaptic connections with adrenergic neurons, which in turn projected back to the neurosecretory cell that innervated it. The idea, then, that neurohormones such as vasopressin and oxytocin would act as "neurotransmitters" is not new, and has been the subject of numerous studies (for review see BARKER, 1976). Relevant to this topic, the last symposium also contained immunohistochemical evidence that vasopressin fibers coursed outside the hypothalamic boundaries (BUPLET et al., 1974). Ultrastructural evidence presented by STERBA (1974) demonstrated peptidergic neurosecretory synapses in contact with neurons of septal and tectal areas of lower vertebrates. This evidence, in addition to a review of peptidergic fibers observed in different regions of the brain of a variety of vertebrates led him to state: "The hypothalamolimbic pathway should be considered as an integral subsystem of the main peptidergic neurosecretory system." Our immunohistochemical studies corroborate this suggestion.

The disposition of immunopositive neurophysin reaction product associated with neurons of limbic system structures, very closely resembles the disposition of γ-aminobutyric acid, a putative neurotransmitter, demonstrated by the elegant immunohistochemical techniques employed by McLAUGHLIN et al. (1975). In their study, the punctate-reaction product for glutamate decarboxylase was seen in contact with somata and dendrites of spinal cord neurons with light microscopy, and corresponded to immunopositive terminals observed with electron microscopy. Similarly, we presume that the punctate-reaction product, visualized with light microscopy for neurophysin associated with limbic system neurons (Figs. 4A,B, 5A,B), has a similar counterpart at the electron microscopic level, viz. the peptidergic neurosecretory terminals discussed by STERBA (1974).

Our studies, although incomplete at this time, indicate that the following structures are associated with neurophysin-containing terminals: olfactory tract, suprachiasmatic (Figs. 5A,B), medial and lateral septal nuclei, medial preoptic nucleus, periventricular area and dorsolateral nucleus of the thalamus, nucleus paratenialis thalami (Figs. 4A,B), central nucleus and lateral-basal part of the amygdaloid body, habenular region (neurons in association with the fasciculus retroflexus), H_1 area of the tegmentum, and lateral mammillary body. Neurophysin-containing fibers were seen to course within the stria terminalis, fornix, fimbria of the fornix, and olfactory tract. Neurophysin-containing cell bodies were distributed singly, or in groups of two or three along neurosecretory hypothalamofugal fibers as they coursed to extrahypothalamic areas (Fig. 1A). These observations are in addition to the major accessory neurosecretory cell groups previously described by PALKOVITS et al. (1974) and ZIMMERMAN (1976). It must be emphasized that several sources of variation exist that account for inconsistencies in tabulating both the course that neurosecretory fibers assume and their terminations on target structures. We have observed variations among species, within animals of the same species, and perhaps according to the physiologic state of the animal. The immunocytochemical procedure is performed in a consistent manner, but unstable reagents and other factors prompt us to consider the possibilities of both false-positive and false-negative results. Interestingly, the results described here closely resemble the distribution of stainable neurosecretory material in a variety of vertebrates studied by BARRY approximately twenty years ago (BARRY, 1954-1958). A parallel exists between his early observation of an extensive distribution of magnocellular elements and their respective peptides, and his later description of an extensive system of parvicellular neurons containing LH-RH (BARRY, 1974). Both systems were courageously described during the time when it was widely accepted that magnocellular and parvicellular neurons resided within limited areas of the hypothalamus.

Since PAPEZ (1937) first ascribed the role of the limbic system to that of providing an anatomic substrate of emotion, much effort has been devoted to elucidating the mechanism of action by which this role is expressed. Clearly, neurosecretory peptides can function in modulating behavior since vasopressin maintains conditioned avoidance behavior when administered to normal rats (DE WIED), 1973) and is able to restore avoidance responses when administered to rats with a heritable deficiency of vasopressin (BOHUS et al., 1975). An increased release of ACTH is seen when vasopressin is administered into the ventral hypothalamus rather than directly into the anterior pituitary (YATES et al., 1971), perhaps implying that neurons containing the appropriate releasing factor are involved. A direct neurosecretory input to limbic system structures speaks in favor of the concept that vasopressin would be acting as a neurotransmitter modulating the electrophysiologic activities of that system. A direct neural input may represent only one pathway by which vasopressin arrives at limbic structures; a ventricular route via CSF may also be involved. If neuropeptides are incapable of crossing the blood-brain barrier (ZAIDI and HELLER, 1974) the question then arises as to the source of vasopressin found in CSF. Both vasopressin and neurophysin have been found in high amounts of CSF (ZIMMERMAN, 1976; ROBINSON et al., 1973) and could arrive there either via peptidergic intraventricular nerve endings (SCOTT et al., 1973) or by being transported from its parenchymal site of release into the ventricle, along with the exchange of fluid that is known to occur between extracellular fluid of brain tissue and the CSF of the ventricle. That is, neurosecretory terminals, either intraventricular or parenchymal, may furnish neurohypophyseal hormones directly into the ventricle via intraventricular nerve endings, or may contribute hormone to the interstitial fluid, which in turn would pass into the CSF for circulation to periventricular structures of the limbic system. In support of the idea that a CSF route may be instrumental in distributing vasopressin to limbic system structures, injections of antiserum to vasopressin, and not to oxytocin, into the lateral ventricle interfere with learning (VAN WIMERSMA GREIDANUS et al., 1975). The possibility that antivasopressin antibodies are acting at synaptic regions of peptidergic terminals of the limbic system remains to be explored.

G. Discussion

The observations and functional considerations resulting from our study of extrahypothalamic neurosecretory projections to the choroid plexus, circumventricular organs, and limbic system indicate a need for more direct confirmation of the chemical and ultrastructural nature of peptidergic synapses. Perhaps this could best be accomplished with immunocytochemical techniques for vasopressin, similar to the preembedding immunocytochemical studies intended to identify the nature of biogenic amine fibers and synapses (PICKEL et al., 1975; MCLAUGHLIN et al., 1975). This technique has the considerable advantage of allowing one

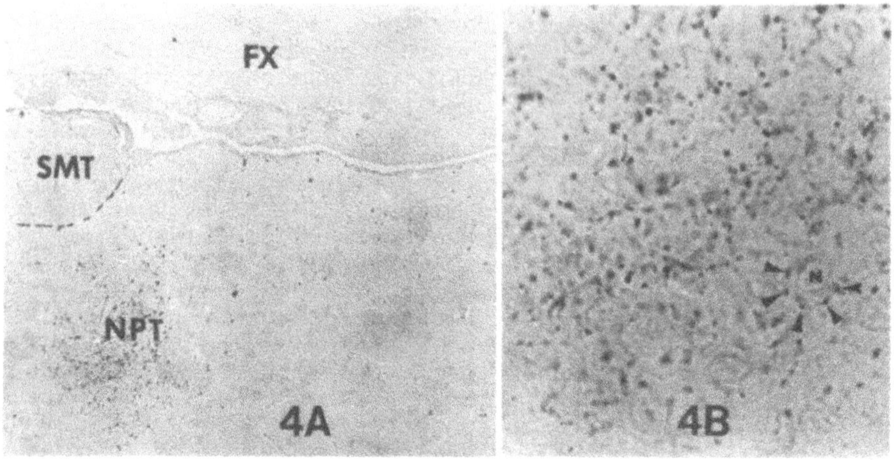

Fig. 4. (A) Cross section of dorsocaudal diencephalon of rat. Nucleus parataenialis thalami (*NPT*), an area especially rich in neurophysin-containing terminals. *SMT* - Stria medullaris thalami, *FX* - fornix. × 130. (B) High magnification of nucleus parataenialis thalami (*NPT*) depicted in Fig. 4A. Nucleus (*N*) and cytoplasm of thalamic neurons are devoid of neurophysin. Punctate areas of neurophysin surrounding cells (*arrows*) are thought to represent peptidergic nerve endings. × 350

to survey large, thick (30-50 μm) sections for immunoreactive areas with the light microscope prior to selection for electron microscopic examination.

A better understanding of the nuclear sites of origin for the extrahypothalamic neurosecretory fiber systems would lead naturally to electrophysiologic studies that could provide evidence as to the functional nature of these pathways and the neuropharmacologic basis for their mechanism of action. Although highly speculative, it is possible that the bipolar nature (Fig. 1B,C) of the cell body and its processes shown by immunocytochemistry represents a morphologic correlate to the concept that each neurosecretory cell could function as a integrative unit, synchronizing activities of various effector sites according to their site of projection and a particular physiologic state of the animal. Thus, an individual neurosecretory neuron may send fibrous projections to septal areas, suprachiasmatic nuclei, and zona externa of the median eminence for mediation of stress responses that result in adrenocorticoid release and the appropriate behavioral response. Whether that same cell provides an intraventricular nerve ending for a wide distribution of hormone via CSF, should remain as difficult to prove as it is to solve the problem of why particular brain structures demand "private" (in the terms of SCHARRER, 1974) peptidergic input versus humorally distributed routes of neuropeptides. It seems probable that elucidation of the morphologic nature and functional significance of extrahypothalamic neurosecretory systems will become one of the most exciting frontiers for future studies by neuroendocrinologists.

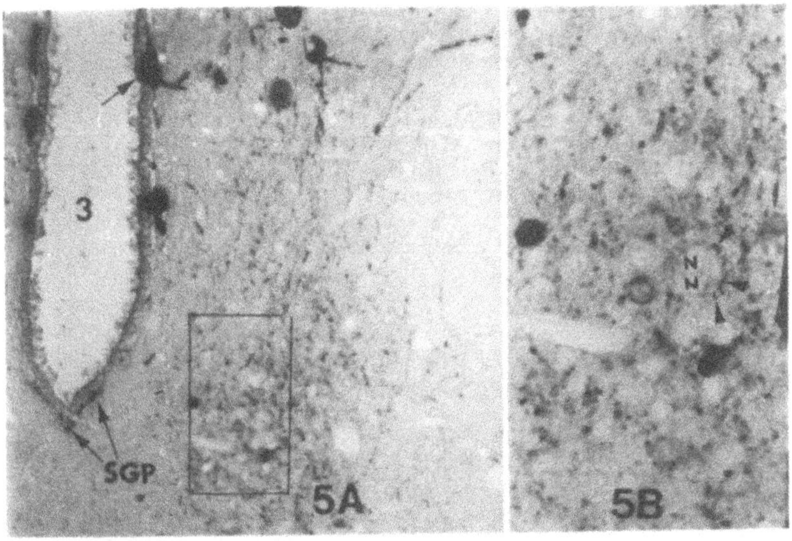

Fig. 5. (A) Ventral portion of suprachiasmatic nucleus exhibits distribution of neurophysin-containing terminals similar to that of limbic system structures. Neurosecretory neurons are in close association with ependymal lining of third (*3*) ventricle, one of which (*arrow*) is intercalated within ependymal lining and is in direct contact with CSF. Neurophysin fibers may form a subependymal glial plate (*SGP*) along different regions of ventricular wall. × 225. (B) High magnification of boxed area seen in Fig. 5A. Two closely adjacent neurons (*N* - nucleus) have neurophysin terminals surrounding their cytoplasm. × 450

Acknowledgments. This work was supported by NIH grant HD-08867. The authors wish to thank Ms. Barbara Paur for her excellent technical assistance. We also wish to express our appreciation to Dr. Earl A. Zimmerman for antibovine neurophysin I and to Dr. Ludwig Sternberger for PAP.

References

BARKER, J.L.: Peptides: role in neuronal excitability. Physiol. Rev. 56, 435-452 (1976)

BARRY, J.: Neurocrinie et synapses "neurosecretoires". Arch. Anat. Microsc. Morphol. Exp. 43, 310-320 (1954)

BARRY, J.: Les voies neurosécrétoires extra-hypophysaires et le problème de l'action nerveuse centrale des hormones posthypophysaires. Jour. Med. Lyon, 1065-1074 (1958)

BARRY, J., DUBOIS, M.P.: Study of the preoptico-infundibular LH-RH neurosecretory pathway in female guinea-pigs during gestation and the oestrous cycle. In: Neurosecretion - The Final Neuroendocrine Pathway. KNOWLES, S.F., VOLLRATH, L. (eds.). Berlin-Heidelberg-New York: Springer-Verlag 1974, pp. 148-153

BOHUS, B., WIMERSMA GREIDANUS T.B. VAN, WIED, D. DE: Behavioral and endocrine responses of rats with hereditary hypothalamic diabetes insipidus (Brattleboro strain). Physiol. Behav. 14, 609-615 (1975)

BURLET, A., MARCHETTI, J., DUHEILLE, J.: Immunohistochemistry of vasopressin: study of the hypothalamo-neurohypophysial system of normal, dehydrated and hypophysectomized rats. In: Neurosecretion - The Final Neuroendocrine Pathway. KNOWLES, S.F., VOLLRATH, L. (eds.). Berlin-Heidelberg-New York: Springer-Verlag 1974, pp. 24-30

CROSS, B.A.: The neurosecretory impulse. In: Neurosecretion - The Final Neuroendocrine Pathway. KNOWLES, S.F., VOLLRATH, L. (eds.). Berlin-Heidelberg-New York: Springer-Verlag 1974, pp. 115-128

DAVSON, H., SEGAL, M.G.: The effect of some inhibitors and accelerators of sodium transport on the turnover of ^{22}Na in the cerebrospinal fluid and the brain. J. Physiol. 209, 131-153 (1970)

HELLER, H., ZAIDI, S.M.A.: The problem of neurohypophysial secretion into the cerebrospinal fluid: antidiuretic activity in the liquor and choroid plexus. In: Ependyma and Neurohormonal Regulation - Proceedings of the Int. Symp. at Smolenice 20-23 September, 1972. MITRO, A. (ed.). Bratislava: Veda 1974, pp. 229-250

KNOWLES, S.F.: Twenty years of neurosecretion. In: Neurosecretion - The Final Neuroendocrine Pathway. KNOWLES, S.F., VOLLRATH, L. (eds.). Berlin-Heidelberg-New York: Springer-Verlag 1974, pp. 3-11

KOZLOWSKI, G.P., NETT, T.M., ZIMMERMAN, E.A.: Immunocytochemical localization of gonadotropin-releasing hormone (Gn-RH) and neurophysin in the brain. In: Anatomical Neuroendocrinology. STUMPF, W.E., GRANT, L.D. (eds.). Basle: Karger 1974, pp. 185-191

KOZLOWSKI, G.P.: BROWNFIELD, M.S., SCHULTZ, W.J.: Neurosecretory pathways to the choroid plexus. Int. Res. Commun. Sys. 4, 299 (1976)

MCLAUGHLIN, B.J., BARBER, R., SAITO, K., ROBERTS, E., WU, J.Y.: Immunocytochemical localization of glutamate decarboxylase in rat spinal cord. J. Comp. Neurol. 164, 308-322 (1975)

PALKOVITS, M., ZABORSZKY, L., AMBACH, G.: Accessory neurosecretory cell groups in the rat hypothalamus. Acta Morphol. Acad. Sci. Hung. 22, 21-33 (1974)

PAPEZ, J.W.: A proposed mechanism of emotion. Arch. Neurol. Psychiatry (Chic.) 38, 725-743 (1937)

PICKEL, V.M., JOH, T.H., FIELD, P.M., BECKER, C.G., REIS, D.J.: Cellular localization of tyrosine hydroxylase by immunohistochemistry. H. Histochem. Cytochem. 23, 1-12 (1975)

ROBINSON, A.G., ZIMMERMAN, E.A.: Cerebrospinal fluid and ependymal neurophysin. J. Clin. Invest. 52, 1260-1267 (1973)

RODRÍGUEZ, E.M., HELLER, H.: Antidiuretic activity and ultrastructure of toad choroid plexus. J. Endocrinol. 46, 83-91 (1970)

SCHARRER, B.: New trends in invertebrate neurosecretion. In: Neurosecretion - The Final Neuroendocrine Pathway. KNOWLES, S.F., VOLLRATH, L. (eds.). Berlin-Heidelberg-New York: Springer-Verlag 1974, pp. 283-287

SCOTT, D.E., KOZLOWSKI, G.P., SHERIDAN, M.N.: Scanning electron microscopy in the ultrastructural analysis of the mammalian cerebral ventricular system. In: Int. Rev. Cytol. 37, 349-388 (1973)

STERBA, G.: Zirkumventrikuläre Organe und Liquor. Bericht über das Symposium in Schloss Reinhardsbrunn vom 13. bis 16. Mai 1968. STERBA, G. (ed.). Jena: Gustav Fischer 1969, pp. 1-309

STERBA, G.: Ascending neurosecretory pathways of the peptidergic type. In: Neurosecretion - The Final Neuroendocrine Pathway. KNOWLES, S.F., VOLLRATH, L. (eds.). Berlin-Heidelberg-New York: Springer-Verlag 1974, pp. 38-47

WIED, D. DE: The role of the posterior pituitary and its peptides on the maintenance of conditioned avoidance behavior. In: Hormones and Brain Function. LISSAK, K. (ed.). New York: Plenum Press 1973

WIMERSMA GREIDANUS, T.B. VAN, DOGTEROM, J., WIED, D. DE: Intraventricular administration of anti-vasopressin serum inhibits memory consolidation in rats. Life Sci. 16, 637-644 (1975)

YATES, F.E., RUSSEL, S.M., DALLMAN, M.F., HEDGE, G.A., MCCANN, S.M., DHARIWAL, A.P.S.: Potentiation by vasopressin of corticotropin release induced by corticotropin-releasing factor. Endocrinology 88, 3-15 (1971)

ZAIDI, S.M.A., HELLER, H.: Can neurohypophysial hormones cross the blood-cerebrospinal fluid barrier? J. Endocrinol. 60, 195-196 (1974)

ZIMMERMAN, E.A.: Localization of hypothalamic hormones by immunocytochemical techniques. In: Frontiers in Neuroendocrinology. MARTINI, L. , GANONG, W.F. (eds.). New York: Raven Press 1976, Vol. IV, pp. 25-62

Ecological and Histophysiological Investigation of the Hypothalamic Peptidergic Centers in Rodents Under Conditions of Hypobaric Hypoxia

I. A. KRASNOVSKAYA and T. V. TAVROVSKAYA
Laboratory of Neuroendocrinology, Sechenov Institute of Evolutionary Physiology and Biochemistry, USSR Academy of Sciences, Leningrad, USSR

The role of the hypothalamo-hypophyseal neurosecretory system (HHNS) in adaptation to various environments in mammals has not been thoroughly studied. Ecological investigations are mainly concerned with the HHNS of desert-dwelling rodents (HOWE and JEWELL, 1959; KHALIL and TAWFIC, 1963; CASTEL and ABRAHAM, 1969; HATTON et al., 1972). There appear to be no publications on the HHNS in animals living at high altitudes.

Adult ground squirrels, *Citellus pygmaeus musicus Men.*, natives of the North Caucasus, living at an altitude of 2200 m, were studied. The closely related species from the plains, *C. pygmaeus planicola Sat.*, were examined for comparison. The relative development of neurosecretory centers was estimated by counting the total number of cells in the supraoptic (NSO), paraventricular (NPV) and postoptic (NPO) nuclei. To make the count of the neurosecretory cells easier, all ground squirrels were injected with 0.5 ml of 0.5% aminazine 6 h before decapitation because it has been shown (POLENOV and BALONOV, 1963) that aminazine administration causes retention of the neurosecretory material (NSM) in the HHNS. All neurosecretory cells were counted in the left or right NSO, NVP, and NPO of one side in alternate sections. The number of cells was multiplied by four, and the result was considered to be the total number of neurosecretory cells in both left and right nuclei.

Male Wistar rats were used for the experimental analysis of some details of adaptation to hypoxia, since the ground squirrels were not available. The rats were exposed in a low pressure chamber for 6 h daily during the course of 3 months. The simulated altitude was 7500 m. The rats were given water *ad libitum*. Such a regime of exposure to hypoxia provoked increased erythropoietic function of the rats to a level similar to that found in the highland ground squirrels (RAVROVSKAYA et al., 1975; BARBASHOVA et al., 1976).

The nucleolar volume of the neurosecretory cells in the NSO, the NVP, and the NPO as well as the nuclear volume of the cells in the suprachiasmatic nucleus were calculated in the rats. In addition, the thyroid gland was studied in both ground squirrels and rats because its great importance for oxidative processes in tissues is well known. The height of the thyroid epithelium was measured. The brain and thyroid gland were fixed in Bouin's fluid; 6 μm serial paraffin sections were stained with Gomori's paraldehyde-fuchsin and counterstained with Heidenhain's Azan.

The number of neurosecretory cells in the NSO was 8898 ± 266 cells in the highland species of the ground squirrels and

Table 1. Number of the neurosecretory cells of the hypothalamic nuclei in the ground squirrels

Nucleus of hypothalamus	Number of animals	*C. pygmaeus musicus Men.*	*C. pygmaeus planicola Sat.*
NSO	8	8898 ± 266[a]	13484 ± 376[a]
NPV	5	3146 ± 103	3322 ± 112
NPO	9	4814 ± 163	4702 ± 116

Values are means ± SE

[a]Difference between the species is significant, $P < 0.001$

13484 ± 376 cells in the lowland species. This difference was not the result of redistribution of the cells between the NSO and the NPO since the number of the NPO cells was equal in both species. There was no significant difference in the number of the NPV cells in *C. pygmaeus musicus Men.* and *C. pygmaeus planicola Sat.* (Table 1).

Three months of training to hypobaric hypoxia did not result in any essential changes of the NSO in rats, though a slight increase of the NSO-cell nucleoli was observed during the first days. The nucleolar volume of the NPV cells also increased during the first week, and the number of cells with multiple nucleoli rose to 19% (4% in control). Later, the diminution of nucleoli and nuclei of NPV cells was observed; these decreased volumes of nucleoli and nuclei persisted till the end of the experiment. Changes in the NPO cells were similar to those in the NPV cells, though the number of nucleoli in the NPO cells did not increase and the rise in nucleolar volume was more prominent during the first week of the experiment (Fig. 1).

Until now, little was known about the NPO function. This nucleus is usually considered part of the NSO (TROYER, 1965; PETERSON, 1966; POLENOV, 1968; BANDARANAYKE, 1971). The present findings indicate some functional peculiarities of the NPO. Functional identity of the NSO and the NPV is also debatable (STUTINSKY, 1974; SWAAB, 1975). Our data reveal a similar character of responses of the NSO, the NPO, and the NPV during short-term exposure to hypoxia, while in the course of prolonged exposure (Fig. 1), or in species adapted to various environments, special reactions of these hypothalamic centers can be seen. The analysis of results of numerous authors supports this point of view.

The thyroid gland revealed signs of high activity during the first week of the exposure in the barochamber (increased mitoses, increased height of thyroid epithelium, and vacuolated colloid). Thereafter the height of the thyroid epithelium was lowered (Fig. 1). These changes in the thyroid epithelium strongly correlated with alteration of nucleolar volume in the NPV (coefficient of correlation $r = 0.81$; $P < 0.01$) and the NPO (coefficient of correlation $r = 0.82$; $P < 0.001$), but not with the NSO ($r = 0.5$; $P < 0.01$) or with the suprachiasmatic nucleus ($r = 0.4$; $P < 0.01$).

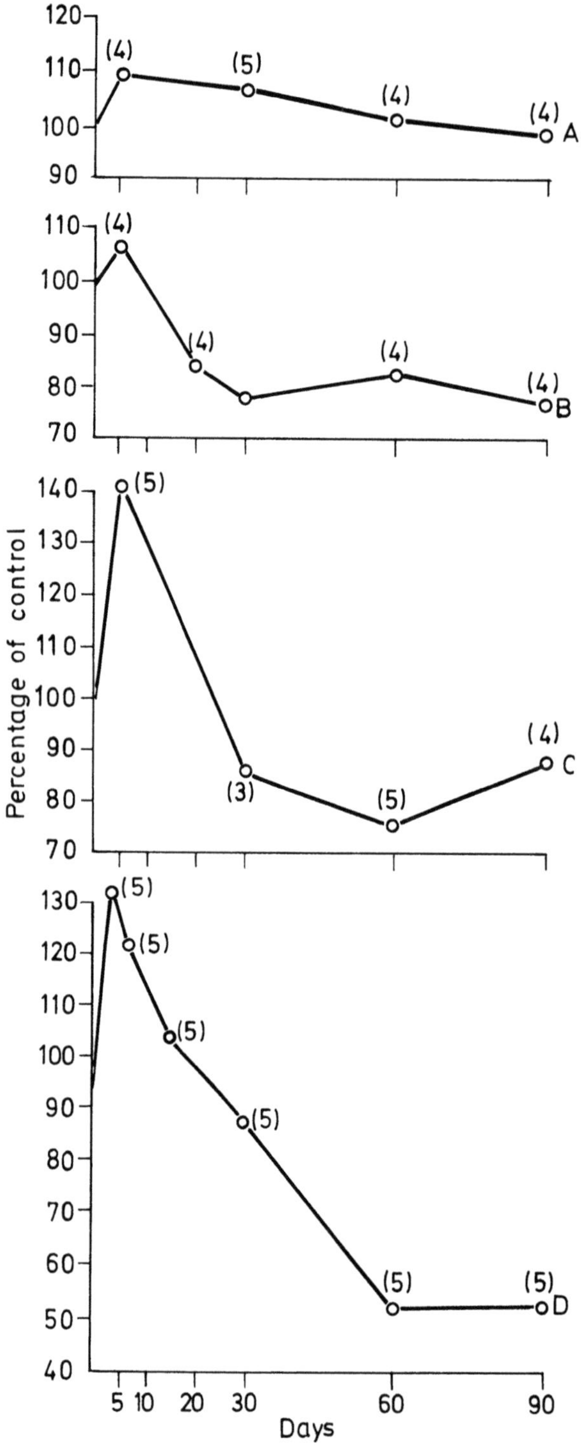

Fig. 1. Volume of neurosecretory-cell nucleoli in NSO, NPV, and NPO and height of thyroid epithelium in rats during hypobaric hypoxia. *A* - NSO, *B* - NPV, *C* - NPO, *D* - height of thyroid epithelium; o - difference is significant, $P < 0.05$; ● - difference is not significant, $P > 0.05$. Figures in parentheses give number of rats

The comparison of two species of ground squirrels has shown that the NSO in *C. pygmaeus planicola Sat.* is nearly 30% larger than that of *C. pygmaeus musicus Men.* (Table 1). It seems likely that this disparity is caused more by the adaptation to water deficiency than by mountain hypoxia. It is known that lowland rodents are more xerically adapted and have higher hematocrit than rodents in mountains (BARBASHOVA et al., 1976). Moreover, it has been found that desert-dwelling rodents have a larger NSO than those adapted to a mesic environment (HATTON et al., 1972). The results of exposure to experimental hypoxia also support this suggestion because no changes of the NSO cells occurred in the rats exposed to prolonged hypoxia under conditions of free access to water. Thus, the decrease of functional activity in the NPV, the NPO, and the thyroid gland apparently play an essential role in adaptation to experimental hypoxia. However, no similar changes have been revealed in the highland ground squirrels.

References

ALESHIN, B.V.: Histophysiology of the Hypothalamo-Hypophysial System. Moscow: Medizina 1971

BANDARANAYKE, R.C.: Morphology of the accessory neurosecretory nuclei and of the retrochiasmatic part of the supraoptic nucleus of the rat. Acta Anat. (Basel) 80, 14-22 (1971)

BARBASHOVA, Z.I., TAVROVSKAYA, T.V., TARAKANOVA, O.I., GEMUCHOVA, E.G., TEMBOTOV, A.K., BELOSHITSKY, P.V., BOGOSLOVA, G.F., PROCHASKA, I.: Comparison of adaptive mechanisms to hypoxia in highland and lowland ground squirrels in the North Caucasus. Ecologiya 2, 63-70 (1976)

CASTEL, M., ABRAHAM, M.: Effect of a dry diet on the hypothalamic neurohypophysial neurosecretory system in spiny mice as compared to the albino rat and mouse. Gen. Comp. Endocrinol. 12 (2), 231-241 (1969)

HATTON, G.I., JONSON, J.I., MALATESTA, C.Z.: Supraoptic nuclei of rodents adapted for mesic and xeric environments: numbers of cells, multiple nucleoli and their distributions. J. Comp. Neurol. 145 (1), 43-60 (1972)

HOWE, A., JEWELL, P.: Effects of water deprivation upon the neurosecretory material of the desert rat (*Meriones meriones*) compared with the laboratory rat. J. Endocrinol. 18 (11), 118-124 (1959)

KHALIL, F., TAWFIC, J.: The hypothalamo-hypophysial neurosecretory system of the desert rodents. J. Exp. Zool. 154 (2), 189-195 (1963)

PETERSON, R.P.: Magnocellular neurosecretory centers in the rat hypothalamus. J. Comp. Neurol. 128 (2), 181-189 (1966)

POLENOV, A.L.: Hypothalamic Neurosecretion. Leningrad: Nauka 1968

POLENOV, A.L., BALONOV, L.Y.: Morphological changes of the rat neurohypophysis in painful stimulation and aminazine injections. Probl. Endocrinol. 9 (5), 40-46 (1963)

STUTINSKY, F.: Morphological and physiological reactions of the supraoptic and paraventricular nuclei. In: Neurosecretion - The Final Neuroendocrine Pathway. KNOWLES, F., VOLLRATH, L. (eds.). Berlin-Heidelberg-New York: Springer-Verlag 1974, pp. 15-24

SWAAB, D.F., NIJVELDT, F., POOL, C.W.: Distribution of oxytocin and vasopressin in the rat supraoptic and paraventricular nucleus. J. Endocrinol. 67 (3), 461-462 (1975)

TAVROVSKAYA, T.V., TARAKANOVA, O.I., BARBASHOVA, Z.I.: Qualitative peculiarities of erythropoiesis in man and animals adapted to prolonged hypoxia. Bull. Exp. Biol. Med. 79 (1), 18-21 (1975)
TROYER, J.R.: Neurosecretion in the hibernating bat, the morphology of the hypothalamo-hypophysial system. Anat. Rec. 151, 77-79 (1965)

Reaction of Rat Hypothalamic, Supraoptic, and Arcuate Nuclei Neurons in Experiment

S. L. KUZNETSOV
The First Moscow Medical Institute, Moscow, USSR

Studies on 65 male rats were made by comparing the activity of supraoptic- (SON) and arcuate (AN)-nuclei neurons after dehydration, unilateral adrenalectomy, and nonspecific-factor effect, i.e., growth of Jensen's-sarcoma conditions. The neuronal activity was assessed by the neuronal-nucleolar optical density (OD) after staining with gallocyanin chromalum (EINARSON, 1951). After 2 days of dry feeding, considerable activation of SON neurons was observed (with OD increasing to 112%, $P < 0.01$). This activation remained until the 5th day, when the level fell. After unilateral adrenalectomy, neuronal activity increased by 109% compared with that of sham-operated rats. In Jensen's-sarcoma growth conditions, the SON neuronal activation was observed on the 21st day of the experiment, and was somewhat lower on the 35th day. AN neuronal activity after 2 days of dehydration was strikingly increased (118.5%, $P < 0.001$) with a negligible decrease on the 5th day. After unilateral adrenalectomy the activity was practically unchanged on the 5th day, but it decreased on the 15th day (94% of control, $P < 0.05$). The AN neurons' response to Jensen's-sarcoma growth was the same as that of the SON neurons, but it was less marked. The data enable us to conclude that the system of magno- and parvocellular hypothalamic nuclei is involved in stress-reaction formation and in aqueous-saline-equilibrium regulation. The increase of SON neuronal activity on the 15th day after adrenalectomy, when there is some decrease of AN neuronal activity, suggests that the SON has a predominant role in compensatory hypertrophy of the adrenal gland.

Neurohypophysis and Thyroid Gland of Fry *Acipenser stellatus* Pallas and *Acipenser güldenstädti* Brandt During Downstream Migration

V. S. LAGUNOVA
Central Scientific Research Institute of the Sturgeon Industry, Astrakhan, USSR

The neurohypophysis and thyroid gland of fry *A. stellatus* and *A. güldenstädti* during downstream migration were studied histologically. The fish were captured at four places on their way down the Volga to the Caspian Sea, where no wide fluctuations of water salinity occurred. The content of neurosecretory material in the neurohypophysis was estimated visually according to an arbitrary 5-unit system. The height of the thyroid epithelium in the thyroid gland was measured. The thyroid gland is moderately active in fry of *A. güldenstädti* captured in the Volga and in the Volga-Caspian channel. The follicles of the thyroid gland contain a large amount of dense colloid vacuolized along the margins; the thyroid epithelium of low prismatic shape is 11.1-11.8 µm high in *A. stellatus*, and 14.0-14.2 µm in *A. güldenstädti*. The neurohypophysis of *A. stellatus* contains 1-3.5 units of neurosecretory material, and that of *A. güldenstädti* 1.5-4.0 units. The thyroid gland in *A. stellatus* fry from the Northern Caspian Sea, where water-chlorine content is 180-920 mg/liter, is more active than at the earlier stages of migration. The colloid is less dense and foamy, the height of the thyroid epithelium, which is of cylindrical shape, increases up to 13.9 µm in *A. stellatus*, and up to 15.2 µm in *A. güldenstädti*. The content of the neurosecretory material in the neurohypophysis decreases to 0.5-2.5 units in *A. stellatus* and to 0.5-2.0 units in *A. güldenstädti*. Thus, the peptidergic hypothalamo-hypophyseal neurosecretory system and the thyroid gland in fry *A. stellatus* and *A. güldenstädti* are rather active during downstream migration; markedly increased activity is most evident when the fish migrate from fresh to salt water. This demonstrates that the hypothalamo-hypophyseal neurosecretory system and the thyroid gland in fry Acipenseridae are concerned with adaptation to changes in their environment.

Alterations of Sex-Differentiation of the Hypothalamus by Sex-Steroids Demonstrated by Ultramorphometric Studies of the Adrenal Cortex in Adult Rats

E. MÄUSLE and G. FICKINGER
Institute of Pathology of the University of the Saarland, 6650 Homburg/Saar, FRG

The zona fasciculata of the adrenal cortex of adult rats was studied by means of ultramorphometry after neonatal administration of 1250 µg testosterone propionate (TP) or 300 µg estradiol benzoate (EB) on the second day of life to four females and four males. Eight females (estrus and diestrus, respectively) and four males served as controls. Application of TP to females brings about a distinct enlargement of cells, with increases in the volumes of nucleus, mitochondria, liposomes, SER, and lysosomes. Mitochondria and liposomes are generally small in size. All these morphometric parameters point towards increased activity of the individual cell, caused by the neonatal alteration of the cyclic female hypothalamic pattern into a monophasic male pattern resulting in permanent estrus. The changes are less pronounced after EB than after TP. In the male, neonatal application of sex steroids results in a similar alteration of the sizes of mitochondria and liposomes; the lipoid content is increased. According to these parameters, fasciculata cells fulfill the morphologic conditions necessary for increased functional reaction. This change is more marked following EB than TP. The sex dimorphism is preserved after neonatal application of sex steroids since the hypothalamic alterations are much more pronounced in females than in males.

Neural Lobe of the Hypophysis of Rats Subjected to Noise

R. MILIN
Institute of Histology and Embryology, Faculty of Medicine, Novi Sad, Yugoslavia

Among aggressive environmental factors, noise should be given special consideration. In this paper, we wish to report the results of our investigations on the morphodynamics of the neural lobe of the hypophysis as influenced by noise. Our preliminary studies on the problem indicate the stress-producing effect of noise on the neural lobe (MILINE and WERNER, 1958).

A. Materials and Methods

Eighty adult white male laboratory rats weighing 150-200 g were used for the experiment. The experimental group consisted of rats exposed to noise for 8 h/day (from 7 a.m. to 3 p.m.) for 14 consecutive days. The source of noise was an electric bell. Physical properties of the noise: (1) 86 dB, (2) 89 dB, (3) 91 dB, (4) 94 dB (Lin), 31.5-31.000 Hz. The animals were killed by decapitation. For light microscopy, organs were fixed in Bouin's fluid. Staining methods: Florentin, Gomori-Bargmann, Gabe, Dominici.
For electron microscopy, tissues were fixed in 6% glutaraldehyde, embedded in araldite according to Parsons, contrasted according to Reynolds and examined in an Iskra Lem 4C electron microscope.

B. Results

In experimental rats subjected to the noise, neurosecretory material was abundant, and hyperplasia of pituicytes was observed. Herring bodies were gradually increased in number. Neurosecretory fibers were distinctly more hypochromatic than in control animals; they were arranged in the shape of a necklace or cockade around the pituicytes. The latter were characterized by proliferation of the processes and by abundant lipid bodies. Mitochondria were hypertrophied, the cisternae of the granular endoplasmic reticulum and the Golgi zone were dilated, and lysosomes were more numerous. Many pituicytes were pervaded by neurosecretory fibers showing signs of disintegration.

Neurosecretory fibers were varied greatly in width; the presence of dark and light axons was very conspicuous. In the former, the neuroplasm was of considerably increased electron density. Elementary granules were variable in size and density. In some nerve endings, the granules were densely aggregated and hyperosmiophilic, in contrast to other axon terminals in which granules were sparse, with considerably less osmiophilia, or devoid of a core.

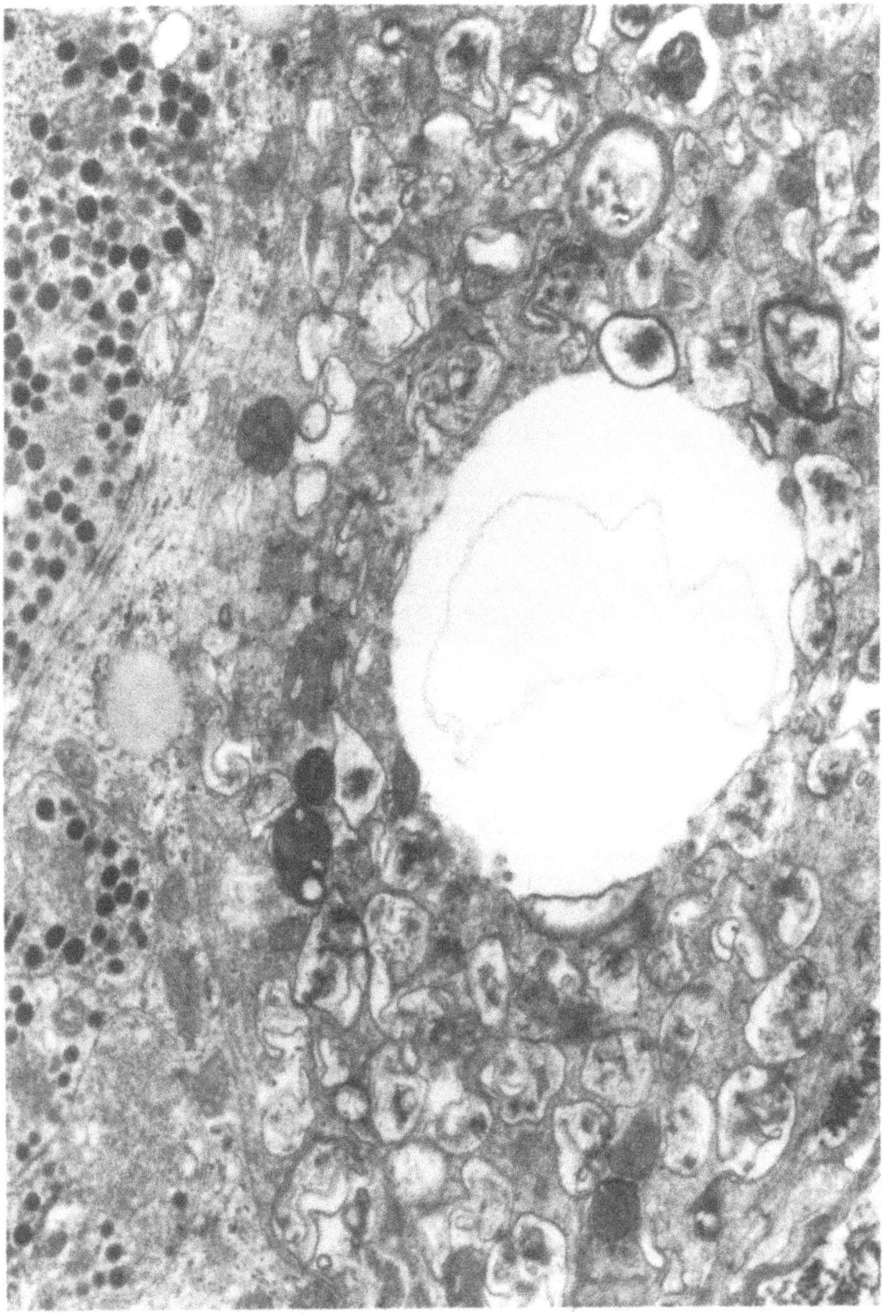

Fig. 1. Posterior pituitary. Dilated part of neurosecretory fiber, displaying large vacuole and polymorphous lamellar and autolytic bodies. Other nerve endings contain numerous microvesicles and single neurosecretory granules. Note part of a Herring body. × 20,000

In dark axons, mitochondria were very polymorphous - wholly or partly devoid of crests, showing wrinkled or ruptured membranes and a confluent matrix. Besides mitochondria, smaller lysosome-like osmiophilic bodies, variable in shape, were observed. Some Herring bodies displayed signs of disintegration. Elementary granules were sparse, with a discontinuous membrane. There were numerous lamellar bodies showing variable degrees of osmiophilia. Dilated parts of neurosecretory fibers may contain a large vacuole or a number of vacuoles lined one below the other (Fig. 1). In the terminals of adrenergic and cholinergic fibers, densely aggregated microvesicles were discernible.

Pericapillary spaces were dilated. The endothelium of capillaries was characterized by numerous microvillar processes, and the cytoplasm was pervaded by numerous micropinocytotic profiles.

C. Discussion

Noise is a neurogenic stressor. Proliferation of pituicytes and their increased phagocytic activity, the depletion and release of secretory granules, the disintegration of neurosecretory fibers, the microvillar processes and the numerous micropinocytotic vesicles in the endothelial cells of capillaries - all these signs speak in favor of a noise-dependent increased activity of the neural lobe of the hypophysis. The morphologic results of this study are in agreement with those obtained under other stress-producing conditions by other authors (POLENOV et al., 1975). They also confirm our previous studies on the influence of noise, and noise and vibration on the nucleus supraopticus and the nucleus paraventricularis. Progressive histophysiologic changes were found in these experiments (MILINE, 1955). They indicate that under auditory stress increased secretion of vasopressin and oxytocin occurs. This is in agreement also with the results of studies on the hypertensive effect of noise (MEDOFF and BONGIOVANNI, 1945), with the results of our previous studies on the influence of noise on the activity of the adrenal gland (MILINE and KOŠAK, 1952) and with the results from studies on the effect of noise on increased secretion of oxytocin (OGLE and LOCKETT, 1966).

References

MEDOFF, H.S., BONGIOVANNI, A.M.: Blood pressure in rats subjected to audiogenic stimulation. Am. J. Physiol. 143, 300-310 (1945)

MILINE, R.: Prilog proučavanju dejstva buke i potresa na hipotalamus. Medicinski Pregled, 90-97 (1955)

MILINE, R.: Contribution à l'étude de l'action du bruit et des vibrations sur le rein. Biol. Prâce 7, 69-82 (1961)

MILINE, R., KOŠAK, O.: Influence du bruit et des vibrations sur les glandes surrénales. C. R. Assoc. Anta. 69, 692-703 (1952)

MILINE, R., WERNER, R.: Effet du bruit sur le lobe postérieur de l'hypophyse. Acta Anat. (Basel) 247 (1958)
OGLE, C.W., LOCKETT, F.: The release of neurohypophyseal hormone by sound. J. Endocrinol. 36, 281-290 (1966)
POLENOV, A.L., UGRUMOV, M.V., BELENKY, M.A.: On degeneration of peptidergic neurosecretory fibres in the albino rat. Cell Tissue Res. 160, 113-123 (1975)

Adenylate-Cyclase Activity in the Neurosecretory Nuclei of Rat Hypothalamus

A. MITRO and J. KNOPP
Institute of Experimental Endocrinology, Slovak Academy of Sciences, 80936 Bratislava, ČSSR

Cyclic adenosine 3'-,5'-monophosphate (cAMP) has various effects in the CNS. The concentration of cAMP in the brain is controlled by the activity of the enzymes catalyzing its formation (adenylate cyclase) and its hydrolysis (phosphodiesterase). Wistar albino rats were used in the experiments. The hypothalamic nuclei (nucleus supraopticus (NSO), nucleus paraventricularis (NPV), nucleus dorsomedialis (NDM), eminentia medialis (EM), and nucleus arcuatus (NA)) were isolated by the method of PALKOVITS (1973). The adenylate-cyclase activity in the nuclei was determined by the method of KRISHNA et al. (1972) with minor modifications. We have found that the adenylate-cyclase activity was different in various nuclei. Similar activity was found in the NSO, NPV, and EM. The highest activity was found in the NA and NDM. In rats exposed to immobilization stress for 20 min, decreased adenylate-cyclase activity in the NPV and NVM and small changes in the NA and EM were seen. It is supposed that variation of the activity of adenylate cyclase, which produces cAMP in the hypothalamic nuclei, may be an important factor for regulation of some hypothalamic functions and is probably involved in the mechanism of stress reactions.

References

KRISHNA, G., HARWOOS, J.P., BARBER, A.J., SAMIESON, G.A.: The glucagon-sensitive adenyl cyclase system in plasma membranes of rat liver. J. Biol. Chem. 246, 1877-1882 (1972)

PALKOVITS, M.: Isolated removal of hypothalamic or other brain nuclei of the rat. Brain Res. 59, 449 (1973)

Immunohistochemical Demonstration of S-100 Protein and GFA Protein in Interstitial Cells of Rat Pineal Gland

M. MØLLER, A. INGLID, and E. BOCK
Anatomy Department A, University of Copenhagen, Universitetsparken 1, DK-2100 Copenhagen Ø, and the Protein Laboratory, Sigurdsgade 32, DK-2200 Copenhagen N, Denmark

The mammalian pineal gland contains different types of cells. The dominant cell is the pinealocyte, which synthesizes the pineal hormones. Another cell is the interstitial cell. Based on electron-microscopic observations of an abundance of microfilaments both in the perikaryon and cell processes, the interstitial cell was considered to be an astroglial cell; however, the cell differs ultrastructurally in many respects from the classical astrocyte in the brain.

Two brain proteins are considered to be present only in glial cells: the S-100 protein and the glial fibrillary-acidic protein (GFA). This study investigated whether these two proteins occur in rat pineal glands. The brains from 35 rats were fixed in 1% formaldehyde for 1 h; 6 µm cryostat or paraffin sections were cut from the pineal gland, cortex cerebri, and cerebellum. The sections were incubated with rabbit antiserum either to the S-100 protein or to GFA protein. The specific antibodies were made visible by the unlabeled antibody-enzyme method (STERNBERGER, 1970). Control sections were treated with antisera that had been adsorbed by S-100 or GFA proteins. Sections reacted with antimicrotubulin serum also served as controls. The specificity of the S-100 antiserum (S-100 protein supplied by Dr. K.G. Haglid, Gothenburg, Sweden) and the GFA antiserum (GFS supplied by Dr. L.F. Eng, Calif., USA) were tested by means of cross-immunoelectrophoresis with intermediate gel.

In the light microscope the S-100 and GFA proteins were located in classical star-shaped astrocytes, both in the cortex cerebri and the cerebellum. In the pineal gland the same proteins were located in a small number of cells scattered throughout the entire gland. Several processes emerged from the cell bodies of the S-100- and GFA-containing cells and approached the perivascular spaces. Based on the morphology and the location in the pineal gland of these S-100- and GFA-containing cells, we believe that they are the interstitial cells. The results support the hypothesis that the interstitial cells are macroglial cells.

Reference

STERNBERGER, L.A., HARDY, P.H., Jr., CUCULIS, J.J., MEYER, H.G.: The unlabelled antibody enzyme method of immunohistochemistry. Preparation and properties of soluble antigen-antibody complex (horseradish peroxidase-anti horseradish peroxidase) and its use in identification of spirochetes. J. Histochem. Cytochem. 18, 315-333 (1970)

Effects of Aldosterone on the Ultrastructure of Rat Hypothalamo-Neurohypophyseal Neurosecretory System

M. MURAKAMI
Department of Anatomy, Kurume University School of Medicine, Kurume, Japan

Recent biochemical data indicate that a close reciprocal relationship exists between vasopressin and aldosterone with respect to water and electrolyte metabolism. The details of this mechanism, however, are still obscure or controversial (GAUNT et al., 1957; HILTON, 1960; PALKOVITS et al., 1974; MÖHRING et al., 1974).

Serial experiments in our laboratory have shown that prolonged administration of synthesized aldosterone (MURAKAMI, 1970), and magnesium deficiency capable of causing a marked but transient increase in plasma concentration of aldosterone (GINN et al., 1976; HELBER et al., 1972; MURAKAMI et al., unpublished data) produce remarkable degenerative changes in the hypothalamo-hypophyseal neurosecretory neurons of rats (MURAKAMI et al., 1970, 1975). The ultrastructural changes of the neurosecretory neurons under these two experimental conditions were essentially similar.

Most of the neurosecretory cells in the nucleus supraopticus and nucleus paraventricularis of the experimental animals underwent a noticeable degeneration. Their cytoplasm was irregularly outlined and became dense because of condensation of cytoplasmic matrix. The cell nucleus was shrunk considerably; it contained occasionally dense inclusions of a spherical shape. In the cytoplasm, not only the cisternae of the rough endoplasmic reticulum but also the perinuclear space were extremely dilated; they often fused to form a large cavity occupying the major part of the cytoplasm. Free and membrane-bound ribosomes were considerably diminished or absent. In addition, elementary (neurosecretory) granules characteristic of this type of cell were significantly depleted in most of the cytoplasm of the neurosecretory cells. Lysosomal bodies were increased in number, and some of them were characterized by the presence of elementary granules or their remnants, probably taken up phagocytotically.

Neurosecretory axon terminals in the neurohypophysis of the experimental animals were more or less swollen and filled with elementary granules of varying density. In these terminals, the increase in the number of lysosomes was as significant as in perikarya. Some of these lysosomes contained isolated elementary granules. The increase in the number of lysosomes probably resulted from a process of crinophagy that has been recently observed by RUFENER (1974) within neurohypophyseal axon terminals of rats after artificial interruption of lactation. RUFENER postulated that this increase represents a mechanism serving the disposal of excess elementary granules. The most striking observation in the neurohypophysis of experimental rats was that dense inclusions of spherical or polygonal shape

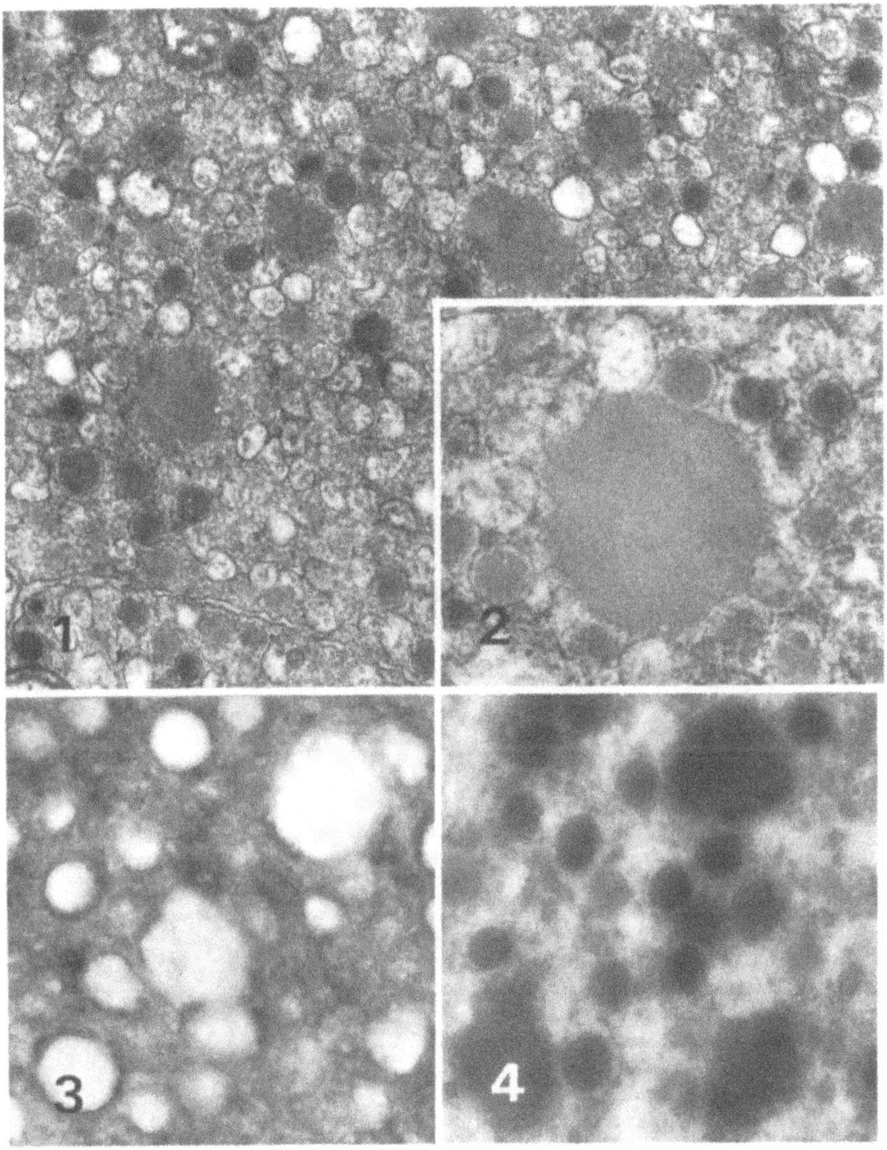

Figs. 1-4. Axoplasm of neurosecretory neuron in neurohypophysis of a magnesium-deficient rat.

Fig. 1. Dense deposits of spherical or polygonal shape are scattered among elementary (neurosecretory) granules. × 28,700

Fig. 2. Dense deposit at higher magnification. × 38,400

Fig. 3. Dense deposits and elementary granules after oxidation with potassium permanganate (method of NAUMANN and STERBA, 1976). × 45,000

Fig. 4. Dense deposits and elementary granules after oxidation with permanganate and subsequent staining with tannic acid. × 48,100 occurred among the axonal elementary granules (Fig. 1). There was no specialized structure, such as a limiting membrane, between the dense, depositlike inclusions and the surrounding axoplasmic matrix (Fig. 2). These deposits consisted of fine granular material and strongly resembled the elementary granules not only in their ultrastructural appearance but also in their ultrahistochemical reactivity. In ultrathin sections oxidized with potassium permanganate to demonstrate neurophysin-containing vesicles (procedure of NAUMANN and STERBA, 1976), the deposits appeared completely lucent and their images were quite similar to the neighboring elementary granules (Fig. 3). After subsequent staining of the ultrathin sections with tannic acid, the deposits and elementary granules, which had disappeared due to the oxidative treatment, again became stainable (Fig. 4). Secretory granules less than 0.1 µm in diameter in amine-containing axons and lipid droplets in pituicytes of the neurohypophysis remained unaltered during these procedures. From these results, it was concluded that each dense deposit represents a conglomeration of degraded elementary granules.

These results suggest that an increase in aldosterone, regardless of its original mechanism, causes an inhibitory effect on the production of neurohormone in the hypothalamic neurosecretory neurons. The detailed mechanism of aldosterone action, however, is still open to discussion.

References

GAUNT, R., LLOYD, C.W., CHART, T.T.: The adrenal-neurohypophysial interrelationship. In: The Neurohypophysin. HELLER, H. (ed.). New York: 1957, p. 233-251

GINN, H.E., CADE, R., MCCALLUM, T., FREGLEY, M.: Aldosterone secretion in magnesium-deficient rats. Endocrinology 80, 969-971 (1976)

HELBER, A., HAYDUK, K., NOWACZYNSKI, W., BRECHT, H.M., KÜCHEL, O., GENEST, J.: Zur Beeinflussung der Aldosteronsekretion des Hundes durch veränderte Plasma-Magnesium-Konzentration. Res. Exp. Med. 157, 336-346 (1972)

HILTON, J.G.: Adrenocorticotropic action of antidiuretic hormone. Circulation 21, 1038-1047 (1960)

MÖHRING, B., MÖHRING, J., DAUDA, G., HAACK, D.: Potassium deficiency in rats with hereditary diabetes insipidus. Am. J. Physiol. 227, 916-920 (1974)

MURAKAMI, M., NAKAYAMA, Y., SHIMADA, T., HIRATA, S.: Ultrastrukturelle Veränderungen des supraoptico-hypophysären Systems der Ratte nach Aldosteronbehandlung. Endokrinologie 56, 18-28 (1970)

MURAKAMI, M., SHIMADA, T., INOKUCHI, T., HIRANO, K.: Ultrastructural changes of the hypothalamo-hypophysial neurosecretory system in the magnesium deficient rats. Endokrinologie 66, 268-278 (1975)

NAUMANN, W., STERBA, G.: Ultrastructural studies on neurophysin-containing vesicles of the neurosecretory system of vertebrates. Cell Tissue Res. 165, 545-553 (1976)

PALKOVITS, M., JONG, W. DE, WIED, D. DE: Hypothalamic control of aldosterone production in sodium-deficient rats. Neuroendocrinology 14, 297-309 (1974)

RUFENER, C.: Autophagy of secretory granules in the rat neurohypophysis. Neuroendocrinology 13, 314-320 (1973/74)

Ultrastructural Method for Identifying Neurophysin-Containing Vesicles of the Neurosecretory System of Vertebrates

W. NAUMANN and G. STERBA
Section of Biosciences of the Karl Marx University Leipzig, GDR

The method described allows the identification of neurophysin-containing vesicles of the magnocellular neurosecretory system of vertebrates. The tissue must be fixed with glutaraldehyde, postfixed in a 2% OsO_4 mixture, and embedded in Mikropal. Ultrathin sections are placed on grids and treated in the following way: oxidation in a sulphuric $KMnO_4$ solution for 20-60 s, treatment with 3% aqueous oxalic acid for 5 s, washing in four changes of double-distilled water, staining for 2-3 min with lead citrate according to REYNOLDS, and washing again in four changes of double-distilled water. After the oxidation of the ultrathin sections, the content of neurophysin vesicles is dissolved specifically in alkaline medium of the contrast mixture. Empty vesicles produced in this way, are electron-microscopically demonstrable in the form of holes. This treatment is without influence on other types of vesicles, e.g., amine-type vesicles, vesicles in all cell types of the adenohypophysis, vesicles in cells of the n. lateralis tuberis and of the urophysis spinalis caudalis of teleosts. In brain areas containing perikarya, axons, or terminals with different types of vesicles in juxtaposition, the neurophysin-containing vesicles can be identified by use of this method.

Reference

NAUMANN, W., STERBA, G.: Ultrastructural studies on Neurophysin-containing Vesicles of the Neurosecretory System of Vertebrates. Cell Tissue Res. 165, 545-553 (1976)

Hypothalamic Structures Responsible for Regulation of Reproduction of Waterfowl

B. G. NOVIKOV, L. M. RUDNEVA, L. S. FELIX, and O. V. DANILOVA
Kiev State University, Kiev, USSR

The discovery of the hypothalamic control of the reproductive function in animals has naturally posed questions about the structural components involved in the regulation of hypophyseal production of gonadotrophins. The present report considers this aspect of the results of our experiments on waterfowl.

Histophysiologic and electron-microscopic investigations demonstrated that the transition of ducks and geese to sexual maturity is associated with an increase in the secretory activity of neurons of the hypothalamic supraoptic, and arcuate nuclei. Simultaneously, a sharp increase in the function of the pituitary gonadotrophs and in FSH and LH concentrations in the peripheral blood are observed.

The seasonal reproduction cycles of these birds are connected with the annual rhythm of the hypothalamo-hypophyseal system. The volume of nuclei of neurons of the supraoptic nucleus and synthesis and secretion of neurosecretory material are significantly increased in the reproduction phase. In the cells of the arcuate area, along with the increase in nuclear volumes, the mitochondria and endoplasmic reticulum are hypertrophied and, on the surface of the latter, the number of ribosomes is noticeably increased. Numerous secretory granules are formed in Golgi bodies. Pituitary gonadotrophs are stimulated and FSH and LH concentration in the peripheral blood is markedly elevated during the reproductive period.

It has been shown by spectrophotometric analysis and light- and electron-microscopic investigations that the eggshell formation and egg laying are associated with the circadian rhythm of the magnocellular hypothalamic nuclei.

The seasonal transition of gonade in the relative physiologic state of rest is accompanied by a decrease in size of the neurons of the supraoptic and arcuate nuclei, with significantly weaker development of endoplasmic reticulum and with a reduction in the density of mitochondrial matrix. Incidentally, gonadotrophs are subject to the destructive changes, and both FSH and LH concentrations in blood decrease.

Histophysiologic evidence shows that age-related changes of the sexual cycle in geese are associated with peculiarities in the functioning of the hypothalamic-hypophyseal system in ontogenesis. In geese in the second year of life, the total productivity increased because of prolongation of the active phase of the hypothalamic-hypophyseal system. Asynchrony of the sexual cycle in male and female geese is also connected with the particular activity of the above-mentioned system. It has been proven in experiments with heterotransplanted testicles that interbreed variations of the final dimensions of gonads are determined by genetically fixed differences in the level of hypothalamic activity (NOVIKOV and PTITZA, 1968).

The importance of the systems of magnocellular and small cells of the hypothalamic nuclei in the regulation of sexual function in birds has been confirmed experimentally. Using a local electrocoagulation technique, it has been established that destruction either of the hypothalamic preoptico-supraoptic or arcuate areas in ducks resulted in complete inhibition of hypophyseal gonadotrophic function (NOVIKOV and RUDNEVA, 1964, 1973; NOVIKOV et al., 1967). In these birds the sexual gland preserves its infantile character for the whole life span and does not respond to the gonad-stimulating effect of light; also, gonadotropin concentrations in the blood plasma have been reduced significantly. The conclusion concerning the dual regulation of gonadal function in birds has been confirmed by the recent experiments of DAVIES and FOLLETT (1974).

It is peculiar that the hypothalamic control of bird reproductive function during the postembryonic period is established relatively late, and that the prefunctional development phase of the gonads progresses independently of the hypothalamus. In Peking ducks, for example the prefunctional period ends at the age of 3 months and is associated with an increase in gonadal dimensions in male and female birds of 20 and 50 times, respectively. The destruction of the median eminence in fledglings does not hamper this growth phase in development of the gonads but it does completely inhibit gametogenesis (NOVIKOV and RUDNEVA, 1973; NOVIKOV et al., 1967).

Consequently, the seasonal reproduction cycle of birds is associated with the annual cycle of activity of the above-mentioned hypothalamic structures. Naturally, the question of the mechanism of seasonal gonadal transitions to the refractory phase has been raised. Our experiments on ducks and sparrows show that the transition of gonads into the refractory phase is associated with a noticeable decrease in hypothalamic secretory activity.

For analyzing the seasonal cycle of bird reproduction we employed the technique of coincubation of testis, hypophysis, and hypothalamus in plastic bags in the cavity of sparrows castrated unilaterally. The transplants were taken from birds that were at different stages of the sexual cycle, caused by the influence of various photoperiods. In these experiments, the recipient bird was always in refractory phase and its preserved right testis was used as the control. The results established that the activation of spermatogenesis could occur provided that the inactive testis, taken out in the refractory phase, had been incubated with the hypothalamus of sparrows of which the activation of the sexual cycle had just been started (RUDNEVA, 1970). Results obtained demonstrate vividly that the refractory period in gonadal function was tied to the change in hypothalamic activity.

The seasonal reproductive cycle in the birds studied was thus related to the annual rhythm of the functional activity of neurons of preoptic, supraoptic, and arcuate nuclei of the hypothalamus. It is not yet clear whether this complicated chain of interrelationships in the system of internal reproductive mechanisms is closed at the hypothalamic level or whether hypothalamic activity is, in its turn, controlled by suprahypothalamic structures.

References

DAVIES, D.T., FOLLETT, B.K.: Changes in plasma luteinizing hormone in the Japanese quail after electrical stimulation of the hypothalamus. J. Endocrinol. 63, 31-32 (1974)

NOVIKOV, B.G., PTITZA, A.N.: Neurohumoral mechanism of phenotypical realization of race differentiations of gonadal dimensions in birds. In: Cytology and Genetics, 1968, Vol. II, No. 6, pp. 522-525

NOVIKOV, B.G., RUDNEVA, L.M.: The dependence of ovarian functions in ducks on the hypothalamus. J. Gen. Biol. 25 (5) (1964)

NOVIKOV, B.G., RUDNEVA, L.M.: Hypothalamic structures participating in the regulation of trophic hypophyseal functions. Probl. Hypothalamic Physiol. (Kiev) 7, 96-106 (1973)

NOVIKOV, B.G., RUDNEVA, L.M., PTITZA, A.N.: The significance of the hypothalamus in the development and gonadal function in birds. Probl. Hypothalamic Physiol. (Kiev) 1, 36-56 (1967)

RUDNEVA, L.M.: Contribution à l'analyse du mécanisme de la phase réfractaire des gonades chez les oiseaux. Ann. Endocrinol. 31 (6), 1065-1069 (1970)

Adrenergic Mechanisms in the Hypothalamic Control of Pituitary Adrenocorticotropic Function

L. A. OUS and B. V. ALESHIN
Institute of Endocrinology and Hormone Chemistry, Kharkov, USSR

The frequent coincidence of the potentiation of pituitary adrenocorticotropic function with increase in the activity of neurosecretory cells of the supraoptic nucleus is sometimes treated as evidence of the participation of Gomori-positive cells in the hypothalamic control of adenohypophyseal hormonopoiesis. We studied the reaction of the supraoptic nucleus in mature male rabbits in which the ACTH secretion had been deliberately increased. This was achieved via a stress reaction evoked by the immobilization of the experimental rabbits with subsequent vibration in a shaking machine for 30 min, or by prolonged stimulation of the sympathetic superior cervical ganglia, or by the combination of both. All the modifications of these experiments showed the potentiation of the neurosecretory activity of the supraoptic nucleus cells. At the same time the estimation of the catecholamine content (performed according to a 3-oxyindole procedure developed by OSINSKAYA, 1957) showed a decrease in norepinephrine concentration in the hypothalamus, and the presence of epinephrine, which is not normally observed in the rabbit hypothalamus. However, norepinephrine depresses the activity of the supraoptic-nucleus cells (see the report by ALESHIN in this volume). Thus, the potentiation of pituitary adrenocorticotropic function (to be exact, the increase of hypothalamic CRH) and the increased activity of the Gomori-positive supraoptic nucleus cells occur simultaneously, for they are induced by the decreased norepinephrine level in the hypothalamus.

Concentrations of the Neurotransmitters in the Supraoptic and Paraventricular Nuclei of the Rat

M. PALKOVITS and M. J. BROWNSTEIN
First Department of Anatomy, Semmelweis University, Medical School, Budapest, Hungary, and Laboratory of Clinical Sciences, NIMH, Bethesda, USA

The supraoptic (NSO) and the paraventricular nuclei (NPV) contain all the presently measurable neurotransmitters. Histofluorescence (DAHLSTRÖM and FUXE, 1964; FUXE, 1965; JACOBOWITZ and PALKOVITS, 1974) and immunohistochemical investigations (HÖKFELT et al., 1973) prove that the neurotransmitters are found not in the magnocellular neurosecretory cells, but in the nerve terminals.

According to quantitative histological studies, the numbers of nerve fibers terminating on the neurosecretory cells, or the cell-synapsis ratio are relatively small in the NSO. The number of the synaptic terminals in the total NSO is 5.19×10^6, which means 600 boutons/cell (LÉRÁNTH et al., 1975). Two-thirds of them are of intranuclear origin. It was found that 32.7% of the extracellular synapses originate from the brainstem (ZÁBORSZKY et al., 1975). They are presumably biogenic amine terminals originating from the brainstem of noradrenaline, adrenaline, dopamine, and serotonin cells. A further 21% of the afferent fibers arise from the medial basal hypothalamus, 13.5-13.5 both from the amygdala and the septum, 8.5% from the hippocampus, and 17% from the olfactory tubercle and other rostral cortical regions (ZÁBORSZKY et al., 1975). Their neurotransmitter functions are not yet known, but their presence proves that direct neuronal connections exist between the above-mentioned brain regions and the neurosecretory nuclei.

By use of enzyme-isotopic micromethods (see PALKOVITS et al., 1976) and a microdissection method (PALKOVITS, 1973) it was possible to determine the concentration of the neurotransmitters and their biosynthesizing enzymes in the individual hypothalamic nuclei, particularly in the NSO and NPV.

The NPV is very rich in noradrenaline; its concentration is one of the highest in the hypothalamus (Table 1). The similarly high dopamine-β-hydroxylase activity indicates that there is also an active local noradrenaline synthesis in the nerve terminals of the NPV. The noradrenaline content and dopamine-β-hydroxylase activity of the NSO are more or less the same as the mean of the values measured in the hypothalamus (Table 1). The noradrenergic nerve terminals of both nuclei originate from the nerve (NE) cells of the brainstem (DAHLSTRÖM and FUXE, 1964). The majority of the fibers arise from the locus coeruleus. Following electrolytic lesions of the locus coeruleus, the NE content of both the NSO (ZÁBORSZKY et al., in press) and the NPV (KOBAYASHI et al., 1974) falls markedly but not completely, indicating that other NE-cell groups of the brainstem (probably A2, A5, A7 cell groups) might also take part in the noradrenergic

Table 1. Concentrations (ng/mg protein) of neurotransmitters and their related enzymes in the rat supraoptic (NSO) and paraventricular (NPV) nuclei

	References	NSO mean ± SEM	NPV mean ± SEM	Hypothalamus (lowest-highest)	CNS (lowest-highest)
		ng/mg protein			
Noradrenaline	18	23.6 ± 5.0	51.0 ± 6.4	12.0 - 54.6	1.1 - 80.2
Adrenaline	9	2.14 ± 0.47	2.16 ± 0.06	ND - 2.52	ND - 2.52
Dopamine	18	3.7 ± 0.6	10.0 ± 1.5	3.4 - 65.0	1.3 - 114.4
Serotonin	23	9.5 ± 2.8	13.5 ± 3.1	7.4 - 37.2	20 - 37.2
Histamine	6	3.0 ± 0.6	2.4 ± 0.5	2.2 - 17.8	0.78 - 11.38
Substance "P"[a]	3	1.58 ± 0.12	3.06 ± 0.21	1.00 - 3.48	0.32 - 38.38
Thyrotropin-releasing hormone	4	0.85 ± 0.17	2.60 ± 0.74	0.70 - 38.38	0.9 - 309.1
Somatostatin	1	3.2 ± 0.6	4.4 ± 1.8	3.2 - 309.1	
		pmol (μg protein) h			
Dopamine-β-hydroxylase (DBH)	21	1.83 ± 0.36	3.55 ± 0.82	0.46 - 4.19	-
Phenylethanol-N-methyltransferase (PNMT)[a]	22	5.2 ± 1.3	15.0 ± 2.5	4.1 - 15.0	ND - 41.5
Tyrosine hydroxylase (TH)	21	0.92 ± 0.14	3.14 ± 0.82	0.42 - 18.03	0.20 -
Tryptophan hydroxylase	5	0.31 ± 0.04	0.32 ± 0.05	0.23 - 1.16	0.10 - 4.31
Choline acetyltransferase	2	8.3 ± 1.1	7.7 ± 0.8	3.6 - 19.5	3.2 - 240.0
Glutamic acid decarboxylase	25	-	609 ± 56	109 - 656	98 - 1110
Catechol-O-methyltransferase	20	0.45 ± 0.11	0.51 ± 0.07	0.18 - 1.21	0.18 - 1.71
Histamine-N-methyltransferase	20	0.75 ± 0.15	1.10 ± 0.19	0.35 - 1.24	0.35 - 1.75
Monoamineoxydase	20	110.5 ± 11.3	69.2 ± 13.9	69.2 - 183.0	52.2 - 304.5

[a]pmol/mg protein; ND = nondetectable

innervation of the neurosecretory nuclei. The NE fibers reach the hypothalamus in dorsal and ventral pathways, which lead to the NSO and NPV in the medial forebrain bundle (UNGERSTEDT, 1971; SACHS et al., 1973; LINDVALL and BJÖRKLUND, 1974).

The adrenaline content of the NPV is relatively high and its phenylethanolamine-N-methyltransferase activity is the highest in the hypothalamus (Table 1). The adrenaline concentration is also high in the NSO, but the enzyme activity is only moderate. By immunohistochemical methods, adrenergic perikarya were located only in the lower part (C1 and C2 regions) of the brainstem (HÖKFELT et al., 1973). Therefore, it is supposed that the adrenaline in the NSO and NPV terminals originates from lower brainstem regions.

There is high dopamine (DA) content and tyrosine hydroxylase activity in the NPV, while those are particularly low in the NSO (Table 1). The origin of the DA located in the nerve terminals of NSO and NPV is uncertain. The A9 and A10 catecholaminergic cell groups (DAHLSTRÖM and FUXE, 1964) do not take part in the dopaminergic innervation of the NSO and NPV, since electrolytic lesions in them do not produce any changes in the dopamine level of the neurosecretory nuclei (KIZER et al., 1976). It is assumed that other DA cell groups - probably located in the diencephalon (A11, A12, A13 cell groups) - innervate NSO and NPV with dopaminergic fibers.

By contrast with the catecholamines the concentrations of serotonin and histamine are low in both nuclei (Table 1). Low tryptophan-hydroxylase activity is also found in the neurosecretory nuclei. Nearly two-thirds of the supraoptic and paraventricular serotonin arise from the mesencephalon. After electrolytic destruction of the dorsal raphe nucleus, or after a brainstem transection at the mesencephalon-diencephalon boundary, a significant fall in the 5-HT level of the NSO and NPV was observable biochemically (PALKOVITS et al., in press). The cellular localization and origin of the histamine found in the magnocellular nuclei, and the role played by it in vasopressin regulation, is not yet known.

The activities of the catabolic enzymes of biogenic amines are different in the NSO and NPV. The catechol-O-methyltransferase activity is moderate in both nuclei, the monoaminooxydase activity is moderate in the NSO and definitely low in the NPV, while the histamine-N-methyltransferase activity is relatively high (Table 1). The physiological importance of these data can be evaluated only after further investigations.

The cholinergic innervation of the magnocellular neurosecretory nuclei indicated by the choline acetyltransferase activity is low (Table 1). Since there are no acetylcholinesterase-containing cells in these nuclei (JACOBOWITZ and PALKOVITS, 1974) the acetylcholine is probably in nerve terminals. There is no direct evidence concerning the location of cholinergic cell bodies innervating the neurosecretory nuclei.

The activity of the glutamic acid decarboxylase, an enzyme important in GABA synthesis, is relatively high in the NPV, but we have no data about that in the NSO. The concentration of the substance "P" is also high in the NPV, but is only half of that in the NSO (Table 1). We have no data about the cellular localization and origins of these substances yet.

Recently, radioimmunoassays have proved that thyrotropin-releasing hormone and somatostatin are found in almost all regions of the brain. Therefore it seems reasonable to assume that they act as neurotransmitters outside the medial basal hypothalamus (see PALKOVITS et al., 1976). Both materials are found in relatively high concentrations in the NPV and in markedly low concentrations in the NSO (Table 1). Their origins, localizations, and physiologic roles are not yet known.

On the basis of the above biochemical data the following conclusions can be drawn:

1. All the neurotransmitters and their biosynthesizing enzymes measured are found in detectable concentrations in the neurosecretory nuclei.

2. The concentrations of neurotransmitters are, with a few exceptions, much higher in the NPV than in the NSO.

3. Among the neurotransmitters found in the nerve terminals of the magnocellular neurosecretory nuclei, the catecholamines seem to be the most important, on the basis of their concentration.

4. The neurotransmitters in the NSO and NPV are found in nerve terminals of neurons that are located in other areas of the CNS. This means that several brain areas are in direct neural connection with the magnocellular neurosecretory neurons and can influence the synthesis of vasopressin and oxytocin in these nuclei.

References

1. BROWNSTEIN, M.J., ARIMURA, A., SATO, T.V., SCHALLY, A.V., KIZER, J.S.: The regional distribution of somatostatin in the rat brain. Endocrinology 96, 1456-1461 (1975)
2. BROWNSTEIN, M.J., KOBAYASHI, R.M., PALKOVITS, M., SAAVEDRA, J.M.: Choline acetyltransferase levels in diencephalic nuclei of the rat. J. Neurochem. 24, 35-38 (1975)
3. BROWNSTEIN, M.J., MROZ, E.A., KIZER, J.S., PALKOVITS, M., LEEMAN, S.E.: Regional distribution of Substance P in the brain of the rat. Brain Res. 116, 299-305 (1976)
4. BROWNSTEIN, M.J., PALKOVITS, M., SAAVEDRA, J.M., BASSIRI, P.M., UTIGER, R.D.: Thyrotropin-releasing hormone in specific nuclei of the brain. Science 185, 267-269 (1974a)
5. BROWNSTEIN, M.J., PALKOVITS, M., SAAVEDRA, J.M., KIZER, J.S.: Tryptophan hydroxylase in the rat brain. Brain Res. 97, 163-166 (1975)

6. BROWNSTEIN, M.J., SAAVEDRA, J.M., PALKOVITS, M., AXELROD, J.: Histamine content of hypothalamic nuclei of the rat. Brain Res. 77, 151-156 (1974b)
7. DAHLSTRÖM, A., FUXE, K.: Evidence for the existence of monoamine-containing neurons in the central nervous system. I. Demonstration of monoamines in the cell bodies of brain stem neurons. Acta Physiol. Scand. (Suppl. 232) 62, 1-55 (1964)
8. FUXE, K.: Evidence for the existence of monoamine neurons in the central nervous system. IV. Distribution of monoamine nerve terminals in the central nervous system. Acta Physiol. Scand. (Suppl. 247) 64, 39-85 (1965)
9. VAN DER GUGTEN, J., PALKOVITS, M., WINJNEN, H.L.J.M., VERSTEEG, D.H.G.: Regional distribution of adrenaline in rat brain. Brain Res. 107, 171-175 (1976)
10. HÖKFELT, T., FUXE, K., GOLDSTFIN, M., JOHANSSON, O.: Evidence for adrenergic neurons in the rat brain. Acta Physiol. Scand. 89, 286-288 (1973)
11. JACOBOWITZ, D.M., PALKOVITS, M.: Topographic atlas of catecholamine and and acetylcholinesterase-containing neurons in the rat brain. I. Forebrain (Telencephalon, diencephalon). J. Comp. Neurol. 157, 13-28 (1974)
12. KIZER, J.S., PALKOVITS, M., BROWNSTEIN, M.J.: The projections of the A8, A9 and A10 dopaminergic cell bodies: evidence for a nigral-hypothalamic-median eminence dopaminergic pathway. Brain Res. 108, 363-370 (1976)
13. KOBAYASHI, R.M., PALKOVITS, M., KOPIN, I.J., JACOBOWITZ, D.M.: Biochemical mapping of noradrenergic nerves arising from the rat locus coeruleus. Brain Res. 77, 269-279 (1974)
14. LÉRÁNTH, Cs., ZÁBORSZKY, L., MARTON, J., PALKOVITS, M.: Quantitative studies on the supraoptic nucleus in the rat. I. Synaptic organization. Exp. Brain Res. 22, 509-523 (1975)
15. LINDVALL, O., BJÖRKLUND, A.: The organization of the ascending catecholamine neuron systems in the rat brain as revealed by the glyocylic acid fluorescence method. Acta Physiol. Scand. (Suppl. 412), 1-48 (1974)
16. PALKOVITS, M.: Isolated removal of hypothalamic or other brain nuclei of the rat. Brain Res. 59, 449-450 (1973)
17. PALKOVITS, M., BRONWSTEIN, M.J., KIZER, J.S.: Effect of total hypothalamic deafferentation on releasing hormone and neurotransmitter concentrations of the mediobasal hypothalamus in rat. In: International Symposium on Cellular and Molecular Bases of Neuroendocrine Processes. ENDRÓCZY, E. (ed.). Budapest: Akadémiai Kiadó, 1976, pp. 575-599
18. PALKOVITS, M., BROWNSTEIN, M., SAAVEDRA, J.M., AXELROD, J.: Norepinephrine and dopamine content of hypothalamic nuclei of rat. Brain Res. 77, 137-149 (1974)
19. PALKOVITS, M., SAAVEDRA, J.M., JACOBOWITZ, D.M., KIZER, J.S., ZABÓRSZKY, L., BROWNSTEIN, M.J.: Serotoninergic innervation of the forebrain: effect of lesions on serotonin and tryptophan hydroxylase levels. Brain Res. (in press)
20. SAAVEDRA, J.M., BROWNSTEIN, M.J., PALKOVITS, M.: Distribution on catechol-O-methyltransferase, histamine N-methyltransferase and monoamine oxidase in specific areas of the rat brain. Brain Res. 118, 152-156 (1976)
21. SAAVEDRA, J.M., BROWNSTEIN, M.J., PALKOVITS, M., KIZER, J.S., AXELROD, J.: Tyrosine hydroxylase and dopamine-β-hydroxylase: distribution in the individual rat hypothalamic nuclei. J. Neurochem. 23, 869-871 (1974a)
22. SAAVEDRA, J.M., PALKOVITS, M., BROWNSTEIN, M.J., AXELROD, J.: Localization of phenylethanolamine N-methyltransferase in the rat brain nuclei. Nature 248, 695-696 (1974b)
23. SAAVEDRA, J.M., PALKOVITS, M., BROWNSTEIN, M.J., AXELROD, J.: Serotonin distribution in the nuclei of the rat hypothalamus and preoptic region. Brain Res. 77, 157-165 (1974c)

24. SACHS, C., JONSSON, G., FUXE, K.: Mapping of central noradrenaline pathways with 6-hydroxy-DOPA. Brain Res. 63, 249-261 (1973)
25. TAPPAZ, M.L., BROWNSTEIN, M.J., PALKOVITS, M.: Distribution of glutamate decarboxylase in discrete brain nuclei. Brain Res. 108, 371-379 (1976)
26. UNGERSTEDT, U.: Stereotaxic mapping of the monoamine pathways in the rat brain. Acta Physiol. Scand. (Suppl.) 367, 1-48 (1971)
27. ZÁBORSZKY, L., BROWNSTEIN, M.J., PALKOVITS, M.: Ascending brain stem pathways from the dorsolateral pontine tegmentum: A biochemical and electronmicroscopical study. Acta Morphol. Acad. Sci. Hung. (in press)
28. ZÁBORSZKY, L., LÉRÁNTH, Cs., MAKARA, G.B., PALKOVITS, M.: Quantitative studies on the supraoptic nucleus in the rat. II. Afferent fiber connections. Exp. Brain Res. 22, 525-540 (1975)

Neurosecretory and Pars-Intermedia Cells of Fish and Mammals

V. PANTIĆ, M. SEKULIĆ, M. LOVREN, and M. ŠIMIĆ
Institute for Biological Research, Belgrade, Yugoslavia

A. Introduction

Since BARGMANN (1967) and SCHARRER (1969) defined neurohormones produced by neurosecretory cells, many papers have dealt with their further elucidation in different species. The study of neurosecretory cells has proceeded using contemporary methods (POLENOV, 1968; SZENTAGOTHAI et al., 1968; DIERICKX and VANDESANDE, 1975; and many others). Current concepts of neurosecretion have been given by SCHARRER (1969). There are still many unanswered questions concerning the differentiation of neurosecretory cells, differences in the development and structure of hypothalamic nuclei in various species, interrelationships between afferents of various brain structures and neurosecretory cells, their efferent terminals in the neurohypophysis and pars intermedia, the site of biosynthesis of releasing factors (RF) and inhibiting factors (IF) and biogenic amines, etc.

The role of neurosecretory cells in the regulation of pituitary-cell activities is still not clear. New data have been obtained concerning the role of the hypothalamus in the control of the release of MSH from the vertebrate pars intermedia (OLIVEREAU, 1971; MacHADLEY et al., 1975; etc.). Involution of the pars intermedia during hypothalamic hyperactivity resulting from water deprivation, continuous illumination, and lactation has been described (LEGAIT, 1962).

During the last few years we have examined the structure of neurosecretory cells in various species: the interrelationship between parvocellular and magnocellular areas, median eminence (ME) and pituitary, the ability of neurosecretory cells to accumulate and transport Gabe- and Gomori-positive (GG+) substances under various experimental conditions, the sites of their terminations, and the nature of pituitary cells. This report is a brief presentation of the structural properties of neurosecretory cells during various seasons, i.e., the sexual cycle, the interrelationship of their terminals with pars-intermedia cells, and some cytologic characteristics of these intermediate cells. For this purpose the following species have been selected: *Torpedo ocellata* (viviparous fish), *Serranus scriba* (hermaphrodite), *Acipenser ruthenus*, *Perca fluviatilis*, and *Carassius carassius* (fresh water fish), and guinea pig and deer (mammals).

B. Methods

The hypothalamus, pituitary, and part of the caudal spinal cord isolated from the animals examined were fixed in Bouin's solution. Sections were stained using Gomori and Gabe Azan methods. Pieces of pars intermedia fixed in 4% glutaraldehyde and postfixed in 1% OsO_4 were embedded in Araldite. Semithin sections, 1 μm thick, were stained with methylene blue and examined using a light microscope.

C. Results and Discussion

Neurosecretory cells of the *nucleus praeopticus* (NPO) of *T. ocellata* appear as stellate cells. The variations of size and shape of these cells were dependent on the age and season, i.e., sexual cycle; they were about twice as large in spring as in autumn. The amount of GG+ substances increased in the spring (Fig. 1a), appearing first in February in the cell bodies, then being transported along the neurites through the ME and infundibulum (Fig. 1b) and terminating in the neurointermediate lobe. The quantity of GG+ substances was highest in the neurites in the region of the ME and in the hypophysis of pregnant females their terminals were closely connected to the intermediate cells (Fig. 1c) (PANTIĆ and SEKULIĆ, 1975).

The nucleus lateralis tuberis (NLT) was slightly developed, with a large population of cell nuclei and poorly developed cytoplasm appearing as Gomori-negative cells. Parvo- and magnocellular cell types, clearly differentiated in *A. ruthenus*, were localized in separate groups. Neurosecretory material was present in the cytoplasm of both cell types as a small amount of finely granulated GG+ substances. A great number of their axons terminated in the neurohypophysis (Fig. 2), as described by POLENOV (1968). Both the parvocellular and magnocellular areas of NPO and NLT of *S. scriba* and other Teleostei examined were hypertrophic, and the amount of neurosecretory material increased in the spring, i.e., before and during the spawning season.

The largest cells in the ventral part of the NPO in *S. scriba* trapped in March were parvocellular, having an area of 22 × 20.2 μm. Their size decreased during the summer. GG+ substances were observed only in fish trapped in March and May, and not from September to February (Fig. 3a). Parvocellular areas of the NLT were more numerous than magnocellular ones. The cells with the largest diameter in the spring decreased their diameter in September by ca. 3.5 times. The largest neurosecretory cells in animals trapped in March were extremely large, an area of 43.8 × 35.2 μm; the smallest in September were 30.4 × 23.3 μm. GG+ substances, located mainly at the peripheral part of the cell-body cytoplasm in March, migrated across the axons towards the NLT and neurohypophysis in May, and only a slight amount of GG+ substances was present in the axons of animals sacrificed from September to February. The fibers of NPO neurosecretory cells, terminating

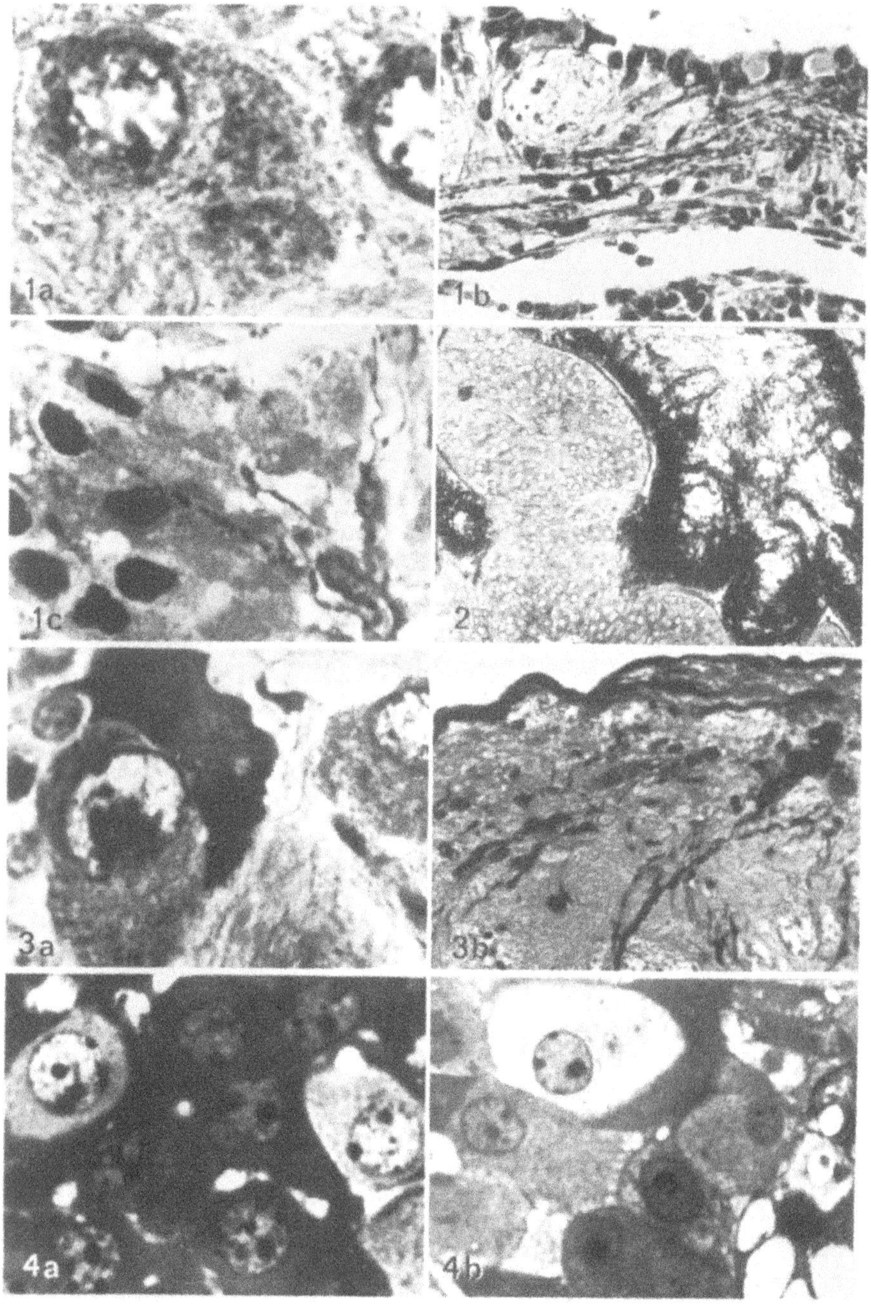
1a
1b
1c
2
3a
3b
4a
4b

Fig. 1. Neurosecretory cells of NPO of *T. ocellata* trapped in March; perikaryon (a), neurites in infundibulum (b), and their terminals in neurointermedia (c). (a) and (c) × 1200, (b) × 190

Fig. 2. Neurohypophysis and pars intermedia in hypophysis of *A. ruthenus*. × 190

Fig. 3. Neurosecretory and glia cells of NPO of *S. scriba* with perikaryon (a) and terminals around NLT cells (b). (a) × 1200, (b) × 480

Fig. 4. Semithin sections of pars intermedia of guinea pig (a) and deer (b). (a) and (b) × 1200

around NLT cells and in the neurohypophysis (Fig. 3b), had the highest quantity of neurosecretory material of animals trapped in May and March.

Caudal neurosecretory cells were more clearly developed, their number and size were large, and more GG+ substances were accumulated in the perikaryon of these cells in *A. ruthenus* than in *T. ocellata*. In the pars intermedia of Teleostei, chromophobes and PAS+ or Pb+ and PAS+ cells were mostly identified (DIMOVSKA, 1971; PAVLOVIĆ and PANTIĆ, 1975). In mammals, however, three cell types have been described (PANTIĆ and SIMIĆ, 1974; LEGAIT, 1962). The staining affinity of pars-intermedia cells differed in the species examined. In *T. ocellata* only Gomori-negative cells were observed; identification of PAS+ at the periphery, and Hpb+ in the central part in *P. fluviatilis* agrees with the observations of DIMOVSKA (1971); chromophobes and PAS+ cells were observed in *C. carassius* as well.

From our examinations of semithin sections of guinea-pig intermediate cells, we consider chromophobes as ACTH and methylene-blue positive as MSH-cells (Fig. 4a); deer chromophobes as ACTH and intermediates as a transitory stage to dark cells that produce MSH (Fig. 4b).

The differences in the structure, appearance, and staining affinity of pars-intermedia cells in various fishes and mammals is undoubtedly closely connected to the evolution of mechanisms regulating the biosynthesis of corticotropinlike intermediate peptide, melanotropins, and lipotropins, as molecules developed from a common ancestral molecule to the structural level characteristic for corresponding species.

D. Summary

Neurosecretory and pars intermedia cells of *T. ocellata*, a viviparous fish; *S. scriba*, a hermaphrodite, *A. ruthenus*, *P. fluviatilis* and *C. carassius*, freshwater fish; and guinea pig and deer, mammals, have been examined. The results obtained can be briefly summarized as follows: the existence of a close interrelationship between the size and structure of neurosecretory cells and the amount of neurosecretory material as they change with the sexual cycle; intimate contact between most of NPO neurosecretory-cell terminals loaded with an enormous amount of Gabe- and

Gomori-positive substances and intermediate cells was observed in *T. ocellata* and between NPO and NLT in *S. scriba*, both trapped in spring; the species characteristics in the structure and staining affinity of pars-intermedia cells are closely connected to the degree of differentiation of specific cells and their ability to synthesize ACTH-, MSH-, and LPH-molecules from the common ancestral molecule.

References

BARGMANN, W., LINDNER, E., ANDRES, K.H.: Über Synapsen an endokrinen Epithelzellen und die Definition sekretorischer Neurone. Untersuchungen am Zwischenlappen der Katzenhypophyse. Z. Zellforsch. Mikrosk. Anat. 77, 282-298 (1967)

DIERICKX, K., VANDESANDE, F.: Identification of the vasopressin- and the oxytocin-producing neurons in the rat hypothalamus. VIII Conf. Europ. Comp. Endcr., Bangor, p. 1 (1975)

DIMOVSKA, A.: Histološko struktura na hipofiza na dojranskata perkija *Perca fluviatilis*. Zavod za Ribarstvo na S R Makedonija, IV, 8, 1-31 (1971)

LEGAIT, E.: Recherches morphologiques et histophysiologiques sur la pars intermedia des Rongeurs. Extrait de la biologie médicale, LI, no. 2 and 3, 125-320 (1962)

LOWRY, P.J., SCOTT, A.P.: The evolution of vertebrate corticotrophin and melanocyte stimulating hormone. Gen. Comp. Endocrinol. 26, 1-16 (1975)

MACHADLEY, E., HRUBY, V.J., BOWER, A., Sr.: Cellular mechanisms controlling melanophore stimulating hormone (MSH) release. Gen. Comp. Endocrinol. 26, 1-24 (1975)

OLIVEREAU, M.: Elaboration d'intermédine par les cellules colorées avec l'hematoxyline au plomb dans la pars intermedia de l'Anguille: preuves nouvelles et controle hypothalamique. C. R. Acad. Sci. (D) (Paris) 272, 102-105 (1971)

PANTIĆ, V., ŠIMIĆ, V.: Pars intermedia of the deer pituitary. Arh. Biol. Nauka (Beograd) 26 (1-2), 15-18 (1974)

PANTIĆ, V., SEKULIĆ, M.: Neurosecretory cells in *Torpedo ocellata*. Arh. Biol. Nauka (Beograd) 26 (3-4), 109-114 (1974)

PAVLOVIĆ, M., PANTIĆ, V.: The adenohypophysis in the Teleostea *Alburnus albidus* and *Alosa fallax* in different phases of sexual cycle. Acta Vet. (Beograd) 25, 4, 163-178 (1975)

POLENOV, A.L.: On the evolution of the median eminence - the proximal neurosecretory contact region in some fishes (Elasmobranchii, Chondrosteoidei). Extrait des Archives d'Anatomie, d'Histologie et d'Embryologie Normales et Experimentales 51, fasc. 118 (1968)

SCHARRER, B.: Neurohumors and neurohormones. Definition and terminology. J. Neurovisc. Relat. 9, 1-20 (1969)

SZENTÁGOTHAI, J., FLERKÓ, B. MESS, B., HALÁSZ, B.: Hypothalamic Control of the Anterior Pituitary. Akadémiai Kiadó. Budapest 1968

Histochemical and Histospectrophotometric Study of PAS-Positive Material in the Hypothalamo-Hypophyseal Neurosecretory Pathway

D. PARENT, V. VILTER, and C. DA LAGE
Laboratoire d'Histologie et Embryologie, Faculté de Médecine Necker-Enfants Malades, Paris 15, France

A. Introduction

In 1952, SCHIEBLER described the neurosecretory substance as being a glycoliprotein. The presence of the protein component was rapidly established, whereas the existence of the glycosidic component has been the subject of some discussion. At first many authors concluded that it was absent, owing to the absence of PAS-positive material. However, in recent studies, the problem has been significantly reinvestigated. Our aim was therefore to localize and, if possible, to identify the glycosidic component by histochemical methods.

B. Materials and Methods

The investigation was done using material obtained from hamsters and from normal and water-deprived rats.

I. Light Microscopy

After decapitation, hypothalamic tissue and pituitaries were fixed and paraffin-embedded. Sagittal serial sections were cut at 7 µm for histochemical tests and at 3 µm for histospectrophotometry. Sections were treated by the following histochemical methods: (1) PAS, (2) toluidine blue at pH 2.4-2.6, (3) alcian blue (G.T. GURR) at two pHs: 0.5 and 2.5, (4) method of Ravetto using alcian blue at pH 0.5 and alcian yellow at pH 2.5, (5) Scott's method, using alcian blue with two concentrations of $MgCl_2$: 0.025 *M* and 0.5 *M*, (6) enzymic digestion: before staining with toluidine blue of alcian blue at pH 2.5, some sections were treated by neuraminidase (from Cl. perfringens, type IV, Sigma). They were incubated at 37°C for 14 h. (7) For the histospectrophotometric study, sections were stained with a 5×10^{-5} *M* pseudoisocyanin solution for 1 h at 0°C. They were then mounted in distilled water and examined with a microscopic device, coupled to a high resolution monochromator.

II. Electron Microscopy

Rats were perfused arterially with Karnovsky's solution. The posterior lobes of their pituitaries were fixed in 2.5% glutaraldehyde for 4 h, postfixed in osmium tetroxide for 1 h and embedded in Epon. Thin sections were stained by two methods: (1) Classic staining with uranyl acetate, (2) a staining procedure developed by THIÉRY (1967) for the detection of carbohydrates.

C. Results

I. Histochemical Study

(1) *The PAS-reaction* is positive in the neural lobe and in the hypothalamic magnocellular nuclei. In the neural lobe the PAS-positive material is distributed in droplets. In the hypothalamus there are many very fine granules in the perikarya of some neurosecretory neurons, whereas others are negative. In water-deprived rats the glycosidic component is depleted from the neural lobe, as is the aldehyde fuchsin-positive material. (2) In the perikarya of the same hypothalamic neurons and in the neural lobe *toluidine blue* gives a metachromatic reaction, which demonstrates the acidic character of the glycosidic substance. (3) *Alcian blue* at pH 0.5 reveals the presence of sulfhydric anions, and at pH 2.5 reveals both sulfhydric and carboxylic groups. Only the second solution stained our sections. (4) Using Ravetto's method, sulfhydric anions are revealed by alcian blue, and carboxylic anions by alcian yellow. The final staining in the neural lobe is yellow. (5) Scott's method demonstrates the distinction between carboxylic and sulfhydric anions. Both are revealed by alcian blue solution containing 2.5 *M* $MgCl_2$, whereas only sulfhydric anions are detected by alcian blue solution containing 0.5 *M* $MgCl_2$. Only the first solution stained our sections. Collectively, these three methods demonstrate that the acidic character of neurosecretory material is due to carboxylic groups. (6) After digestion with neuraminidase the metachromatic staining with toluidine blue disappears, as well as the staining with alcian blue at pH 2.5 g. Thiéry's staining enables detection of a glycosidic component inside the neurosecretory granules, the center of which remains less stained.

II. Histospectrophotometric Study

A new test for cell basophilia developed by VILTER et al. (1973) is used for histospectrophotometric study. The method can be used histochemically for the identification of acidic groups in carbohydrate material. Its application to the analysis of PAS-positive neurosecretory substance reveals a single absorption peak, with a wavelength characteristic of sialic acid. The peak is found in hypothalamic nuclei, as well as in the posterior pituitary of golden hamsters and rats. After digestion with neuraminidase, this peak disappears.

D. Discussion

These results show the presence of PAS-positive material in the neurosecretory pathway. This problem has often been discussed. HOWE and PEARSE (1956) did not accept the view of SCHIEBLER (1952), whereas GABE (1960) claimed that the intensity of the reaction varied according to the species. Regarding the rat, our findings are not in accord with those of GABE, who mentioned a negative reaction. However, the main problem is the significance of the glycosidic component. The enzymic digestion with neuraminidase shows clearly that sialic acid was present. Nevertheless, this is not in agreement with the data of HOLWERDA (1972a,b), who isolated a glycopeptide from the pituitary of the pig. According to this author, however, the glycopeptide contains no sialic acid. One must bear in mind the question of species variation. We observed that in the hypothalamic nuclei only certain neurons are PAS-positive. There are two likely interpretations: either the neurons are not all in the same state of secretion, or certain neurons synthesize a glycosidic molecule, whereas the others do not. This last interpretation is compatible with the results from TASSO (1973; TASSO and RUA, 1975). He presented evidence that neurons which synthesize vasopressin contain granules showing a glycopeptide halo just beneath their membrane, whereas those that synthesize oxytocin do not have this feature. One might think the glycosidic material is bound in some manner to the hormone - at least for vasopressin - because it disappears after dehydration, as does the neurosecretory substance. However, JONES and SWANN (1974) have shown that the glycoprotein isolated from rat neurosecretory granules is distinct from both neurophysin and hormone, which are known to have a nonglycosidic composition.

In summary, our results demonstrate that the neurosecretory pathway of rats and hamsters contains sialic acid located inside the elementary granules, probably attached to the inner face of their membrane, and therefore transported from perikarya to nerve endings. In this view, there is no contradiction between these observations and what is known about the biochemical composition of the granules' content.

References

GABE, M.: Présence de glucides décelables par la réaction à l'acide periodique-Schiff dans le produit de neurosécrétion hypothalamique chez quelques vertébrés. C. R. Acad. Sci. (D) (Paris) 250, 937-939 (1960)
GABE, M.: Neurosécrétion. Paris: Gauthier-Villars 1967, p. 1091
HOLWERDA, D.A.: A glycopeptide from the posterior lobe of pig pituitaries. I. Isolation and characterization. Eur. J. Biochem. 28, 334-339 (1972a)
HOLWERDA, D.A.: A glycopeptide from the posterior lobe of pig pituitaries. II. Primary structure. Eur. J. Biochem. 28, 340-346 (1972b)
HOWE, A., PEARSE, A.G.E.: A histochemical investigation of neurosecretory substance in the rat. J. Histochem. Cytochem. 4, 561-569 (1956)
JONES, C.W., SWANN, R.W.: A glycoprotein in the neurosecretory granules of neurohypophysis. J. Physiol. (Lond.) 245, 45 (1974)
SCHIEBLER, H.T.: Die chemischen Eigenschaften der neurosekretorischen Substanz in Hypothalamus und Neurohypophyse. Exp. Cell Res. 3, 249-250 (1952)
TASSO, F.: Localisation cytochimique ultrastructurale de glycoprotéines dans les granules neurosécrétoires de la posthypophyse. J. Microsc. (Paris) 18, 115-118 (1973)

TASSO, F., RUA, S.: Étude cytochimique ultrastructurale des glycoprotéines dans le complexe hypothalamo-post-hypophysaire du rat. Arch. Anat. Microsc. Morphol. Exp. 64, 247-260 (1975)
THIÉRY, J.P.: Mise en évidence des polysaccharides sur coupes fines en microscopie électronique. J. Microscop. (Paris) 6, 987-1018 (1967)
VILTER, V., TREMBLAY, P., CHARTON, G.: Recherches histospectrophotométrique sur la métachromasie bathochrome de la pseudo-isocyanine. C. R. Soc. Biol. (Paris) 167, 406-411 (1973)

Functional Morphology of the Synaptic Apparatus of Peptidergic Neurosecretory Cells in the Nucleus praeopticus of Carp *Cyprinus carpio* L.

L. T. PLUZHNIKOV, YU. I. SENCHIK, and A. L. POLENOV
Laboratory of Neuroendocrinology, Sechenov Institute of Evolutionary Physiology and Biochemistry of the Academy of Sciences of the USSR, Leningrad, USSR

Electron-microscopic observations of the nucleus praeopticus (NP) of Teleostei have revealed two main types of synaptic boutons (SB) on the perikarya and the processes of the neurosecretory cells (NSC). Type-I SB contain synaptic vesicles (SV) and small (60-110 nm) dense-core vesicles, while type-II SB possess only SV (FOLLENIUS, 1963; WEISS, 1970; EKENGREN, 1973). It was supposed that axons forming type-I SB belong to monoaminergic neurons (BAUMGARTEN and BRAAK, 1967). The origin of type-II SB is not yet clear.

The ultrastructure, arrangement, and distribution of SB on the perikarya, and the processes of the NSC of the NP in adult carp under normal and experimental conditions have been studied. The carp is most convenient for the purpose of this investigation because polarity in the arrangement of the NP cells of different sizes is pronounced in this fish: small poorly differntiated NSC occur in the ventral zone and highly differentiated large and "aged" NSC are seen in the dorsal zone (POLENOV, 1954).

Four adult female carp sacrificed in winter were examined. The neurosecretory material is accumulated by the NSC of the NP at this time of year (POLENOV, 1959).

The two types of SB described in other species exist also in the carp. To elucidate the functional state of the synaptic apparatus of the NP, SB were classified into subtypes, according to the content of SV and their ratio to the dense-core vesicles. Thus, type-I SB were subdivided into five subtypes. In intact fish, Ia SB comprise 15.2%; Ib, 27.2%, Ic, 17.8%; Id, 10.5%; Ie, 1.6%. Comparing our data with those of SENCHIK and PISUGIN on mammals (1974) we have come to the conclusion that subtypes Ia and Ib (a small number of SV and dense-core vesicles) represent a state of moderate activity, subtype Ic (a large number of SV and a small number of dense-core vesicles) are functionally most active, subtype Id (a large content of dense-core vesicles) are in a state of accumulating a neurotransmitter, and subtype Ie (presence of degenerating structures) demonstrates degeneration of organelles and, possibly, of the nerve ending itself (Fig. 1).

Our results show that type-I SB (72.3%) predominate in the NP. They are most frequent on the small NSC of the NP ventral zone. Type-II SB are less numerous (27.7%; IIa, 14.1%; IIb, 13.6%) and are seen on the large NSC of the dorsal zone of the NP, which suggests a high functional activity of the large NSC. Distribution of the SB in the neuropil in the zones of the NP is similar to that on the NSC perikarya in the initial parts of their pro-

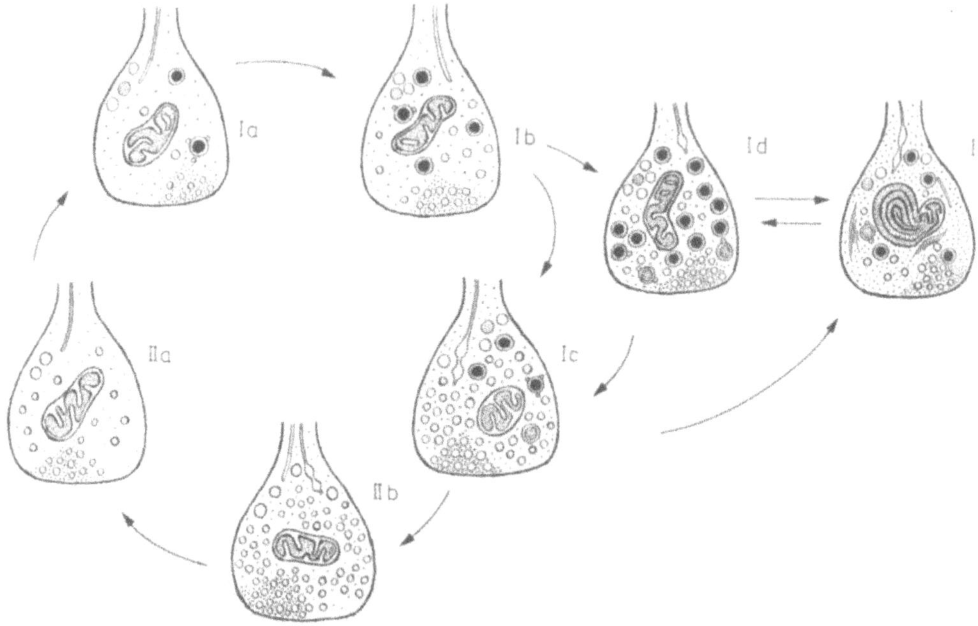

Fig. 1. Morphofunctional types of SB of a monoaminergic nature on NSC of carp NP. Types *Ia* and *Ib* reflect state of moderate activity; type *Ic* - high activity, *Id* - accumulation of neurotransmitter, *Ie* - degeneration of organelles, type *IIa* - state of exhaustion after release of neurotransmitter, type *IIb* maximum activity

cesses. Moderately active SB prevail on the NSC in both zones. This observation correlates with the state of moderate activity of neurosecretory processes in the NP in winter (POLENOV, 1959; POLENOV et al., 1973).

Density of SB on the NSC perikarya is inversely proportional to the size of the NSC, being ~ 1.7 ± 0.2 SB on a profile of a small, 1.4 ± 0.2 - of a medium-size, and 1.0 ± 0.1 - of a large NSC ($P = 0.05$). SB are especially numerous on the initial parts of the processes of the large cells. The latter have more processes than the small NSC. Thus, SB are more numerous on the large NSC than on the small ones.

Four tentative types of relationships between the surface of SB with that of the NSC are distinguished. The axosomatic-type SB are seen: (1) on the smooth surface of the plasmalemma, (2) in invaginations, (3) on evaginations of the plasmalemma, and (4) on the axodendritic-type SB in the initial parts of the processes (Fig. 2). Sometimes SB occur among accumulations of cilia in deep invaginations of the plasmalemma of the large NSC (Fig. 3). This complex seems to represent a peculiar receptor apparatus of the cell (PLUZHNIKOV and SENCHIK, 1975). As it is shown in Figure 2, the number of SB on the processes of the NSC as well as in the invaginations and evaginations of the plasmalemma of the perikarya tend to increase from the small to the

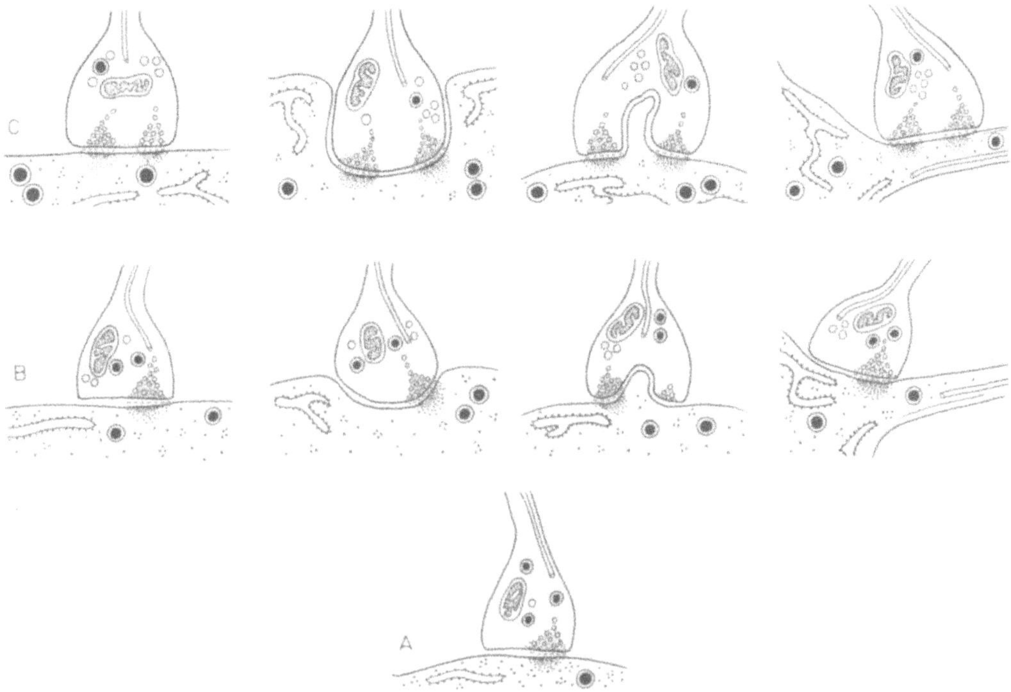

Fig. 2. Relations of SB with surface of perikarya and processes of (A) small, (B) medium-sized, and (C) large NSC of carp NP

large NSC. This complication of relations between the surfaces of the NSC and SB reflect a different degree of differentiation of the NSC as well as intensification of their functional activity (SENCHIK et al., 1976).

Type-I SB seem to be monoaminergic in nature. It is quite possible that type-II SB are also monoaminergic and that their morphology reflects active discharge of monoamines (Fig. 1). Alternatively, the plane of the profiles may not display the dense-core vesicles. However, the possibility of a cholinergic character of these SB cannot be excluded. Thus, morphologic observations of the synaptic apparatus of the NP in normal carp are not sufficient to give any definitive answer concerning the innervation of these NSC.

To examine this question, nialamid was injected into three sexually mature female carp. Two hours after the first intramuscular injection of nialamid (300 mg/kg) the number of dense-core vesicles in the SB on the processes of the NSC increases significantly (Fig. 3). Type-II SB practically disappear (only 0.1% persist). The number of subtype-Ia SB increases up to 40.8%, that of subtype 1d and 1e up to 24.8% and 4.1%, respectively; that of 1b decreases by a factor of 2. Similar changes are seen in the neuropil. These results agree with the increased green monoamine fluorescence of the neuropil around the NSC perikarya

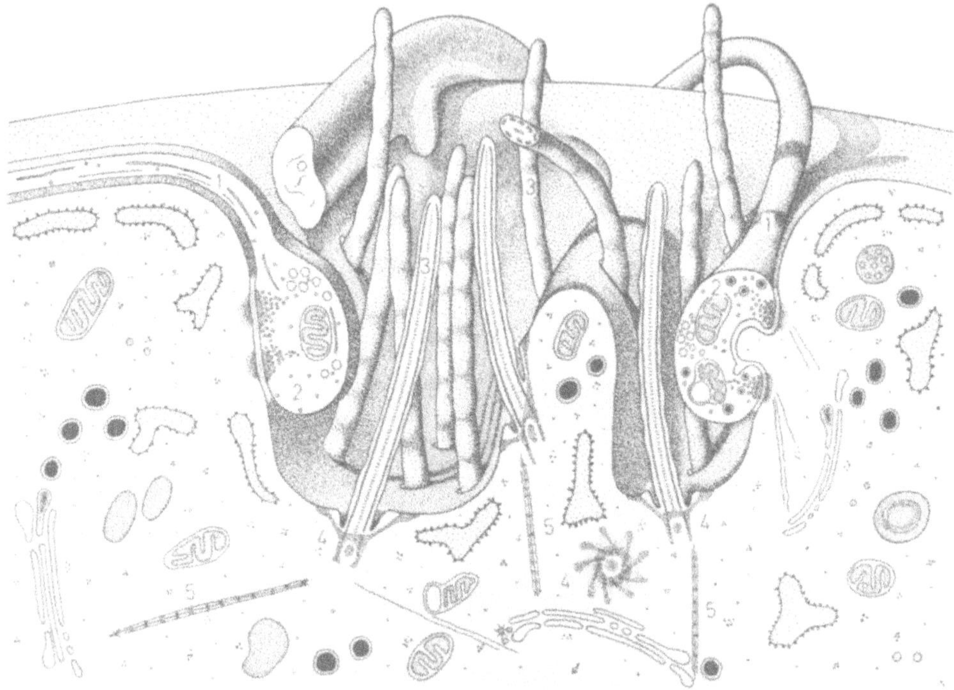

Fig. 3. Complicated "receptor apparatus" on perikaryon of a large highly differentiated NSC. *1*, afferent fibers; *2*, synaptic boutons (SB); *3*, cilia; *4*, basal bodies; *5*, rootlets

(ZAMBRANO, 1968). The number of neurosecretory granules decreases markedly in the perikarya and in the initial parts of the NSC processes. This seems to be due to their evacuation into the axons. Thus, the quantity of type-II SB in intact fish represent a degree of inhibition of the transport of secretory material from the NSC perikarya to the processes.

On the basis of the present data it is concluded: (1) Development of the synaptic apparatus is due to growth and differentiation of the NSC of the NP in the adult carp; (2) The synaptic apparatus is moderately active in carp during the winter; (3) The synaptic apparatus on the large NSC of the dorsal zone is in a more active state than that on the small NSC of the ventral zone; (4) The NSC of the NP of the carp receive predominantly, and perhaps exclusively, adrenergic innervation that seems to be responsible for inhibition of release of neurosecretory granules from the perikarya.

References

BAUMGARTEN, H.G., BRAAK, H.: Catecholamines im Hypothalamus vom Goldfisch *(Carassius auratus)*. Z. Zellforsch. 80, 248-263 (1967)

EKENGREN, B.: The nucleus preopticus and nucleus lateralis tuberis in the roach, *Leuciscus rutilus*. Z. Zellforsch. 140, 369-388 (1973)

FOLLENIUS, E.: Etude comparative de la cytologie fine du noyau préoptique (NPo) et du noyau latéral du tuber (Nlt) chez la truite *(Salmo irideus* Gibb.) et chez la perche *(Perca fluviatilis)*. Comparaison des deux types de neurosécrétion. Gen. Comp. Endocrinol. 3, 66-85 (1963)

PLUZHNIKOV, L.T., SENCHIK, Yu.I.: Morpho-functional types of synapses in the neurosecretory cells of the Nucleus preopticus in *Cyprinus carpio* L. Tsitologiya (Leningrad) 17, 891-897 (1975)

POLENOV, A.L.: On physiological degeneration and restoration of the neurosecretory cells of the Nucleus praeopticus in sazan and the mirror carp. Dokl. Akad. Nauk SSSR 99, 625-628 (1954)

POLENOV, A.L.: The preoptico-hypophysial Gomori-positive neurosecretory system of sazan and the mirror carp. Dokl. Akad. Nauk SSSR 129, 1413-1416, (1959)

POLENOV, A.L., PLUZHNIKOV, L.T., SENCHIK, Yu.I.: Ultrastructure of neurosecretory cells of the Nucleus praeopticus in *Cyprinus carpio* L. before and during spawning. Paper Abstracts, IV European Ichthyological Congress, p. 119. Sarajevo 1973

SENCHIK, Yu.I., PISUGIN, I.I.: Functional morphology of synapses on the neurosecretory cells of the Nucleus supraopticus in the white rat. In: Proc. I All-Union Conference on Neuroendocrinology. POLENOV, A.L. (ed.). Leningrad 1974, pp. 159-160

SENCHIK, Yu.I., PLUZHNIKOV, L.T., POLENOV, A.L.: Peculiarities of the ultrastructure and distribution of synapses on the neurosecretory cells of different size of the Nucleus preopticus in *Cyprinus carpio* L. Tsitologiya (Leningrad) 18, 275-283 (1976)

WEISS, I.: Saisonale Veränderungen des Enzymmusters and des Neurosekretgehaltes sowie die Innervation des Nucleus praeopticus der Bachforelle (*Salmo trutte* Fario) unter besonderer Berücksichtigung der hypothalamischen Hydrencephalokrinie. Morphol. Jahrbuch 115, 444-486 (1970)

ZAMBRANO, D.: The effect of nialamide and L-dopa on the synaptic endings of the neurosecretory neurons of the supraoptic nucleus of the rat. Neuroendocrinol. 3, 99-106 (1968)

Seasonal Dynamics of the Activity of the Hypothalamo-Pituitary Neurosecretory System, Thyroid and Adrenal Cortex in Lemmings (*Dicrostonyx torquatus* Vinogradovi Ognev, 1948)

T. V. POPOVICH, A. V. TKACHEV, and A. A. ARDASHEV
Institute of Arctic Biology FESC AS USSR, Magadan, USSR

The seasonal changes in the activity of endocrine glands seem to play an important role in the ecology of lemmings. Some aspects of special interest are: (1) topography of the hypothalamus and its structure, (2) neurosecretory activity of the nucleus supraopticus (NSO), n. paraventricularis (NPV) and n. postopticus (NPO) evaluated by cytophotometry, (3) the structure and function of the thyroid gland, (4) the level of 11-hydroxysteroids (11-OCS) in the blood as an index of adrenal function.

It was found that the NSO in lemmings is located in a more dorsocaudal position while the NPV is located in a more dorsal position than the comparable structures in albino rats. In *Dicrostonyx torquatus* these differences were more distinct than in *Lemmus obensis*.

The hypothalamus of both lemmings contains additional groups of neurosecretory cells, and the number of cells comprising these groups is greater than that observed in other species of rodents. Extrahypothalamic pathways are well-formed in lemmings.

It was found that functional activity of hypothalamic nuclei has biphasic fluctuations. The first coincides with the period of reproduction of the animals. The volume of cells, nuclei, and nucleoli is increased. The relative number of degenerating cells is increased and the quantity of neurosecretion in that system decreases. The second phase of increased activity of the hypothalamo-hypophyseal neurosecretory system (HHNS) in *D. torquatus* was observed in late July and early August, at the time of reduced reproductive activity. Unlike the first phase, the increased activity of HHNS during the second phase is not accompanied by a decrease of neurosecretory substances in the cells. Inhibition of the release of neurosecretory substance may account for these findings of HHNS activity in lemmings, and this may be caused by shedding of hair and by increasing aggressivity of these animals during autumnal migration.

The dynamics of neurosecretory activity in *L. obensis* is generally the same as in *D. torquatus*, although the time sequences are different. These differences may be attributed to the fact that reproduction in these species begins at different times.

In addition to the magnocellular nuclei, we have studied the changes in the n. arcuatus, which is known to be very important in the regulation of sex function. The greatest activity in these nuclei was found in June, both in *D. torquatus* and *L. obensis* males. This activity coincides with maximum reproductive activity. When reproductive activity is decreased, the neurosecretory activity of n. arcuatus in males also decreases. It does not increase even in autumn, when the activity of the hypothalamus increases.

In females, the changes of neurosecretory activity in n. arcuatus, as in magnocellular neurosecretory nuclei, also exhibit a biphasic character determined by seasonal factors. This activity does not depend upon the stage of the estrus cycle, and maximum activity was observed in late July and in the first 10 days of August. In pregnant and lactating females, the neurosecretory activity of n. arcuatus from July until mid-August gradually increases in a linear manner. The highest activity was observed in the second half of August.

These data indicate that the n. arcuatus takes part in a feedback mechanism of the hypothalamo-hypophyseal-gonadal system. Together with magnocellular peptide neurosecretion of the hypothalamus, it plays an important role in the adaptive reaction to environmental conditions.

The absolute and relative weight of the thyroid gland in *D. torquatus* is greatly increased at the onset of reproductive activity; it then slowly decreases. The structure of the thyroid is, as a rule, quite stable up to the time of reproduction. When the sexual activity of these animals increases, the morphology of the gland changes considerably. The epithelial wall of the follicles thickens, with evidence of papillary hyperplasia. Later, desquamation of epithelial cells into the follicular space occurs. At the time of greatest sexual activity in these animals the gland actually loses its follicular structure. Only stroma, with extensive spaces filled with colloid and desquamated epithelial cells, is observed. When the reproductive period is completed, the thyroid parenchyma and follicular walls are partially restored. The newly formed follicles have a hypoplastic appearance, indicating the weak function of that gland.

All these data show that stimulation of neurosecretory processes and gonadotrophic function at the time of reproduction is accompanied by exhaustion of hormonal activity of the thyroid gland. It was also found that the weight of the adrenal glands and the quantity of 11-hydroxycorticosteroids in the blood greatly increased at the time of reproduction in these species. When the sexual activity of lemmings decreased, the weight of the adrenals and level of their hormones also decreased.

These findings suggest that seasonal changes in endocrine function in *D. torquatus* and *L. obensis* are determined by a number of factors, including the rate of reproduction, density of population, and perhaps by climatic factors.

Reaction of Magnocellular Hypothalamic Nuclei to Unilateral and Full Thyroidectomy During Early Ontogenesis

A. N. PTITSA and M. A. STEZENKO
Kiev State University, Kiev, USSR

It was determined that compensatory hypertrophy of the thyroid gland shows itself 3-7 days after unilateral thyroidectomy of ducklings, irrespective of their age (ducklings at the ages of 1 day, 1 month, and 3 months were examined). This process is followed by distinct alterations in the hypothalamo-hypophyseal system, showing themselves in increased secretory and excretory activity of neurons of the paraventricular nucleus and of thyrotrophs of the hypophysis. The response of the neurosecretory system to unilateral and full thyroidectomy was also investigated in the embryo of rabbits operated during the 21st day of their development. It was found that within 3 days after unilateral thyroidectomy the embryos showed both an increase in the height of secretory epithelium and the formation of resorptional vacuoles in thyroid-gland follicles, together with a response of the neurosecretory system to the experimental procedure. Nuclei of neurons in the supraoptic nucleus increase in size from 6.7 μm to 8.1 μm; those in the paraventricular nucleus increase from 6.8 to 8.2 μm. Bilateral thyroidectomy causes constantly increasing activation of magnocellular hypothalamic nuclei. In the median eminence and in the neural lobe of the hypophysis, the accumulation of neurosecretory material at unilateral and full thyroidectomy is formed 5 days earlier than in normal embryos. The data allow us to conclude that the neurosecretory system of rabbits even in embryo reacts distinctly to changes in the quantity of circulating thyroid hormones.

Effect of Intracranial Hypertension on Glycogen Accumulation in the Neurohypophysis

Z. M. RAP
Department of Neuropathology, Medical Research Center, Pol. Acad. Sci., Warsaw, Poland

Comparative histochemical and electron-microscopic studies were performed on the effect of intracranial hypertension on glycogen accumulation in the neurohypophysis of human beings and animals. Increased intracranial pressure in humans was evoked by spontaneous cerebrosubarachnoid hemorrhage, and in animals (rabbits, cats, dogs) it was produced experimentally by injection of blood into the subarachnoid space and by cerebral compression. In all cases, but particularly in subarachnoid hemorrhage, an increase of glycogen in the neurohypophysis was observed. Grains of glycogen were found disseminated and in compact aggregates - resembling Herring bodies - in the neuropil of the median eminence, stalk and the neural lobe of the hypophysis. Electron-microscopic studies showed the presence of glycogen in neurosecretory axons. Sometimes glycogen grains completely filled the enlargements of the axons (in animals) or accompanied residual fragments of neurosecretory axons in phagocytic forms of pituicytes (in human beings). The occurrence of glycogen in the neurosecretory system was probably the result of ischemic changes and damage to the CSF barrier.

References

RAP, Z.M., SZUMAŃSKA, G., GAJKOWSKA, B.: Neuropatol. Pol. 13, 33-47 (1975)

RAP, Z.M., STASZEWSKA-BARCZAK, J.: VIIth Internat. Congr. of Neuropathology. Budapest, Hungary, 1-7 Sept. 1974; Exc. Med. Amsterdam, Akad. Kiado Budapest, 623-626 (1975)

STERBA, G., BRÜCKNER, G.: Z. Zellforsch. Mikrosk. Anat. 93, 74-83 (1969)

WOLF, H.: Z. Zellforsch. Mikrosk. Anat. 88, 228-261 (1968)

Significance of the Mediobasal Hypothalamus in Regulation of Gonadal Functions in Birds

L. M. RUDNEVA and B. G. NOVIKOV
Kiev State University, Kiev, USSR

We have investigated the influence of implantation of estradiol, testosterone, and actinomycin-D into the mediobasal hypothalamus (MBH) of Peking ducks in their reproductive phase, on the functional state of testes and ovaries, on egg-laying, and on the content of folliculotropin (FSH) and luteotropin (LH) in the blood plasma. In birds with estradiol and actinomycin-D implanted into the MBH, egg-laying ceased completely 3 days after the operation and the gonads were reduced in size. The testes of drakes became inactive as a result of testosterone implantation. Small cannulae were localized either in the arcuate nucleus or terminating in the cavity of the third ventricle. The development of glial elements inside the cannulae confirmed the presence of a contact between the hormone and the tissues. The functional activity of follicle-stimulating and luteinizing gonadotropocytes decreased considerably under the influence of implantation of sexual steroids into the MBH. Under the effect of estradiol or actinomycin-D implantation into the arcuate region, the content of FSH in the blood plasma decreased four- and seven-fold respectively. After the implantation of testosterone-8 the content of LH in the plasma decreased 6, 8, and 8.5 times, respectively. No appreciable changes were seen in the structures of gonadotropocytes or in the level of gonadotropic hormones in the blood plasma after implantation of the substances mentioned above into the rear part of the hypothalamus or after implanting empty cannulae into the MBH. These data confirm our previously obtained data concerning the participation of the arcuate hypothalamic region in the regulation of reproductive function in birds.

Autoradiographic Localization of ^{3}H-Oxytocin in the Rat Brain

H.-J. RÜHLE and A. ERMISCH
Section of Biosciences, Karl Marx University, Leipzig, GDR

Labeled oxytocin and labeled vasopressin, injected into the general circulation, cross the blood-brain barrier (AROSKAR et al., 1964; WILLUMSEN and BIE, 1969; ÅGMO, 1974; STIBAL et al., 1974). In these studies radioactivity was detected in the brain by liquid-scintillation counting. Using this method, only approximate statements of the topographic distribution of the label are possible. Microautoradiographic methods ensure a more exact localization of accumulated tissue radioactivity. Thus SOLOFF et al. (1975) showed in vitro the localization of ^{3}H-oxytocin radioactivity in the rat mammary gland and oviduct. We tried to investigate autoradiographically the distribution of radioactivity in the rat brain following systemic administration of ^{3}H-labeled oxytocin.

Urethane-anesthetized male Wistar rats were injected with 0.1 mCi ^{3}H-tyrosyl-oxytocin (1.2 Ci/mmol) (prepared by Dr. I. MEZÖ of the Semmelweis University, Budapest). Four animals received the hormone intravenously and were killed after 90 s. For comparison, three animals received intracarotid injections, with a survival time of 15 s. The autoradiographs were prepared using a thaw-mount technique (STUMPF, 1971). The exposure time was between 7 and 13 months. The autoradiographs were evaluated quantitatively by grain counting over selected brain areas. The silver grains were counted in each brain region over not less than 10,000 μm^2.

The autoradiographs of the brain cross sections showed a heterogeneous distribution of silver grains. The grain concentrations were highest over the lumina of brain blood vessels (Fig. 1a), over the meninges and the choroid plexus. The radioactive material had obviously also crossed the blood-brain barrier as it was accumulated in the brain parenchyma. The largest number of silver grains, however, was localized over the circumventricular organs lacking a well-developed blood-brain barrier. The heaviest labeling was observed in the pineal gland (Fig. 1b), followed by the subfornical organ, the vascular organ of the lamina terminalis, the median eminence, and the neurohypophysis. Furthermore, besides the generalized nonspecific distribution of silver grains, single neurons in the median eminence, probably arising in the arcuate nucleus, were constantly observed to concentrate the radioactive material. Surprisingly, a high concentration of radioactivity was found also in the arcuate nucleus (Fig. 1c), although this region has, to our knowledge, a tight blood-brain barrier. The arcuate nucleus thus stands in contrast to other hypothalamic nuclei, including the magnocellular supraoptic and paraventricular nuclei, the grain density over which is significantly lower (Fig. 1d). Moreover, it was observed throughout the brain that groups of glia-like cells, mostly adjacent to a

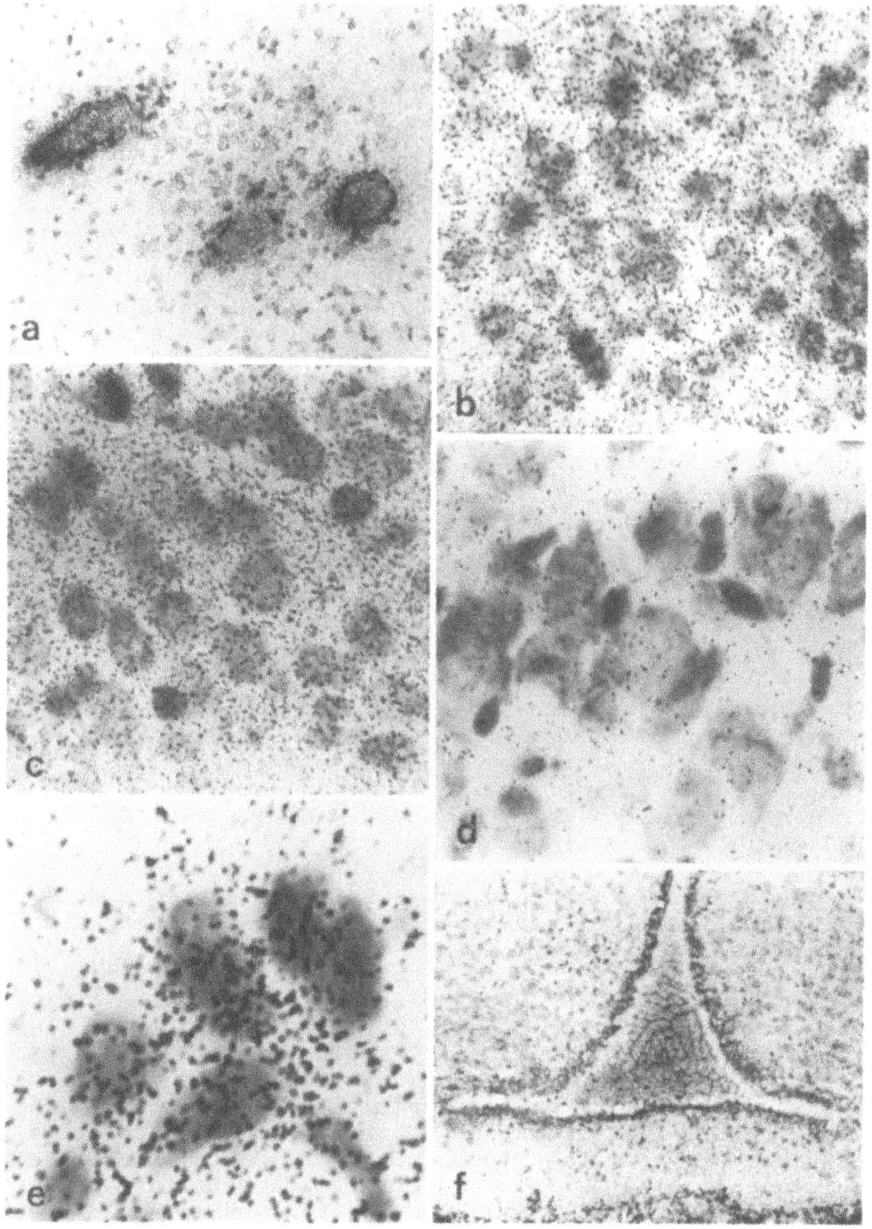

Fig. 1a-f. Autoradiographs of different regions of rat brain, stained with toluidine blue. (a) Heavily labeled lumina of blood vessels in the region of the interpeduncular nucleus. (b) Labeled parenchyma of the pineal body. (c) High grain density over the arcuate nucleus. (d) Sparsely scattered grains over cells of paraventricular nucleus. Grain density over most brain areas was of the same magnitude. (e) Hypothalamic group of labeled glial cells. (f) Strong labeling of CSF in the infundibular recess

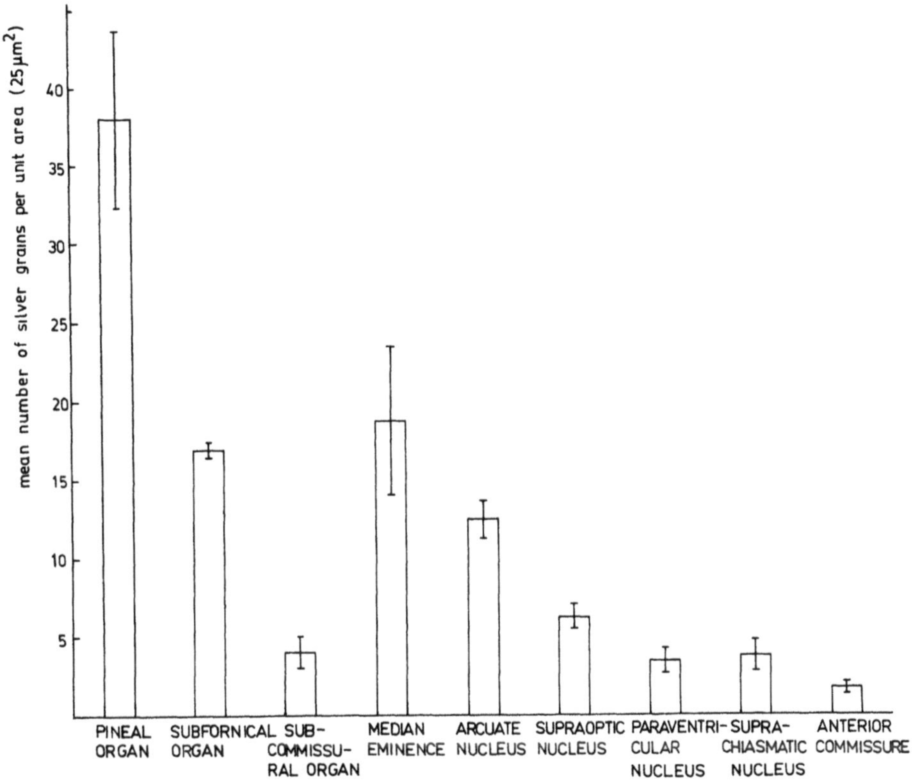

Fig. 2. Uptake of radioactivity by different brain regions of rat 90 s after intravenous injection of 0.1 mCi (35.8 IU) ^{3}H-tyrosyl-oxytocin, n = 4

vessel, are able to concentrate the radioactive material (Fig. 1e). Another interesting observation concerns the high concentration of radioactivity found in the ventricular cavities (Fig. 1f). Particularly after intracarotid injections, the CSF was almost as heavily labeled as the blood.

Figure 2 presents the results of grain counts over selected brain areas of the four animals that received the labeled oxytocin intravenously. Pineal gland, subfornical organ, and median eminence, i.e., the circumventricular organs lacking a blood-brain barrier, showed the highest concentrations of radioactive label. However, the subcommissural organ, with its functioning blood-brain barrier, the hypothalamic supraoptic, paraventricular, and suprachiasmatic nuclei, and the anterior commissure are in striking contrast to them. On the other hand, the arcuate nucleus can be regarded as an exception because it was heavily loaded with the radioactive label and did not, in spite of its blood-brain barrier, differ significantly from the median eminence, which is outside the barrier.

No firm conclusions can be made about the nature of the radioactivity. During the process of enzymatic breakdown of oxytocin the tyrosine residue, carrying the label of the oxytocin molecule used in our experiments, may be set free soon after the beginning of the step-by-step degradation of the molecule (WALTER, 1974). Therefore, we were comparing the distribution of radioactivity from ^{3}H-oxytocin with that from ^{3}H-tyrosine administered under the same conditions. The comparison revealed a different uptake pattern for both labeled molecules. Thus, we suggest that the labeled oxytocin underwent no profound metabolic changes; the possibility cannot be excluded that the autoradiographically detected radioactivity is, at least in part, still associated with the intact hormone molecule, especially after the very short survival time of only 15 s.

Summarizing the results of the present investigation, we should like to emphasize that in the rat we have been able to show, by means of autoradiography, that the radioactive label originating from ^{3}H-oxytocin, injected into the circulation, actually enters the brain tissue and the CSF. The tissue radioactivity was highest in structures lacking the blood-brain barrier, but the label was also heavily accumulated in the hypothalamic arcuate nucleus. Besides the presence of labeled single neurons, showing a specific cellular uptake of the tracer, the grain density over this nucleus attained two to four times the level found in other hypothalamic areas including the magnocellular neurosecretory nuclei. There appears to be no correlation between the degree of vascularization of the above-mentioned brain nuclei and the extent of their labeling. Therefore, it may be assumed that the arcuate nucleus might be a specific target for the intracerebral action of oxytocin, and that a direct feedback relation between oxytocin and the neurons synthesizing it apparently does not exist.

References

ÅGMO, A.: Uptake of iodinated oxytocin by some tissues and organs in the male rat. Acta Physiol. Scand. 91, 330-338 (1974)

AROSKAR, J.P., CHAN, W.Y., STOUFFER, J.E., SCHNEIDER, C.H., MURTI, V.V.S., VIGNEAUD, V. DU: Renal excretion and tissue distribution of radioactivity after administration of tritium-labeled oxytocin to rats. Endocrinology 74, 226-232 (1964)

SOLOFF, M.S., REES, H.D., SAR, M.: STUMPF, W.E.: Autoradiographic localization of radioactivity from [^{3}H]oxytocin in the rat mammary gland and oviduct. Endocrinology 96, 1475-1477 (1975)

STIBAL, S., BIGL, H., STERBA, G.: Bestimmung der Radioaktivität nach intravenöser Injektion von H^{3}-markiertem Oxytocin im Hirn der Ratte. Endokrinologie 63, 33-42 (1974)

STUMPF, W.E.: Autoradiographic techniques for the localization of hormones and drugs at the cellular and subcellular level. Acta Endocrinol. (Suppl.) (Kbh.) 153, 205-222 (1971)

WALTER, R.: Oxytocin and other peptide hormones as prohormones. In: Psychoneuroendocrinology. Workshop Conf. Int. Soc. Psychoneuroendocrinology, Mieken 1973. HATOTANI, N. (ed.). Basle: S. Karger 1974, pp. 285-294

WILLUMSEN, N.B.S., BIE, P.: Tissue to plasma radioactivity in the rat hypothalamo-hypophyseal system after intravenous injection of ^{3}H-lysine^{8}-vasopressin and ^{3}H-mannitol. Acta Endocrinol. (Kbh.) 60, 389-400 (1969)

Hypothalamo-Pituitary Neurosecretory System of Rats After a 22-Day Space Flight

E. A. SAVINA, V. K. PODYMOV, and E. I. ALEKSEEV
Academy of Medical Sciences, Moscow, USSR

The purpose of this investigation was to do a morphologic study of the hypothalamus-pituitary system of rats flown for 22 days on board the biosatellite "Cosmos-605." The animals were sacrificed 2 and 27 days postflight. The functional state of the hypothalamus-pituitary system was assessed by histologic, histochemical, and morphometric methods. On the 2nd postflight day, morphologic signs of an increase in the functional activity of neurons of the supraoptic nuclei of the hypothalamus were found. These comprise (1) increase in the nuclear volume and neuronal size, (2) decrease in the intensity of neuronal staining of chromatophilic substance, (3) uniform distribution of neurosecretory granules in the neuronal bodies, and (4) reduction of their content in axons at the level of the supraoptic nuclei and in terminals of the posterior pituitary. The lack of such changes in control rats not subjected to space flight suggests that they were induced by that flight, or were postflight responses of the hypothalamus-pituitary system. Two days seems to be a sufficient period of time for morphologic reactions to develop in response to the gravity change. The changes found in the hypothalamus-pituitary neurosecretory system of rats 2 days postflight are indicative of an increased production of ADH-vasopressin and are in agreement with the evidence on increased antidiuretic activity in the blood of cosmonauts during the 1st postflight day.

Hormonal Regulation of Catecholamine Metabolism in the Rat Brain

V. G. SCHALYAPINA, C. B. MILUSCHEVA and V. V. RAKITSKAYA
Pavlov Institute of Physiology of the USSR Academy of Science, Leningrad, USSR

A. Introduction

The central adrenergic system plays an important role in the release of corticotropin-releasing hormone (CRH; corticoliberin) and ACTH (FUXE et al., 1970; SCHALYAPINA and RAKITSKAYA, 1976). This system also participates in the transmission of nerve signals to the hypothalamus. The histochemical-fluorescence technique has revealed the presence of monoaminergic neurons and terminals in several hypothalamic areas. Corticosteroids penetrate and are bound in the hypothalamus, in the limbic system, and in the cortex. Their presence in the latter has an inhibitory effect on the pituitary-adrenal system either by modulation or by negative feedback. The mechanism of this effect is not yet clear.

It has been found that intraperitoneal injection of dexamethasone, hydrocortisone, or corticosterone into rats results in a decrease in the catecholamine level in the brain. This effect depends on inhibition of steroidogenesis rather than on the absolute level of corticosteroids (SCHALYAPINA, 1970). The brain catecholamine content decreased after bilateral adrenalectomy, provided it was accompanied by a disturbance in ionic and protein metabolism (RAKITSKYA and SCHALYAPINA, 1974). However, information on the mechanism of the corticosteroid effect on catecholamine metabolism is only fragmentary.

In the present work we analyzed the effect of hydrocortisone on the incorporation, synthesis, and release of catecholamines in the rat brain.

I. Effect of Hydrocortisone on L-Dopa Incorporation and Dopamine Synthesis in the Rat Brain

Levels of dopamine and dopa in rat brain 30 and 180 min after intraperitoneal injection of 5 mg/100 g L-dopa were higher, if simultaneously 1 mg/100 g hydrocortisone was administered. No significant changes in the noradrenaline concentration of the brain were observed. Hydrocortisone also was effective when administered before the L-dopa. If the hormone was injected three times in doses of 5 mg/100 g, 180 min after the last injection, the catecholamine content of the blood decreased. Finally, the concentration gradient of L-dopa and dopamine in the brain and blood increased. We believe that the uptake of L-dopa by the brain tissue is a major factor in the effects of hydrocortisone.

II. Effect of Hydrocortisone on the Incorporation, Synthesis, and Release of Catecholamines in Rat Brain Cortex Slices and Hypothalamus

Only recently has attention been given to the role of corticosteroids in the incorporation of catecholamines. The results reported by MAAS and MEDNIEKS (1971) have demonstrated that hydrocortisone increased incorporation of H^3-noradrenaline into cortex slices. In our experiments hydrocortisone (10^{-6} - 10^{-4} g/ml) inhibited the uptake of the H^3-noradrenaline by the cortex slices and hypothalamus. In other series of experiments the cortex slices and hypothalamus were first incubated in the medium with H^3-noradrenaline and after that in another medium containing hydrocortisone 10^{-4}- 10^{-6} g/ml. After this, the concentration of H^3-noradrenaline in the tissue was lower than in the control.

Synthesis of catecholamines from H^3-tyrosine by cortical slices and hypothalamus in rats was also studied. After 30 min of incubation, noradrenaline and dopamine content was determined by differentiation on Dowex-50 (MANUCHIN and PUSTOVOITOVA, 1969). No significant increase in concentration of catecholamines occurred after incubation of tissues with hydrocortisone alone, but when iproniazid was added to the medium with the hormone, the concentration of catecholamines increased. The data obtained demonstrate that corticosteroids have an inhibitory effect on the noradrenaline incorporation and a stimulatory effect on the release and synthesis of catecholamines in the adrenergic neurons.

III. Effect of Hydrocortisone on Catecholamine Fluorescence in the Hypothalamus

An increase in fluorescence of catecholamines in the lateral areas, and paraventricular and dorsomedial nuclei of the hypothalamus after intraperitoneal injection of L-dopa and hydrocortisone into rats was shown using a histochemical method (FALCK and OWMAN, 1965).

B. Conclusion

By analogy with its effect on peripheral organs (AVAKIAN and CALLINGHAM, 1968; LANDSBERG and AXELROD, 1968; WURTMAN and AXELROD, 1967) the participation of hydrocortisone in regulation of catecholamine metabolism in the brain might be suggested. It was established that the adrenocortical hormones influence catecholamine metabolism in the brain. Corticosteroids increased the incorporation of L-dopa and synthesis of catecholamine. Hormones inhibited uptake of noradrenaline and intensified the oxidative desamination of catecholamines. This effect may have a physiologically significant role in the regulation of the pituitary-adrenal system.

References

AVAKIAN, V.M., CALLINGHAM, B.O.: An effect of adrenalectomy upon catecholamine metabolism. Br. J. Pharmocol. 33, 211-215 (1968)

FALCK, B., OWMAN, Ch.: A detailed methodological description of the fluorescence method for the cellular demonstration of biogenic monoamines. Acta Univ. Lund II, 3-31 (1965)

FUXE, K., HÖKFELT, T., JONSSON, G.: Participation of central monaminergic neurones in the regulation of anterior pituitary secretion. In: Neurochemical Aspects of Hypothalamic Regulation, 1970

LANDSBERG, L., AXELROD, J.: Influence of pituitary, thyroid and adrenal hormones on norepinephrine turnover and metabolism in the rat heart. Circulat. Res. 22, 559-563 (1968)

MAAS, J., MEDNIEKS, M.: Hydrocortisone-mediated increase of norepinephrine uptake by brain slices. Science 171, 178-179 (1971)

MANUCHIN, B.N., PUSTOVOITOVA, Z.E.: Determination of adrenaline, noradrenaline, dopamine and dopa in tissues. Lab. Dela 2, 102-105 (1969)

RAKITSKAYA, V.V., SCHALYAPINA, V.G.: The noradrenaline content in the brain of adrenalectomized animals. Physiol. J. USSR 59, 1337-1339 (1973)

SCHALYAPINA, V.G.: Adrenal cortex hormones and brain catecholamines. In: Adrenal Cortex Hormones and the Central Nervous System, Leningrad, 1970

SCHALYAPINA, V.G., RAKITSKAYA, V.V.: Participation of brain monoamines in hypothalamic regulation of ACTH secretion. Usp. Physiol. Nauk. 7, 145-160 (1976)

WURTMAN, R., AXELROD, J.: Control of enzymatic synthesis of adrenaline. Inhibition of enzymatic synthesis of epinephrine by low doses of glucocorticoids. Endocrinology 80, 825-828 (1967)

Efferent Oxytocinergic Projections from the Hypothalamus to the Hindbrain in Rats and Pigeons

F. SCHOBER, W. NAUMANN, and G. STERBA
Section of Biosciences of the Karl Marx University Leipzig, GDR

It has been confirmed by fluorescence- and light-microscopic techniques that the neurosecretory system of the rat and the pigeon comprises exohypothalamic pathways besides the fibers of the hypothalamo-neurohypophyseal tract. The targets of the exohypothalamic pathways are the habenular region, the subfornical organ, and the reticular formation. We were able to demonstrate, by the immunohistochemical technique and by the pseudoisocyanine technique, that the hypothalamus-hindbrain connection known from lower vertebrates is also present in the pigeon and the rat. These fibers follow known pathways through the mesencephalic reticular formation to the hindbrain. Most of the fibers are found in the medial cuneate nucleus and in the gracile nucleus. Fewer fibers are seen in the lateral cuneate nucleus, in the nucleus solitarius and also in the area postrema. Using the electron microscope, the neurosecretory fibers in the dorsal-columns region are seen to contain neurophysin vesicles that are of the same type as the neurophysin vesicles of the classic neurosecretory system. First, the diameter of these vesicles ranged from 90 to 150 nm in the pigeon and from 130 to 200 nm in the rat. Secondly, using the method of NAUMANN and STERBA (1976) we were able to show that the content of these vesicles is indeed neurophysin. Furthermore, synaptic terminals of such oxytocinergic fibers were shown to exist.

Reference

NAUMANN, W., STERBA, G.: Ultrastructural Studies on Neurophysine-containing Vesicles of the Neurosecretory System of Vertebrates. Cell Tissue Res. 165, 545-553 (1976)

Changes in Hypothalamic Multiunit Activity After Hemorrhage in Anesthetized Rabbits

H. SCHULZ, H. SCHWARZBERG, and H. UNGER
Institute of Physiology, Medical Academy Magdeburg, GDR

Hemorrhage is a specific stimulus for release of antidiuretic factors into the blood or CSF (SCHRIER et al., 1968; VORHERR et al., 1968; ROCHA E SILVA and ROSENBERG, 1969; CLAYBAUGH and SHARE, 1973), and the neuronal activity of the paraventricular neurons is increased (WAKERLEY et al., 1975). The effect of hemorrhage on mean hypothalamic-neuronal activity of supraoptic (SON) and preoptic (POA) neurons was studied in anesthetized rabbits. A rapid hemorrhage of 15-20% of blood volume produced increased SON discharge, but generated an inhibition of POA activity. The neuronal-spike discharge in the lateral hypothalamic area (LHA) remained unchanged. The cortical EEG was desynchronized and showed a decreased amplitude.

The mean content of antidiuretic factors in the CSF in the same animals rose to 18.8 ± 3.8 µU/ml ($n = 8$) 15 min after bleeding, but in sham-operated animals the mean antidiuretic content in the CSF was 2.8 ± 1.1 µU/ml ($n = 8$). The differences between the two groups were highly significant ($p < 0.001$).

On the basis of these data and those of other investigators, it may be possible to explain the connection between increasing antidiuretic activity in the CSF and electrophysiologic alterations in the CNS.

References

CLAYBAUGH, J.R., SHARE, L.: Vasopressin, renin, and cardiovascular responses to continuous slow hemorrhage. Am. J. Physiol. 224, 519-523 (1973)

ROCHA E SILVA, M., ROSENBERG, M.: The release of vasopressin in response to hemorrhage and its role in the mechanism of blood pressure regulation. J. Physiol. (Lond.) 202, 535-557 (1969)

SCHRIER, R.W., VERROUST, P.J., JONES, J.J., FABIAN, M., LEE, J., DE WARDENER, H.E.: Effect of isotonic saline infusion and acute haemorrhage on plasma oxytocin and vasopressin concentrations in dogs. Clin. Sci. 35, 433-443 (1968)

VORHERR, H., BRADBURY, M.W.B., HOGHOUGHI, M., KLEEMAN, C.R.: Antidiuretic hormone in cerebrospinal fluid endogenous and exogenous changes in its blood level. Endocrinology 83, 246-250 (1968)

WAKERLEY, J.B., POULIN, D.A., DYBALL, R.E.J., CROSS, B.A.: Activity of phasic neurosecretory cells during haemorrhage. Nature 258, 82-84 (1975)

Effect of Intraventricular Administration of Oxytocin and Vasopressin on Self-stimulation and Reaction Time in Rats

H. SCHWARZBERG, G. HARTMANN, and G. TELEGDY
Institute of Physiology, Medical Academy, Magdeburg, GDR, and Institute of Physiology, Medical University, Pécs, Hungary

There is ample evidence that the neurohormones oxytocin and vasopressin may alter several functions of the CNS in mammals. The purpose of the experiments reported here was to administer oxytocin (500 μU) and vasopressin (50 μU) into the third brain ventricle of male rats, and to examine the effects on hypothalamic self-stimulation and reaction time of a *switch-off* response. The methods have been described previously (SCHWARZBERG and UNGER, 1970; SCHWARZBERG et al., 1976). Oxytocin injection increased the self-stimulation rate by 40.2% ± 12.3% (Student's t-test, $p < 0.02$ versus control), while vasopressin injection decreased it by 23.4% ± 8.1% (Student's t-test, $p < 0.05$ versus control) when tested 10-20 min following application.

Oxytocin showed a tendency to shorten reaction time (10.3% difference versus control, no significance), while vasopressin caused a longer reaction time (47.2% difference versus control, Wilcoxon's test, $\alpha = 0.025$) investigated 45 min after intraventricular injection. Our data demonstrated that intraventricular administration of oxytocin and vasopressin was able to influence different functions of the CNS. On the other hand, it has been found recently (SCHWARZBERG et al., 1977) that oxytocin and vasopressin levels are altered as a result of endogenous and exogenous factors (seasons, labor). Thus, a regulatory role of the neuropeptides in the CNS appears likely.

References

SCHWARZBERG, H., UNGER, H.: Änderung der Reaktionszeit von Ratten nach Applikation von Vasopressin, Oxytocin und Na-Thioglykolat. Acta Biol. Med. Germ. 24, 507-516 (1970)

SCHWARZBERG, H., HARTMANN, G., KOVÁCS, G.L., TELEGDY, G.: The effect of intraventricular administration of oxytocin and vasopressin on self-stimulation in rats. Acta Physiol. Acad. Sci. Hung., 1976 (in press)

SCHWARZBERG, H., MIEHLKE, B., SCHUTZ, H., UNGER, H.: Der Einfluß von Narkose, Jahreszeit und Geburtsvorgang auf die Oxytocinaktivität des Kaninchens, 1977 (in press)

Secretory Function of Neurons of the Suprachiasmatic Nucleus in the White Mouse and Rat

YU. I. SENCHIK, N. BOGDANOVIĆ-STOŠIĆ, and A. L. POLENOV
Sechenov Institute of Evolutionary Physiology and Biochemistry, Leningrad, USSR, and Institute of Biological Research, Belgrad, Yugoslavia

The suprachiasmatic nucleus (SCN) of adult male and female white mice and rats has been studied light- and electron-microscopically. Four types of neurons have been recognized in the SCN. Type-I neurons predominate in the SCN. They are very small, have a round and folded nucleus, one or two nucleoli, and a thin rim of cytoplasm. The latter contains numerous loosely arranged polysomes, free ribosomes, single narrow and short canaliculi of the rough endoplasmic reticulum (RER), poorly developed Golgi complex (GC), solitary lysosomes, and very rare small granules (d = 65-110 nm) resembling secretory granules. Type-II neurons are few and generally similar to those of type I. Unlike type-I neurons, however, those of type II contain a great number of larger secretory granules (d = 72-192 nm). Images of forming granules are frequent in the GC. Accumulations of the neurons are often seen near the capillaries, which are of the brain type. The neurons occur in female rats especially after opening of the vagina. Type-III neurons are rare and are seen in the periphery of the SCN. They are small, poor in cytoplasm, and contain few polysomes. Canaliculi of the RER are longer and more branched compared with those of type-I and -II neurons. The size and structure of the granules are similar to those of type-I neurons, the number of granules is about equal in both types. Type-IV neurons are rare and are observed mainly in the periphery of the SCN. They are markedly larger than those of types I-III. All their organelles are prominent. Canaliculi of the RER are concentrated in the periphery, and GC, mitochondria, and lysosomes are in the central zone of the cytoplasm. Small granules (d = 65-110 nm) are rare. Single cilia, basal bodies, rootlets, and synaptic boutons are often observed in the neurons of all four types. Oligodendrocytes and protoplasmic astrocytes are seen among the neurons. The SCN is poor in blood capillaries. Type-I and -II neurons are thought to be one functional type, producing a neurohumoral substance that is active in the regulation of reproduction.

Localization of LH-RH-containing Neurons in the Rabbit Brain

G. SÉTÁLÓ[1], B. FLERKÓ[1], S. VIGH[1], A. ARIMURA[2], A. V. SCHALLY[2,3]
[1]Department of Anatomy, Pécs University Medical School, 7643 Pécs, Hungary, [2]Department of Medicine, Tulane University School of Medicine, New Orleans, Lousiana 70112, USA and [3] Endocrine and Polypeptide Laboratories, Veterans Administration Hospital, New Orleans, Lousiana 70146, USA

In the last three years immunohistologic methods have successfully been used to localize the hypophysiotrophic (releasing and inhibiting) hormones. The first releasing hormone localized by immunohistologic methods in the guinea pig by LEONARDELLI et al. in 1973 was luteinizing hormone-releasing hormone (LH-RH). The species studied so far for the histologic localization of LH-RH include guinea pig, rat, mouse, duck, toad, cat, dog, and greenfinch (BARRY and CARETTE, 1975; SÉTÁLÓ, 1976).

With the use of rabbit anti-LH-RH serum, we described a system of delicate nerve fibers and terminals that contain immunoreactive LH-RH in the median eminence (SÉTÁLÓ et al., 1975), presuprachiasmatic area and periventricular gray matter (SÉTÁLÓ et al., 1976a), and in the organum vasculosum of the lamina terminalis (SÉTÁLÓ et al., 1976b) of rat. Preoptic-anterior hypothalamic localization of the LH-RH cells is characteristic for rat (SÉTÁLÓ, 1976a), guinea pig, and cat (LEONARDELLI et al., 1973). In dog, about 40% of the cells are found in the tuberal-premammillary regions, while in primates, the majority of LH-RH cells are found in these regions (BARRY and CARETTE, 1975). The other major difference between the species is that LH-RH perikarya are easily detected in dog, cat, and primates, whereas in rat and in guinea pig, stimulation of LH-RH synthesis and/or the blockage of its axoplasmic transport or release are required to locate the cells synthesizing the hormone. This finding suggested that in animals having a relatively short estrous cycle, LH-RH cells do not participate in the storage of the hormone. No data are available for rabbit, which in contrast to the former species, ovulates, i.e., releases an ovulatory dose of LH-RH, only in response to genital stimuli. It was reasonable to assume that in the absence of such stimuli relatively large amounts of LH-RH are stored in the system. Therefore, we studied mature virgin rabbits and rabbits mated within 1-48 h before fixation.

Rabbit antiserum generated against synthetic LH-RH adsorbed to polyvinylpyrrolidone (No. 422) was used for the study. Our observations are summarized in Figure 1. On the drawing (Fig. 1a) showing a paramedian-sagittal section of the rabbit brain, Roman numerals indicate the areas containing LH-RH positive neural elements. Perikarya containing LH-RH were detectable both in the suprachiasmatic (V-VIII) and tuberal (I-III) regions of virgin female rabbits. LH-RH positive fibers are easily found in the tuberoinfundibular (I,II) and praeoptico-infundibular (III-V) tract. In addition, a plexus of LH-RH fibers was found in the periventricular area (XIII) immediately under the ependymal layer, carrying axons, probably from the preoptic-suprachismatic

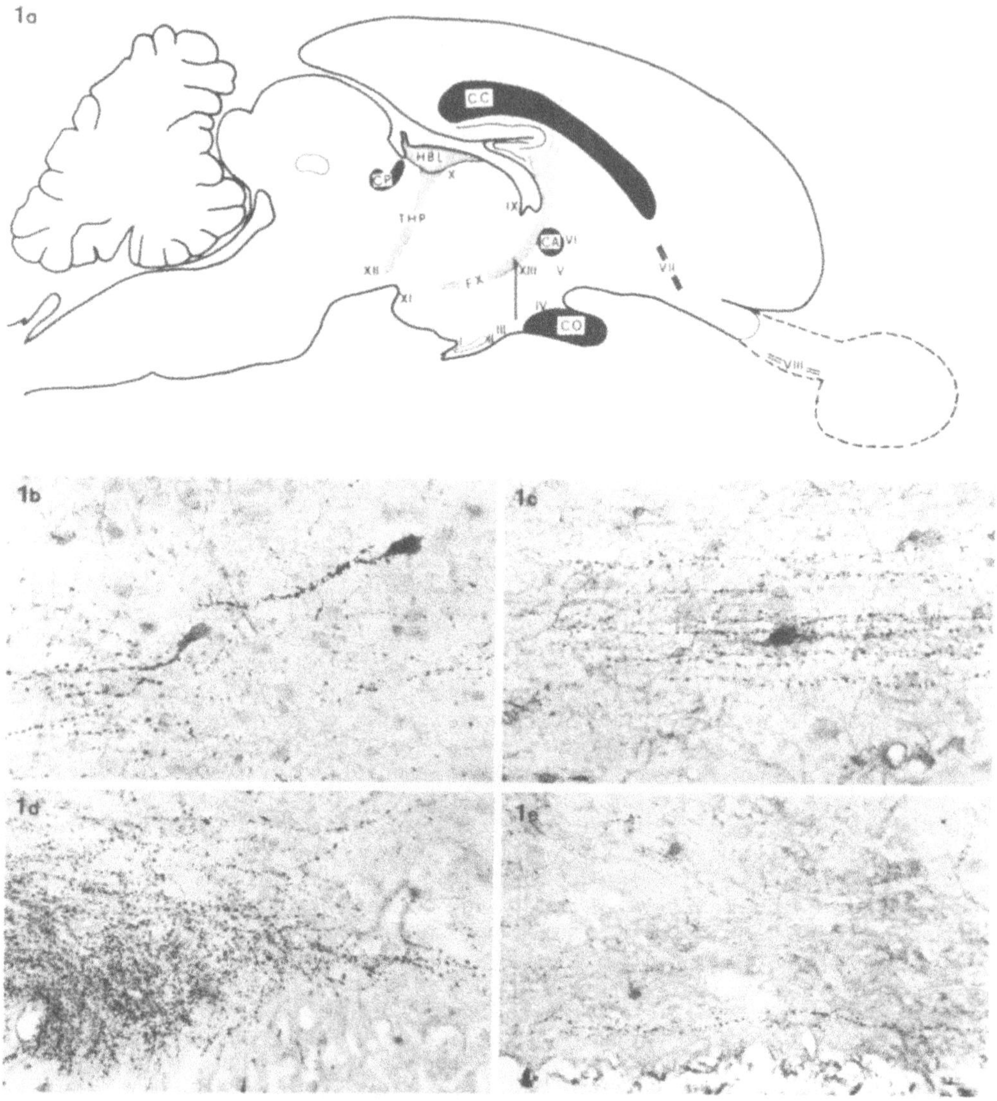

Fig. 1. (a) Schematic drawing of paramedian-sagittal section of rabbit brain. *CC* - corpus callosum, *CA* - commissura anterior, *CO* - chiasma opticum, *FX* - fornix, *HBL* - nucleus habenulae medialis, *THP* - tractus habenulopeduncularis. LH-RH perikarya and axons in area III (b) and VII (c). Sagittal sections from anterior part of median eminence of virgin (d) and mated (e) rabbit. N.B., many more axons are filled with LH-RH in virgin than in mated animals

area towards the median eminence. LH-RH axons were found in and behind the mammillary nuclei (XI), at the mesencephalic end of the tractus habenulopenduncularis (XII), in the medial habenular nucleus, around the emerging fibers of the habenulopeduncular tract (X), in the stria terminalis, and in the stria medullaris thalami (IX). An unusually compact tract of LH-RH axons was found in rabbit in the vicinity of the diagonal band of Broca

(VII, VIII). Among the fibers of this tract, LH-RH perikarya could also be detected. The fibers of this tract were followed towards the dorsal part of the septum pellucidum, where they intermingled with other fibers. The other end of this bundle was traced along the olfactory tract close to the ventral surface up to the olfactory bulb. Nothing definite can be said about the origin and destination of these extrahypothalamic fibers until experiments with lesions of these tracts are made. Although quantitative measurement of the LH-RH content of the brain was not performed, its amount seemed to be reduced shortly after copulation (Fig. 1d, e). LH-RH axons were only detected in the tuberal and habenular regions 1-48 h after copulation.

References

BARRY, J., CARETTE, B.: Immunofluorescence study of LRF neurons in primate. Cell Tissue Res. 164, 163-178 (1975)

BARRY, J., DUBOIS, M.P.: Immunofluorescence study of LRF-producing neurons in the cat and the dog. Neuroendocrinology 18, 290-298 (1975)

LEONARDELLI, J., BARRY, J., DUBOIS, M.-P.: Mise en évidence par immunofluorescence d'un constituant immunologiquement apparenté au LH-RF dans l'hypothalamus et l'éminence médiane chez les mammifères. C. R. Acad. Sci. (D) (Paris) 276, 2043-2046 (1973)

SÉTÁLÓ, G.: Anatomy, using new immunohistological methods. In: Proc. Fifth Int. Congr. of Endocrinology. Hamburg, July 18-24, 1976

SÉTÁLÓ, G., VIGH, S., SCHALLY, A.V., ARIMURA, A., FLERKÓ, B.: LH-RH containing neural elements in the rat hypothalamus. Endocrinology 96, 135-142 (1975)

SÉTÁLÓ, G., VIGH, S., SCHALLY, A.V., ARIMURA, A., FLERKÓ, B.: Immunohistological study of the origin of LH-RH-containing nerve fibers of the rat hypothalamus. Brain Res. 103, 597-602 (1976)

SÉTÁLÓ, G., VIGH, S., SCHALLY, A.V., ARIMURA, A., FLERKÓ, B.: Changing immunoreactivity of the LH-RH-containing nerve terminals in the organon vasculosum of the lamina terminalis. Acta Biol. Acad. Sci. Hung., 1976 (in press)

Seasonal Changes in the Structure of the Neurohypophysis and Thyroid Gland of the Great Spotted Woodpecker, *Dendrocopos major* L.

A. V. SIROTKIN
State University of Leningrad, USSR

A maximal amount of neurosecretory material (NSM) is found in the median eminence (ME) and posterior pituitary (PP) of adult woodpeckers in winter. Most of the NSM in the PP is located along the capillaries and around the recessus hypophyseus. Intensively stained Herring bodies are present. A smaller amount of NSM is seen in the PP in the spring during migration, the mating season, and the beginning of gonadal development; NSM is not found in the external layer of the ME. In the latter, NSM disappears first from the zone surrounding the recessus hypophyseus, suggesting the release of neurohormones, mostly into the CSF. A minimal amount of NSM is found in the neurohypophysis (Nh) in the summer, during nesting, and the first stages of molting. NSM in the highly hyperemic PP disappears from the zone around the recessus hypophyseus and the capillaries. No stained Herring bodies are seen. This suggests an intensive release of neurohormones, into both the CSF and the general circulation. In the period from summer to winter, accumulation of NSM is observed in the Nh; Herring bodies appear, and the degree of hyperemia decreases. There is a difference between the annual cycle of the thyroid gland (TG) and that of the Nh. Moderate TG activity (epithelium colloid - E/C = 0.803) is seen in later winter. A significant increase of TG activity is found during the mating season and spring migration. A lower activity of the TG (up to a moderate level) is observed during nesting and the beginning of molting (E/C = 0.499); it is minimal by the end of molting, during autumn migration, and in early winter (E/C = 0.343). The annual cycle of TG activity differs greatly from that of other passerine birds. Neither conspicuous correlation with seasonal, photoperiodic, and temperature changes nor considerable activation of the TG during molting is observed.

Morphofunctional Activity of the Hypothalamo-Hypophyseal Neurosecretory System (HHNS) After Destruction of the Median Eminence in Cold Stress

E. M. STABROVSKY and L. S. SHPANSKAYA
Kirov Institute for Physicians' Perfection, Leningrad, USSR

We have studied the functional activity of the neurosecretory cells (NSC) of both the supraoptic and paraventricular nuclei (NSO and NPV, respectively) of male white rats 14-15 days after electrolytic destruction of the median eminence (ME) in conditions of cold stress (5°C). Electrocoagulation of the ME was performed according to the coordinates of E. Fifkov's and J. Marshal's atlas, with histologic control. The morphofunctional state of the HHNS was assessed by karyometry of the NSC, NSO, and NPV and by counting the percentage of the NSC types on those nuclei. The destruction of the ME leads to the following morphofunctional changes: reduction of the proportion of NSC with high functional activity in both the NSO and NPV; reduction of the volume of NSC nuclei in the NPV; retrograde degeneration of NSCs in the NSO, which we observed mostly on one side, while on the other side we observed a compensatory increase of neurosecretory activity. Investigations of the thermoregulatory reactions showed a 30% reduction of thermoproduction and an increase of thermorelease (reduction of skin and rectal temperatures by 1.5-2°C). Regarding endocrine functions, we observed considerable reduction (70%) of the functional activity of the hypophyseal-adrenal system and a smaller reduction (30%) of the activity of the enterochromaffine system and the thyroid. Thus, the destruction of the ME in conditions of cooling was accompanied by a reduction of the functional activity of the HHNS and a weakening of the thermoregulatory and hormonal reactions.

Effects of Posterior-Pituitary-Lobe Peptides on the Maintenance of a Conditioned Avoidance Response in Rats

H. STARK, H. BIGL, and G. STERBA
Section of Biological Sciences of the Karl-Marx-University Leipzig, Leipzig, GDR

Peptides of the posterior pituitary lobe increase the resistance to extinction of active avoidance behavior in intact rats (see D. DE WIED: Peptides and Behavior. In: Memory Transfer of Information. Ed. by H. ZIPPEL, 1973).

The active avoidance behavior was studied using a pole-jumping situation. Male Wistar rats (180-220 g) were used. The sound of a buzzer served as the conditioned stimulus (CS) which was presented for 4 s. Rats that failed to jump onto the pole within 4 s after CS onset received an electric shock (length 16 s, 8 mA) applied through the grid floor. Ten acquisition trials were given daily for 3 days with intertrial intervals averaging 60 s. Nonreinforced extinction trials (sound for 20 s max.) were given ten per day on the following 2 successive days.

Single subcutaneous (s.c.) injections of pitressin (0.5 IU; Fa. Sandoz, Switzerland), synthetic Lys-vasopressin (0.06 or 0.5 IU) or Arg-vasopressin (0.5 IU) into rats 1 h before the third acquisition session leads to a prolongation of the retention time of the conditioned avoidance reaction. Similar results were obtained in rats after intrahippocampal administration of 0.002 or 0.01 IU Lys-vasopressin. Subcutaneous injection of oxytocin or octapressin (2-Phe-Lys-vasopressin) have no influence on the retention of this reaction. The combination of both Lys-vasopressin (0.5 IU) and oxytocin (0.5 IU or 20 IU) affects the retention time in a way that suggests a competition between both hormones. Corresponding effects were obtained in rats treated with pitressin or Lys-vasopressin and trained to brightness discrimination in a Y-chamber.

Oxytocinergic Extrahypothalamic Neurosecretory System of the Vertebrates and Memory Processes

G. STERBA
Department of Cell Biology and Regulation, Section of Biosciences, Karl Marx University, Leipzig, GDR

A. Definition

The term "oxytocinergic" as used in this paper refers to peptidergic neurons that synthesize oxytocin-type neurohormones, as oxytocin itself, or vasopressin, or vasotocin, as well as other nonapeptides. The specific transport organelles of the oxytocinergic neurons, the elementary vesicles or neurosecretory vesicles, are termed "neurohphysin vesicles."

B. Extrahypothalamic Part of the Classic Neurosecretory System

It is now fairly certain that the classic neurosecretory system of the vertebrates producing oxytocin-type neurohormones is considerably more differentiated than has been supposed. The descending hypothalamo-neurohypophyseal subsystem is well-known. But as yet we know very little about the ascending subsystem and its functional importance. Most of the neurons of the descending subsystem release their products into the circulation; most of the neurons of the ascending subsystem are not connected to capillaries, but make true synapses with other neurons. The targets of these ascending neurons are different structures of the limbic system, as the medial septum region, the habenular region and, in higher vertebrates, also the subfornical organ (Fig. 1). Further targets are situated both in the midbrain and hindbrain. Apart from these sites present in all vertebrates, additional targets exist in individual species or in taxonomic groups (STERBA, 1974; WEGELIN et al., 1976).

One of the most interesting extrahypothalamic pathways is the hypothalamo-hindbrain connection. Primarily known only from lower vertebrates, this pathway was shown during the past year to exist also in pigeons and rats. In both species, the terminals of the hypothalamo-hindbrain pathway are arranged within the area of the nuclei cuneatus and gracilis, the first relay station of the dorsal spinal tracts, which in mammals also conduct receptor fibers of the mammilla (Fig. 3).

The existence of an extrahypothalamic subsystem opens up an interesting new field of neurosecretory research. The ascending axis makes clear that the classic neurosecretory system is not merely a one-way system represented mainly by receptors, signal transfer to the magnocellular neurons, neurohormone release, and humoral transfer of information to the targets, the outcome being

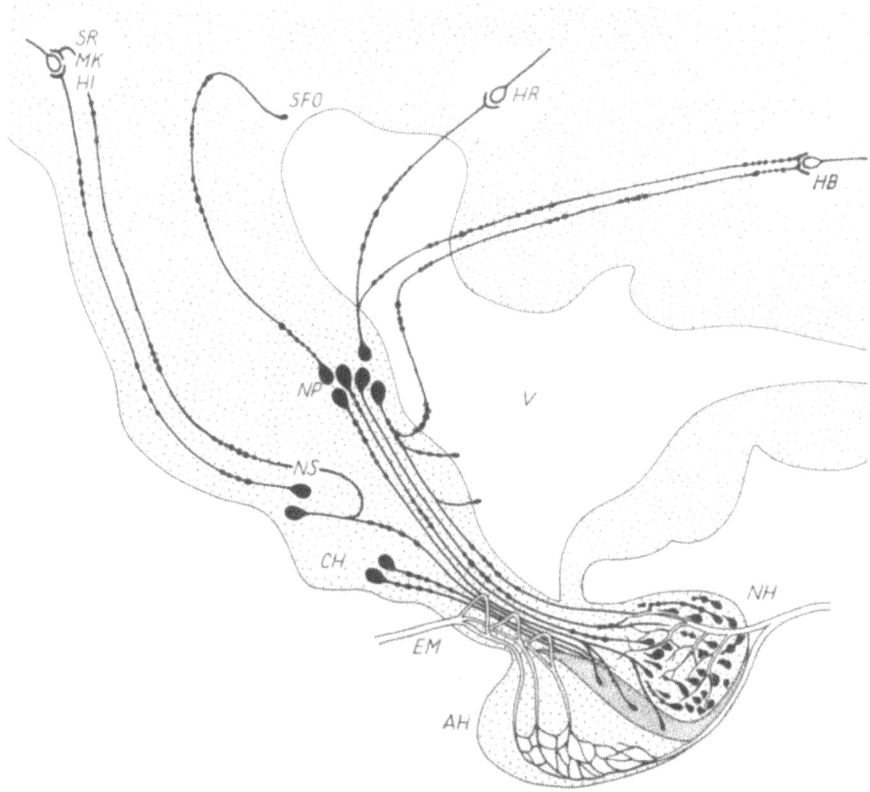

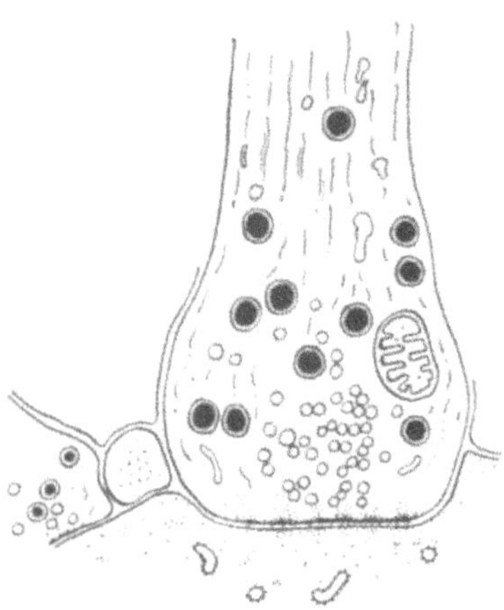

Fig. 1. Classic neurosecretory system of vertebrates with its descending and ascending parts: *AH* - adenohypophysis, *CH* - chiasma, *EM* - median eminence, *HB* - hindbrain connection, *HI* - hippocampus connection, *HR* - habenular region, *MK* - amygd. nuclei, *NH* - neurohypophysis, *NP* - nucleus paraventricularis, *NS* - nucleus supraopticus, *SFO* - subfornical organ, *SR* - medial septum region, *V* - third ventricle

Fig. 2. Oxytocinergic neuroneuronal synapse with microvesicles and neurophysin vesicles

conditioned by the internal and external environment. Rather, we believe the neurosecretory system also affects other subsystems of the brain by direct neuronal intervention in a specific manner, and thus takes part in various cerebral functions.

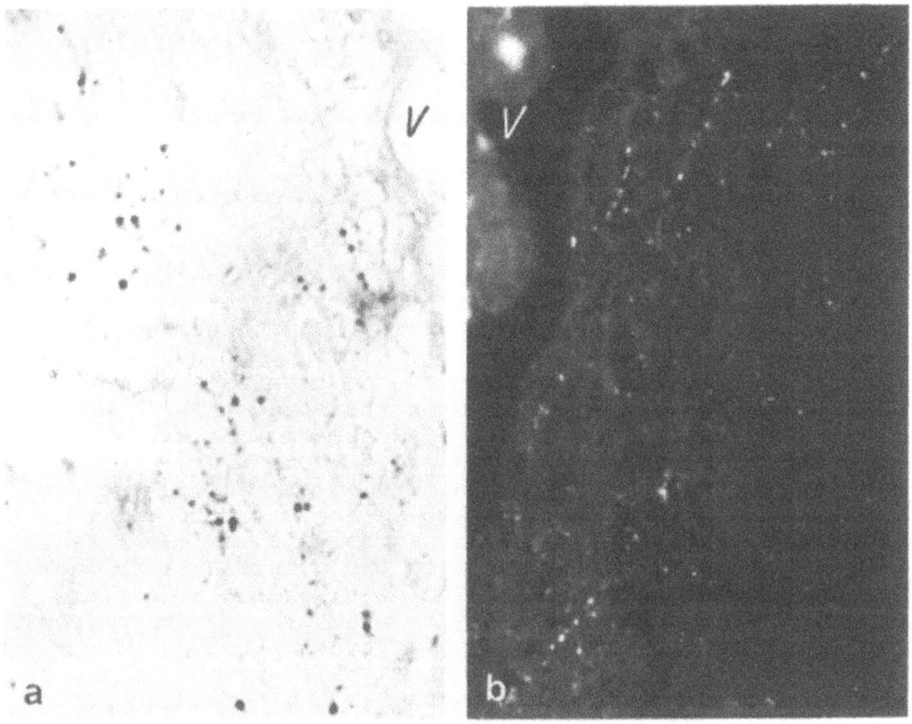

Fig. 3a and b. Neurosecretory oxytocinergic fibers within area of nucleus cuneatus medialis of rat. *V* - fourth ventricle. (a) Immunoperoxidase technique with rabbit antineurophysin antiserum. (b) Pseudoisocyanine-fluorescence technique

C. The Oxytocinergic Synapses

BARGMANN et al. (1967) described "peptidergic synapses" between neurosecretory peptidergic fibers and epithelial cells of the cat's pars intermedia. But these very interesting findings were only understood to be an exception to the widely accepted view that neurosecretory neurons form no synapses with other neurons. KNOWLES, for example, certainly held this view, stating at the last Symposium of Neurosecretion in London: "It (the neurosecretory neuron) receives synaptic efferents but itself makes no efferent synapses with other neurones." Interestingly enough, however, he remarked in a footnote of his printed paper: "This may need to be modified (see CROSS, this volume, p. 115)," (KNOWLES and VOLLRATH, 1974, p. 11). CROSS postulated such synapses from the results of electrophysiologic recordings, especially from the evidence of recurrent inhibition of neurosecretory cells. "Generation of the neurosecretory action potentials in the hypothalamus is facilitated by cholinergic (nicotinic receptors) mechanisms and inhibited by adrenergic (β-receptors) mechanisms but the morphologic and neurotransmitter basis for the recurrent inhibition of neurosecretory cells' discharges remains obscure" (CROSS, 1974, p. 126). BARRY (1975) demonstrated neurons in Golgi-preparations of the paraventricular region of the mouse, which perhaps correspond to the unknown Renshaw-like units (KOIZUMI and YAMASHITA, 1972) in the recurrent inhibition of neurosecretory cells.

The synapses formed by the axons of oxytocinergic neurons ascending from the magnocellular nuclei to different regions of the brain are probably not identical with the postulated synapses with interneurons, but they are suitable to serve as a model. Up to now we have demonstrated such synapses in different brain regions of lamprey (*Lampetra planeri*), salamander (*Pleurodeles waltli*), frog (*Rana temporaria*), pigeon (*Columba livia*), and rat (Wistar line). In all species investigated, the terminals of the oxytocinergic axons are differentiated in the same manner. They represent the presynaptic component of axosomatic and axodendritic synapses with other neurons. The enlarged terminals are bulbiform, the contacting membrane is thickened, and inside the presynaptic membrane numerous microvesicles are present. But the most conspicuous structures are the neurophysin vesicles (Figs. 2, 4). The oxytocinergic synapses pose the question as to whether or not neurohormones are released from the terminals. If this is the case, the question arises as to whether they are released alone, or together with an unknown neurotransmitter. With our present knowledge these questions cannot be answered. It might only be stated that oxytocinergic synapses and monoaminergic synapses, in some cases also cholinergic synapses, can be seen to be arranged side by side at one effector neuron (Fig. 3). Therefore we assume that the oxytocinergic synapses are in fact a new type of synapse releasing nonapeptides in a fairly precise way caused by volleys of action potentials, and that these peptides effect a long-term action in the postsynaptic neuron.

Since the oxytocinergic synapse is the first peptidergic synapse demonstrated morphologically, it is a model of general importance for brain research.

D. The Extrahypothalamic Oxytocinergic Subsystem and Its Assumed Relationship with Memory Processes

DE WIED et al. (1972, 1975) have demonstrated the effects of vasopressin, its analogs, and fragments thereof on the consolidation of memory processes after subcutaneous and cerebroventricular administrations. "These peptides under certain conditions facilitate acquisition of active avoidance behaviour, increase resistance to extinction of active and passive avoidance behavior and of sexually motivated approach behaviour" (VAN WIMERSMA GREIDANUS and DE WIED, 1976, page 36). Arginine vasopressin (AVP), followed by lysine-vasopressin (LVP), are the most potent peptides in rats. Oxytocin and vasotocin possess about 20% of the AVP-activity. The desglycinamide fragment of both vasopressins, which lacks antidiuretic, pressor, oxytocin,

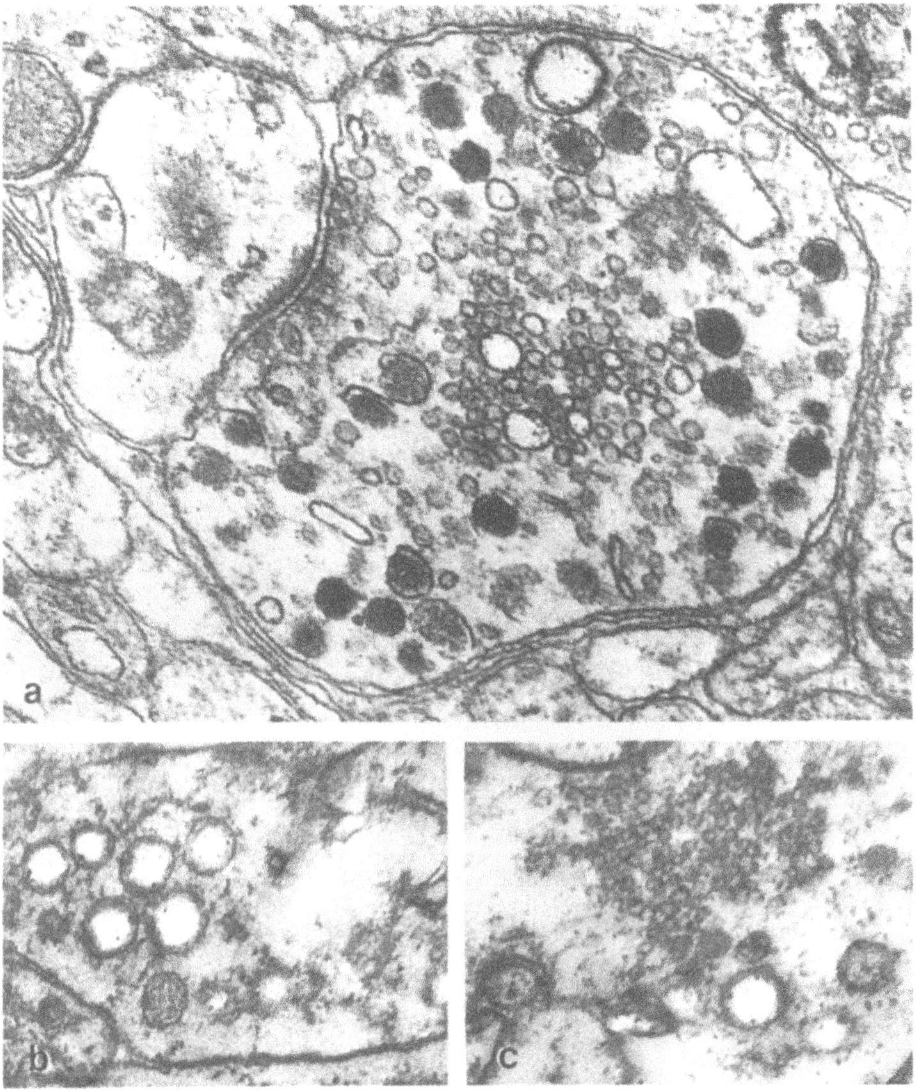

Fig. 4a-c. Neurosecretory structures within area of nucleus cuneatus, a target region of hypothalamo-hindbrain pathway. (a) Electron-microscopic demonstration of oxytocinergic synapse (pigeon). (b) Ultrahistochemical demonstration of neurosecretory fiber with neurophysin vesicles (rat). (c) Ultrahistochemical demonstration of synapse with neurophysin vesicles (rat). × 35,000

and ACTH-releasing activity, decreases the potency of the behavioral effect only by approximately 50% (DE WIED et al., 1972). These findings indicate that the mechanisms by which vasopressin acts on the classic target tissues and on the brain may be different. It is supposed that the receptor in the brain interacts only with a part of the molecule located in the ring structure. The cerebroventricular route of administration is much more effective than subcutaneous injection. Conversely, severe memory disturbances could be demonstrated in homozygous Brattleboro rats with hereditary diabetes insipidus due to the complete lack of vasopressin (DE WIED et al., 1975).

Furthermore, DE WIED et al. determined the location of the areas sensitive to AVP and LVP. Their results point to an important role of midbrain limbic structures, mainly the rostral septal region and dorsal hippocampal region, in vasopressin-induced effects on avoidance behavior (VAN WIMERSMA GREIDANUS and DE WIED, 1976). These results correspond to our present knowledge on septal and hippocampal areas in relation to behavior and learning processes. From the situation in peripheral target organs we know that the effects of vasopressin involve activation of the adenyl cyclase (3',5'-cyclic AMP) system, which initiates the synthesis of specific proteins. As MATTHIES (1975) demonstrated, long-term memory processes might be generally accompanied by protein synthesis. The observation that vasopressin influences memory consolidation rather than learning processes points in this direction (VAN WIMERSMA GREIDANUS and DE WIED, 1976).

One of the main problems is the physiologic route involved in causing the effects of AVP and LVP on memory processes. We assume that the extrahypothalamic-oxytocinergic subsystem participates in these processes. This conception is predicated upon the idea that the behavioral actions of these peptides are effected by neuronal transmission or modulation and not by endocrine operations alone. I think it is time to recognize the classic peptidergic neurosecretory system as being a part of the brain, not only involved in the control of the endocrine system but also acting on the nervous system. The same molecules acting as neurohormones might also perform this second function. In this sense the oxytocin-type neurohormones have a dual potency, a principle well known from the duality of monoamines. As SCHARRER (1974a,b), SCHARRER and WURZELMANN (1974) and GERSCH (1975) indicated, this principle might be realized also in invertebrates.

References

BARGMANN, W., LINDNER, E., ANDRES, K.H.: Über Synapsen an endokrinen Epithelzellen und die Definition sekretorischer Neurone. Untersuchungen am Zwischenlappen der Katzenhypophyse. Z. Zellforsch. 77, 282-298 (1967)

BARRY, J.: Essai de classification, et technique de Golgi, des diverses catégories de neurones du noyau paraventriculaire chez la souris. C. R. Soc. Biol. (Paris) 169, 978 (1975)

CROSS, B.A.: The neurosecretory impulse. In: Neurosecretion - The Final Neuroendocrine Pathway. KNOWLES, F., VOLLROTH, L. (eds.). Berlin-Heidelberg-New York: Springer-Verlag 1974, pp. 115-128

GERSCH, M.: Prinzipien neurohormonaler und neurohumoraler Steuerung physiologischer Prozesse bei wirbellosen Tieren und Versuch einer ersten komplexen Charakterisierung. Wiss. Beiträge der Friedrich-Schiller-Univ. Jena 1975, pp. 1-151

KNOWLES, F.: Twenty years of neurosecretion. In: Neurosecretion - The Final Neuroendocrine Pathway. KNOWLES, F., VOLLRATH, L. (eds.). Berlin-Heidelberg-New York: Springer-Verlag 1974, pp. 3-11

KOIZUMI, K., YAMASHITA, H.: Studies of antidromically identified neurosecretory cells of the hypothalamus by intracellular and extracellular recordings. J. Physiol. (Lond.) 221, 683-705 (1972)

MATTHIES, H.: The biochemical basis of learning and memory. Life Sci. 15, 2017-2031 (1975)

SCHARRER, B.: New trends in invertebrate neurosecretion. In: Neurosecretion - The Final Neuroendocrine Pathway. KNOWLES, F., VOLLRATH, L. (eds.). Berlin-Heidelberg-New York: Springer-Verlag 1974a

SCHARRER, B.: The spectrum of neuroendocrine communication. In: Recent Studies of Hypothalamic Function. Basle: Karger 1974b, pp. 8-16

SCHARRER, B., WURZELMANN, S.: Observation on synaptoid vesicles in insect neurons. Zool. Jb. Physiol. 78, 387-396 (1974)

STERBA, G.: Ascending neurosecretory pathways of the peptidergic type. In: Neurosecretion - The Final Neuroendocrine Pathway. KNOWLES, F., VOLLRATH, L. (eds.). Berlin-Heidelberg-New York: Springer-Verlag 1974a, pp. 38-47

STERBA, G.: Das oxytocinerge neurosekretorische System der Wirbeltiere. Beitrag zu einem erweiterten Konzept. Zool. Jb. Physiol. 78, 409-423 (1974b)

WIED, D. DE, BOHUS, H.M., LANDE, S., WITTER, A.: Dissociation of the behavioral and endocrine effects of lysine vasopressin by tryptic digestion. Br. J. Pharmacol. 45, 118-122 (1972)

WIED, D. DE, BOHUS, B., VAN WIMERSMA GREIDANUS, T.B.: Memory deficit in rats with hereditary *diabetes insipidus*. Brain Res. 85, 152-167 (1975)

WIMERSMA GREIDANUS, T.B. VAN, WIED, D. DE: The physiology of the neurohypophysial system and its relation to memory processes, 1976 (in press)

Functional Significance of Two Types of Neurosecretory Granules in the Posthypophysis: Ultrastructural and Cytochemical Approach

F. TASSO, J. L. BOUDIER, and D. PICARD
ERA-CNRS n° 322-Laboratoire d'Histologie I, Faculté de Médecine, 13385 Marseille Cedex 4, France

Since elementary neurosecretion granules and two neurohormones, vasopressin and oxytocin, have been shown to occur in the hypothalamo-posthypophyseal system, the question has been raised whether different types of granules, fibers, and neurons correspond to each of the two hormones. This view was initially supported by biochemical data from ultracentrifuged cellular fractions; two types of granules and fibers containing vasopressin and oxytocin respectively could be separated.

By means of light-microscopic immunocytochemistry, VANDESANDE and DIERICKX (1975) have clearly demonstrated the existence and distribution of two types of neurons and fibers containing vasopressin or oxytocin. However, at the ultrastructural level, such a distinction is not so clearly established. Previous studies on a variety of species including fishes, amphibians, reptiles, birds, and mammals have shown in each particular case at least two types of granules; the granule classification is based either on size, or electron density, or shape. In some instances, the findings suggested a possible correlation between the structural aspects and the hormonal content of the granules. However, several reports on the granules are contradictory, and the differential characteristics are not always sufficiently clear-cut. A better criterion for granule classification might be provided by differences in their structure, as observed e.g. in guinea pig, hedgehog, and cat.

Our own observations (BOUDIER, 1976) on the garden dormouse (*Eliomys quercinus*) suggest a relationship between the ultrastructure and the hormonal content of the granules. In the posterior pituitary lobe of this species, a clear distinction is seen between the two types of fibers on the basis of their granule structure (Fig. 1). In one type of fiber, the granules are round, with a homogeneous dense core separated from the granular mem-

→

Fig. 1. Posthypophysis of garden dormouse in active rats at end of winter. Col. UR + Pb. On *right*, in two axons, granules with amorphous content. On *left*, axon containing paracrystalline-cored granules with great diversity of images due to variation of the plane of section. × 36,000

Figs. 2 and 3. Uranyl acetate and periodic acid-thiocarbohydrazide-silver proteinate method.

Fig. 2. Secretory axons in neural lobe of normal rat; *upper axon* contains nonreactive granules; in *lower axon*, granules show ring-shaped electron density. × 35,000

Fig. 3. Nonreactive granules in neurohypophysis of Brattleboro rat. × 42,000

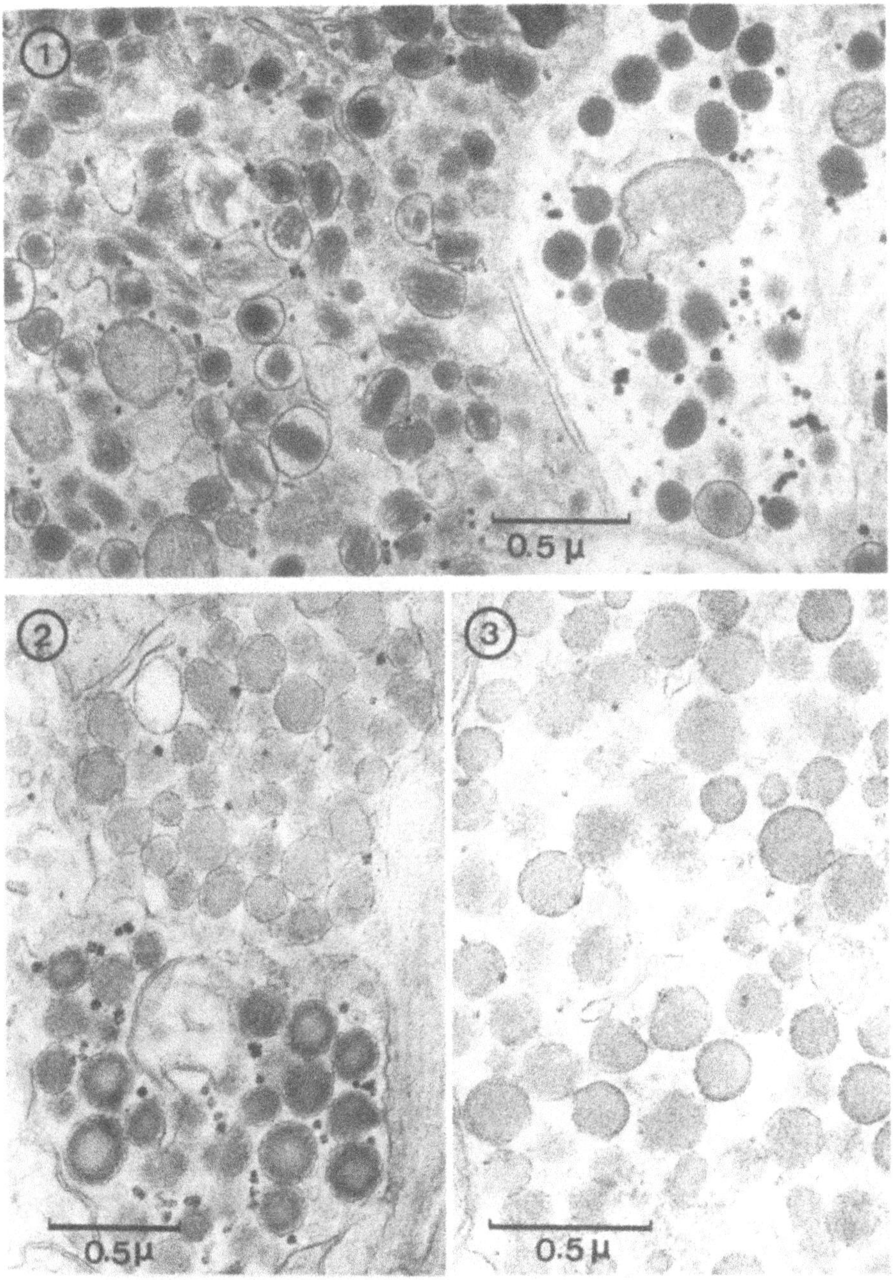

brane by a narrow electron-lucent zone. In the other type, sections of granules show a great variety of profiles, ranging from circular to elongated rodlet shapes. The dense core, circumscribed by a wide electron-lucent halo, is heterogeneous and reveals paracrystalline organization; the latter is characterized either by periodically alternating dense and clear layers or by bundles of tubules, as determined by tilting of a goniometric stage.

Further evidence was obtained from cytochemical studies characterizing glycoproteins in the posterior pituitary of Sprague Dawley and Long Evans rats; two types of axons were identified containing either homogeneous, nonreactive granules, or granules supplied with a ring-shaped deposit of silver proteinate (TASSO, 1973). The contrast between these two aspects of granules could be enhanced by combining the periodic acid-thiocarbohydrazide-silver proteinate method with prestaining by "en bloc" impregnation with uranyl acetate (Fig. 2). Uranyl acetate per se induced in some fibers a ring-shaped dense area in granules. This method enabled us to distinguish not only different types of fibers, but also to classify magnocellular perikarya of the supraoptic and paraventricular nuclei on the basis of cytochemical granule features.

Both morphologic duality of elementary granules in the garden dormouse and cytochemical duality of their composition in the rat are highly suggestive of a correlation of fine structure with the hormonal content. This hypothesis has been further examined in the rat by use of the Brattleboro mutant of the Long Evans strain, which is known to be characterized by a complete deficiency of vasopressin and neurophysin II. Recently, in cooperation with J.J. DREIFUSS (TASSO et al., 1976), the authors examined the posterior lobe and the hypothalamic magnocellular nuclei of Brattleboro rats. While many neurons and axon terminals in these animals contained no granules, the granules found in the other neurons and terminals were all of the nonreactive type, i.e., devoid of the ring-shaped dense area and glycoprotein localization observed in normal rats (Fig. 3). Thus, we feel justified in correlating the "reactive type" granules with vasopressin, and in distinguishing at the ultrastructural level two types of fibers and neurons in accordance with the findings of VANDESANDE and DIERICKX (1975) using the light microscope findings.

The authors have also demonstrated a similar cytochemical duality in the mouse, although it is less distinct than in the rat. As to the garden dormouse, a slight deposit of silver proteinate was obtained only on the membrane of the "highly organized granules"; although this reaction is too weak to have a high significance, it favors the hypothesis of a relation between morphologic peculiarities and hormonal content of granules in this species.

References

BOUDIER, J.L., BURLET, C.: On presence and distribution of two types of neurosecretory granules in the neurohypophysis of the garden dormouse. J. Microsc. Biol. Cell 27, 69-70 (1976)

TASSO, F.: Localisation cytochimique ultrastructurale de glycoprotéines dans les granules neurosécrétoires de la posthypophyse du rat. J. Microsc. (Paris) 18, 115-118 (1973)

TASSO, F., DREIFUSS, J.J., PICARD, D.: Ultrastructural identification of granules containing oxytocin and vasopressin. Nature 260, 21-22 (1976)

VANDESANDE, F., DIERICKX, K.: Identification of the vasopressin-producing and of the oxytocin-producing neurons in the hypothalamic magnocellular neurosecretory system of the rat. Cell Tissue Res. 164, 153-162 (1975)

Functional State of the Praeoptico-Hypophyseal Neurosecretory System (PHNS) of the Prespawning Lake Whitefish, *Coregonus autumnalis migratorius* G.

N. I. TISHCHENKO and A. L. POLENOV
Institute of Cytology and Genetics, Novosibirsk, and Sechenov Institute of Evolutionary Physiology and Biochemistry, Leningrad, USSR

Activity of the PHNS was estimated morphologically in prespawning male and female lake whitefish - stenohaline (lake) anadromous migrants. Only euryhaline fish (sea anadromous migrants) have previously been analyzed in this respect. In spring (March) there is an accumulation of neurosecretory material (NSM) both in the secretory cells and in the neurohypophysis (NH). This is characteristic of an inactive functional state. The synthesis of the NSM is slightly increased in the neurosecretory cells of the fish during the period of active life (July). The NSM is transported along the axons of the preoptico-hypophyseal tract and accumulates in the NH. No obvious signs of neurohormone discharge are seen in the NH. NSM synthesis and transport is greatly activated in the PHNS of the fish during the prespawning and spawning migrations (August-September). Peptide neurohormones seem to be released into the blood circulation at this stage in both sexes, but especially in females. This is probably due to the greater energy expenditure needed to complete ovogenesis. The phenomenon of the neuronal hydroencephalocriny is pronounced in prespawning lake whitefish. This supports the idea of a possible influence of the peptide neurohormones on the CNS (neurotropic effect). Thus, the PHNS of the lake whitefish appears to be involved with prespawning activities of the fish.

Oxytocic Activity of the Cerebrospinal Fluid and Changes in the EEG Before and During Pregnancy and Labor in the Rabbit

H. UNGER, B. MIEHLKE, H. SCHWARZBERG, and H. SCHULZ
Institute of Physioloy, Medical Academy, Magdeburg, GDR

A. Introduction

Oxytocin is mainly produced in the paraventricular nucleus and intra-axonally transported to the neurohypophysis. Specific stimuli (suckling stimulus, vaginal dilation) cause the release of oxytocin into the blood. Moreover, oxytocin is released into the cerebrospinal fluid (CSF) through special neurosecretory pathways (STERBA, 1966; SCHWARZBERG, 1968; UNGER and SCHWARZBERG, 1970).

The oxytocin content of the blood of man and mammals is greatly increased during parturition, reaching its maximum when the head disengages (FOLLEY and KNAGGS, 1965). The oxytocic activity of the human CSF varies, e.g., it is extremely high during epileptic fits and extremely low in cerebral atrophy and infantile brain damage (UNGER et al., 1971). So far, nothing has been reported of changes in oxytocic activity of the CSF during delivery. From the CSF, oxytocin is capable of influencing the activity of hypothalamic neurons (SCHULZ et al., 1971). Therefore, we studied the oxytocic activity in the CSF of waking nonpregnant rabbits and of animals during and immediately after labor. Moreover, we examined the state of activity of the CNS during these periods by EEG recorded on waking animals.

B. Material and Methods

The experimental animals were 150 rabbits of various breeds, between 10 and 15 months old and weighing 2.5-3.5 kg. They were given standard feed and water *ad libitum*. CSF was obtained by suboccipital puncture after local anesthesia using procaine. The oxytocic activity was determined by means of the rat-uterus test against synthetic oxytocin (Richter/Budapest) as a standard. To inactivate the oxytocin, standard and test solutions containing equivalent amounts of 0.1 *N* Na-thioglycolate were incubated.

To record the EEG, four silver electrodes were epidurally and chronically implanted in 42 animals.

C. Results and Discussion

The annual mean of oxytocic activity in the CSF of 80 female and 19 male rabbits was found to be 349 ± 43 μunits/ml. The

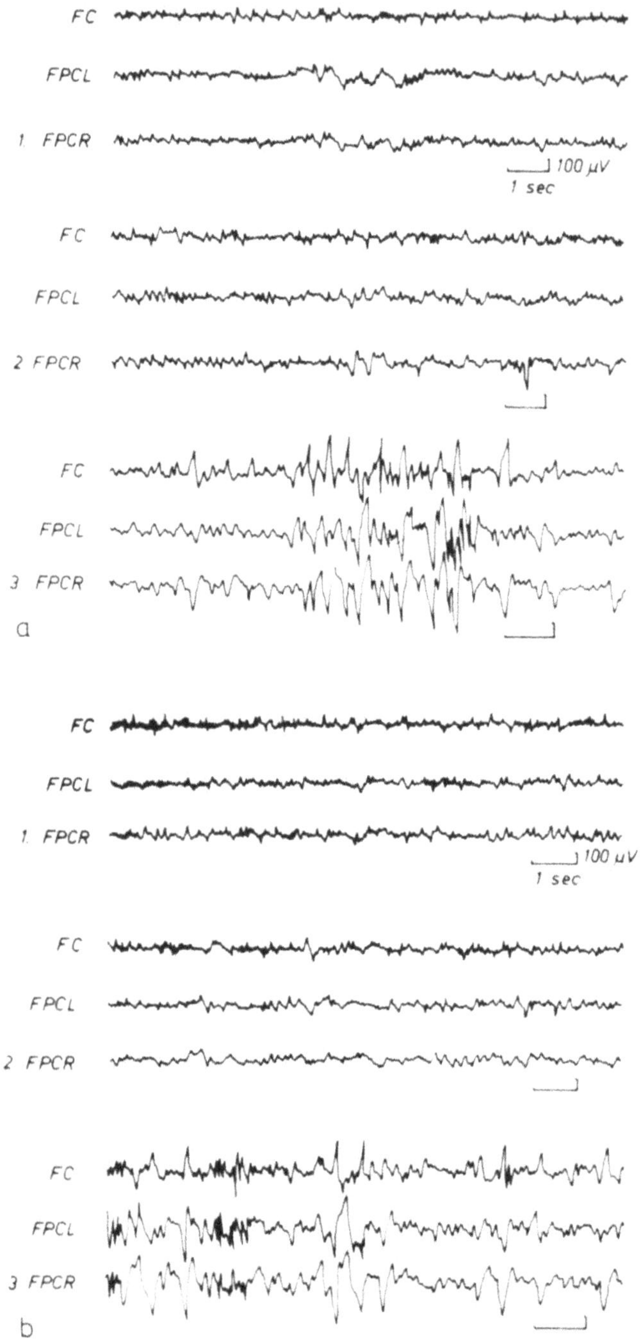

Fig. 1a and b. EEG from rabbits. (a) *1* nonpregnant, *2* pregnant; *3* 5 min after labor. (b) *1* nonpregnant; *2* pregnant; *3* 3 h after labor average oxytocic activity of the CSF from May to August was 90 ± 21 μunits/ml. In the course of 1 year, the oxytocic activity of the CSF revealed no sexual differences: male (n = 19) = 344 ± 56 μunits/ml; female (n = 80) = 349 ± 52 μunits/ml. In addition to the lowest values of 90 μunits/ml observed from May to August, there were two peaks, one in the spring at 340 μunits/ml and one in autumn at 630 μunits/ml. A correlation with daily photoperiod, reproduction, and food uptake was assumed to exist.

In 12 rabbits, the oxytocic activity of the CSF during and immediately after labor in the period from May to August was determined to be 644 ± 135 μunits/ml. For seven animals, determination of the oxytocic activity of the CSF was successful both in normal conditions (106 ± 36 μunits/ml) and during labor (667 ± 164 μunits/ml).

EEG recordings were obtained from five animals during pregnancy as well as during and immediately after delivery. The EEG recorded during pregnancy did not reveal any particular trends. Immediately postpartum, at the time of maximum oxytocic activity of the CSF, pronounced synchronization effects appeared that were observed as long as 3 h postpartum (Fig. 1). During this phase, the EEG was similar to that of a fully relaxed human being when falling asleep. Oxytocin was assumed to exert a sedative influence on certain structures and functions of the CNS.

References

FOLLEY, S.J., KNAGGS, G.S.: Levels of oxytocin in the jugular vein blood of goats during parturition. J. Endocrinol. 33, 301-315 (1965)

SCHULZ, H., UNGER, H., SCHWARZBERG, H., POMMRICH, G., STOLZE, R.: Neuronenaktivität hypothalamischer Kerngebiete von Kaninchen nach intraventrikulärer Applikation von Vasopressin und Oxytocin. Experientia 27, 1482 (1971)

SCHWARZBERG, H.: Untersuchungen über den Einfluß des Wasserentzuges auf das periphere und zentralnervöse Geschehen an Ratten. Acta Biol. Med. Germ. 21, 23-49 (1968)

SCHWARZBERG, H., SCHULZ, H.: Zur Methodik chronisch implantierter Hinventrikelkanülen und Subokzipitalpunktion bei Kaninchen. Acta Biol. Med. Germ. 31, 609-611 (1973)

STERBA, G.: Zur cerebrospinalen Neurokrinie. Zool. Anz. (Suppl.) 29, 393-440 (1966)

UNGER, H., SCHWARZBERG, H.: Untersuchungen über Vorkommen und Bedeutung von Vasopressin und Oxytocin im Liquor cerebrospinalis und Blut für nervöse Funktionen. Acta Biol. Med. Germ. 25, 267-280 (1970)

UNGER, H., POMMRICH, G., BECK, R.: Der Oxytocingehalt im menschlichen pathologischen Liquor. Experientia 27, 1486 (1971)

The Hypothalamic Influence on Secretion of the Adenohypophysis Cultured in the Anterior Chamber of the Eye

E. P. VOLODINA and A. A. STADNIKOV
Department of Histology, Orenburg Medical Institute, USSR

The adenohypophysis is one of the powerful effectors assisting in homeostatic mechanisms. The present uncertain location of the hypothalamic zones responsible for production of releasing factors acting on the adenohypophysis, and the indistinct understanding of the interaction of hypothalamic regions in regulating the process of hormone formation have prompted a reinvestigation of this issue. The aim of this report is to reveal cytologic reactions in adenohypophyseal cells, resulting from direct contact with different hypothalamic zones, alone and in combination, in tissue culture in vivo.

The experiments were carried out on mature and immature rabbits. A method of adenohypophyseal implantation (LASARENKO, 1934), allotransplantation of the organ into a peritoneal sac formed from the intestinal mesentery, and allotransplantation into the anterior chamber of the eye were used.

Regardless of the site of the transplantation, four series of experiments were carried out. In the first, a transplant consisting solely of adenohypophyseal tissue was performed. In the second series of experiments, adenohypophyseal parenchyma was transplanted along with supraoptic nuclei. In the third series, adenohypophyseal tissues were combined with the mediobasal zone of the hypothalamus. In the fourth series, adenohypophyseal tissues were transplanted together with both the mediobasal zone and supraoptic nuclei of the hypothalamus simultaneously. Transplants were studied for periods ranging from 6 h to 60 days. In sections of the transplanted adenohypophyseal tissues, RNA was stained by methyl-green pyronin and proteins revealed by Danielli's reaction. In order to distinguish the different types of acidophil and basophil adenohypophyseal cells, the PAS reaction was used, with additional orange staining, and combined staining with Azan-aldehyde fuchsin. Neurosecretory substance was revealed by the Gomori method. In total, over 500 transplants were studied. In immature animals the structure of the sex glands was also studied.

In control experiments (first series), regardless of the site of transplantation of adenohypophyseal cells, general trends of changes were observed proceeding in stages: destruction and adaptation, activation and proliferation, functional differentiation, and death of the tissues. The distinctness and duration of these stages varied, but they were nevertheless present in all four series.

In the new conditions, adenohypophyseal cells either adapted themselves and thereafter proliferated, or they died. A gradual and continued degranulation of the basophils (Fig. 1a) was noted during the first 4 days (ACTH cells reacted first, then gonadotrophs, and later thyrotrophs). Highly loaded with secretory products, adenohypophyseal cells did not undergo degranulation and progressive transformations. In cultivation of adenohypo-

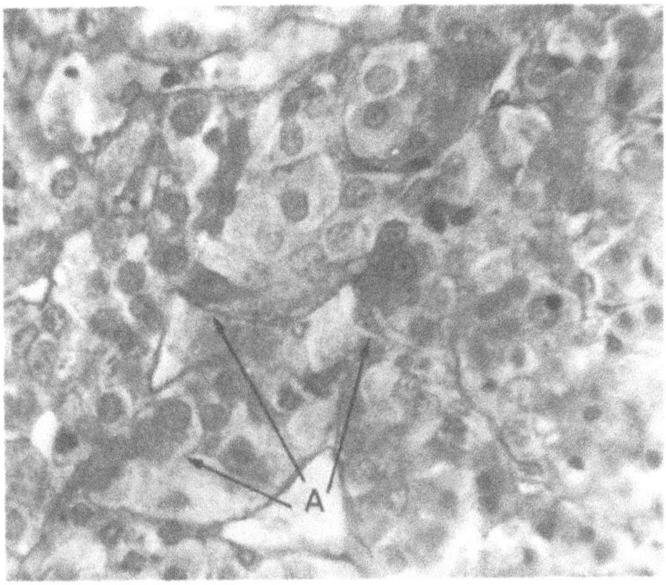

Fig. 1. Tissue culture of adenohypophysis in anterior chamber of eye of rabbit. Stage: 1 day; Zenker-formol; PAS reaction. × 630. *A* - basophilic adenocytes

physeal cells in the anterior chamber of the eye, the cell degranulation and activation were more prolonged.

Joint cultivation of the adenohypophyseal tissue with supraoptic nuclei produced a rapid discharge of the secretory granules from the basophils in the course of the first day (Fig. 2a). The principal mass of the adenohypophyseal cells were degranulated, but the cellular RNA was increased prior to synthesis of the protein component of the hormones. Degranulated chromophils in control experiments displayed their histiotypic properties, proliferating into layers, cords, and cyst formations. Differentiation of epithelium was depressed and often abortive. It was noted that the degranulated basophils in the second series of experiments survived longer than in the first one.

In joint transplantations of the adenohypophysis with mediobasal nuclei of the hypothalamus, a prolonged survival of thyrotropes and gonadotropes has been revealed (Fig. 3a), such cells being found even after 30 days. Moreover, newly formed epithelium differentiated in an organospecific direction. In the stage covering over 30 days, a large number of the cysts filled with colloid arose in the adenohypophyseal tissue.

The study of the structure of the sex glands in the control and experimentally immature recipients showed that the basophils preserved in the adenohypophyseal parenchyma are hormonally active. They synthesize gonadotropins that penetrate into the recipient's bloodstream.

The results of cultivation of the adenohypophysis in the anterior chamber of the eye in the presence of both supraoptic and mediobasal nuclei does not enable us to completely reject the significance of the magnocellular nuclei in the regulation of hormon-

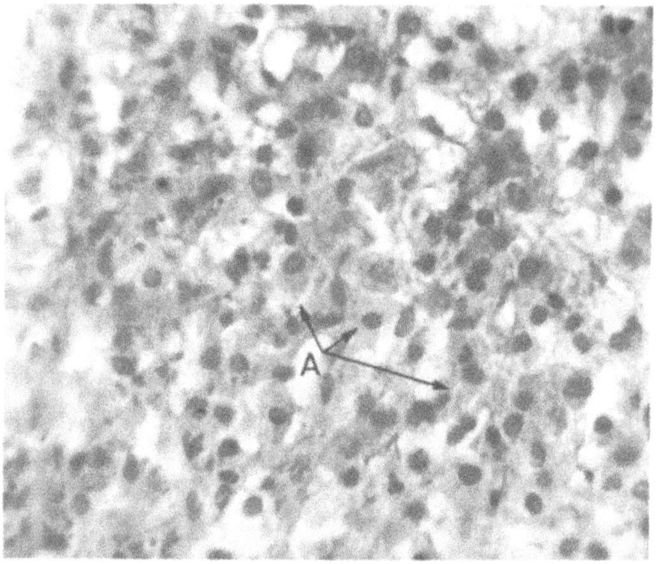

Fig. 2. Tissue culture of rabbit adenohypophysis combined with supraoptic nuclei of hypothalamus in anterior chamber of eye. Stage: 1 day; Zenker-formol; PAS reaction. × 630. *A* - degranulated adenocytes

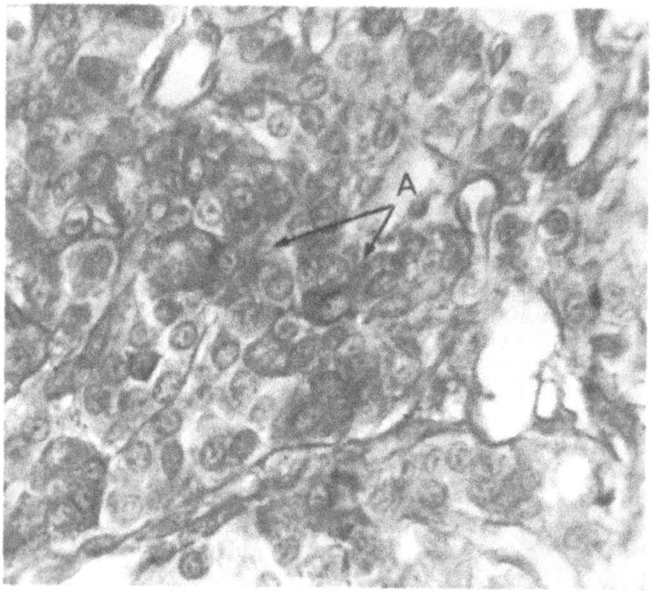

Fig. 3. Tissue culture of rabbit adenohypophysis combined with mediobasal hypothalamus in anterior chamber of eye. Stage: 6 days; Bouin's solution; PAS reaction - orange. × 630. *A* - basophilic adenocytes

opoiesis in the anterior lobe of the pituitary gland. In this series, chromophilic adenohypophyseal cells never acquire hyperchromic staining (which indicates the accumulation of the hormones in the cells), as was noted in the previous series of experiments.

The results of this investigation indicate that, in the regulation of the adenohypophysiotropic hormonopoiesis "Gomori-positive" neurosecretory material influences the rate of hormone release, whereas the mediobasal zone is able to carry out more specific roles connected with synthesis of adenohypophyseal hormones.

References

ALESHIN, B.V.: Histophysiology of the Hypothalamo-Hypophysial System. Moscow: Medicina 1971

ALESHIN, B.V.: Mechanisms of hypothalamic control of adenohypophyseal functions. Uspekhi Physiol. Nauk (Moscow) 5, 48-81 (1974)

LAZARENKO, F.M.: Application of a new method to the experimental study of tissues; some preliminary results. Arkh. Biol. Nauk (Moscow) 34, 88-97 (1934)

POLENOV, A.L.: Hypothalamic Neurosecretion. Leningrad: Nauka 1968

SZENTÁGOTHAI, J., FLERKÓ, B., MESS, B., HALÁSZ, B.: Hypothalamic control of the Anterior Pituitary. Budapest: Academiai Kiadó 1965

ZIMMERMAN, E.: Localization of gonadotropin-RF (Gn-RH) in the hypothalamus of the mouse by immunoperoxydase technique. Endocrinology 95, 1-8 (1974)

Distribution of Vasopressin, Oxytocin, Neurophysin, Somatostatin, and Luteinizing Hormone Releasing Hormone-Producing Neurons*

A. WEINDL, M. V. SOFRONIEW, and I. SCHINKO
Anatomisches Institut (Histologie) der Universität München, Pettenkoferstraße 11, 8000 München 2, FRG

The use of immunohistochemical techniques has confirmed the presence of neurohypophyseal and adenohypophysiotropic hormones within axons and axon terminals of the median eminence (see ZIMMERMAN, 1976). The magnocellular perikarya of the supraoptic (SON) and paraventricular nuclei (PVN) have also been confirmed as the sources of the neurohypophyseal hormones (BURLET et al., 1974; VANDESANDE et al., 1975). However, the location of the perikarya of origin of the "releasing and inhibiting hormones" remains a source of controversy. Using antisera capable of detecting somatostatin perikarya in normal animals, and LRH perikarya in castrated rats, we have begun a study on the topical neuroanatomy of neuroendocrine cells. We have taken the approach of using the magnocellular neurons of the hypothalamo-neurohypophyseal system as regional landmarks against which to compare the distribution of perikarya containing releasing and inhibiting hormones. We have also been able to identify a substantial amount of arginine vasopressin (AVP), oxytocin (OT), and neurophysin (NPh) containing fibers in several areas of the brain outside the hypothalamus.

The procedure for the fixation and preparation of tissue, the details of the immunoperoxidase method employed, and the control tests conducted, have been described (SOFRONIEW et al., 1978), for AVP, OT, and NPh. Luteinizing hormone releasing hormone (LRH) antiserum was raised in our laboratory in a manner similar to that described for AVP and OT (SOFRONIEW et al., 1978). Antiserum to bovine NPh I was provided by Dr. E.A. Zimmerman, Columbia University, New York, N.Y., and Dr. A.G. Robinson, University of Pittsburg, Pa. Antiserum to somatostatin was provided by Drs. Knigge and Sorrentino, University of Rochester, N.Y. Peroxidase-anti-peroxidase complex was provided by Dr. L. Sternberger, Edgewood Arsenal, Maryland.

In the zona interna of the median eminence as well as in the stalk and neural lobe, fibers positive for AVP or OT are inter-

*Supported by the Deutsche Forschungsgemeinschaft (SFB 51-C/21 and C/27).

Fig. 1a-h. Sagittal sections through hypothalamus of a castrated rat. (a-e). Immunoperoxidase reaction with antisera to (a) *LRH*, (b) oxytocin, (c) somatostatin, (d) neurophysin, (e) arginine-vasopressin; × 38. (f) detail of (b); oxytocin-producing perikarya, (g) detail of (c); somatostatin-producing perikarya. (h) detail of (d); neurophysin- (and vasopressin-)producing parvocellular perikarya of SCN; × 160. Note differences in size of perikarya in (f-h). *AC*, anterior commissure; *ME*, median eminence, *OCh*, optic chiasm; *PVN*, paraventricular nucleus; *SCN*, suprachiasmatic nucleus. ↓ points to location of perikarya; ‡ points to location of fibers

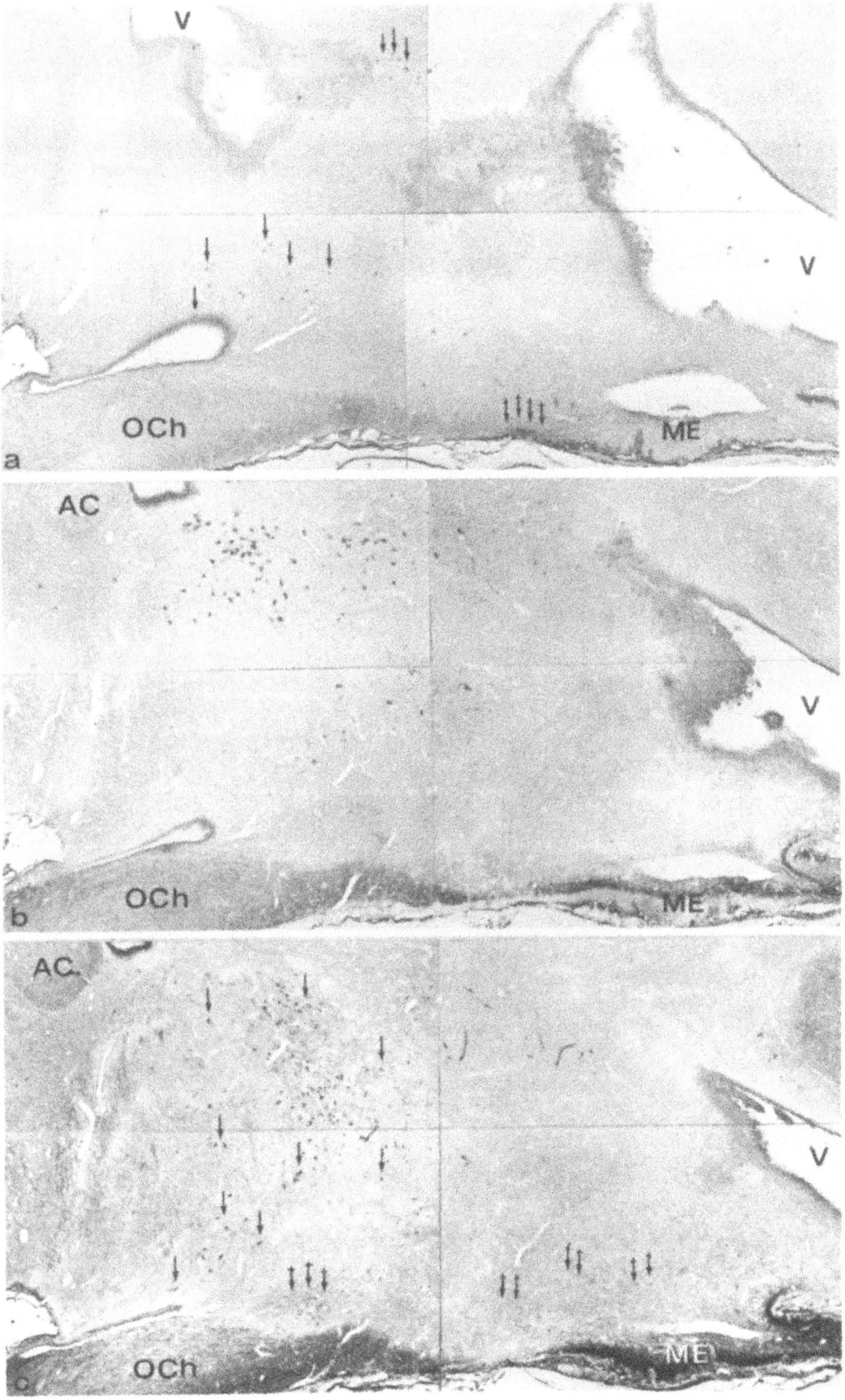

Fig. 1a-c

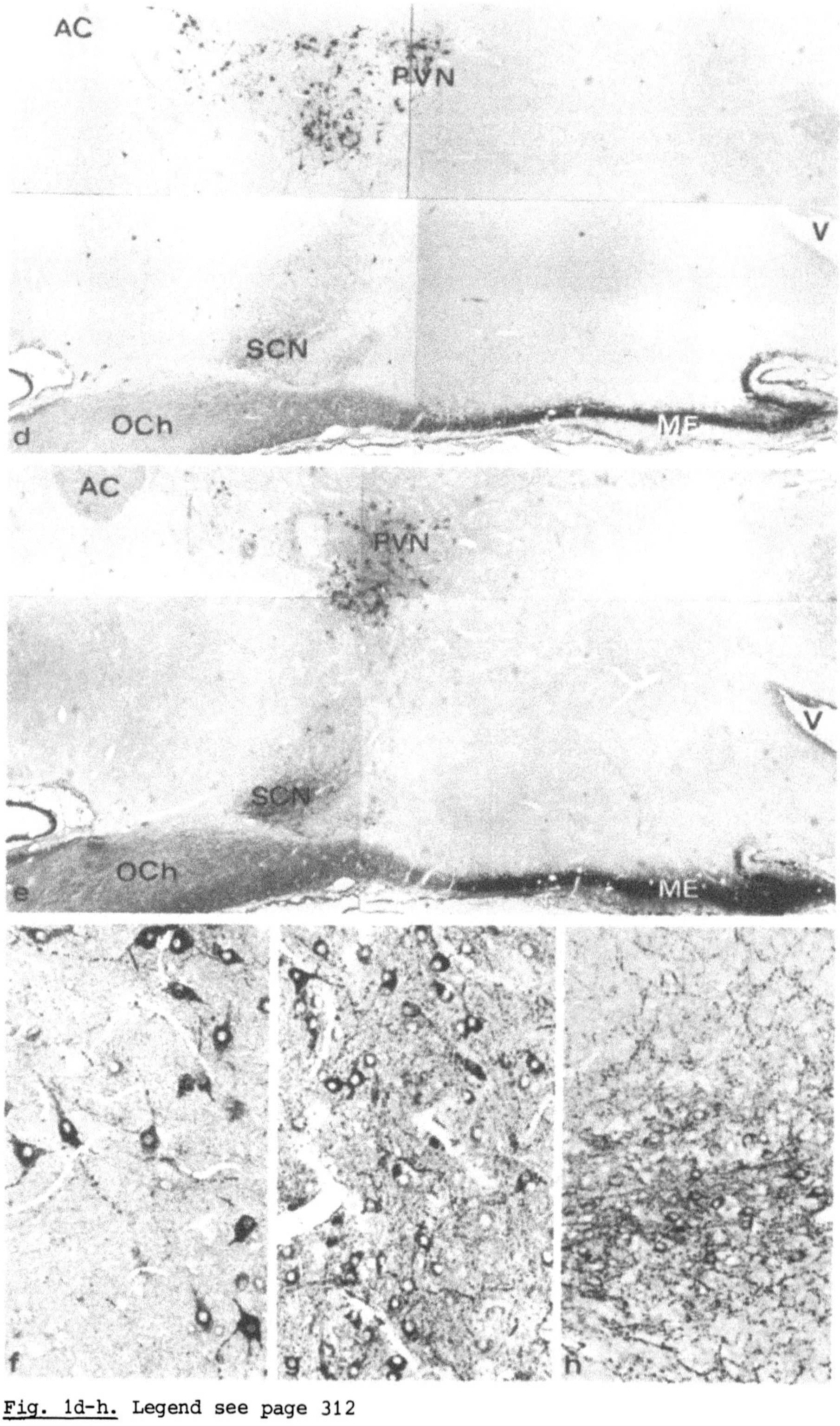

Fig. 1d-h. Legend see page 312

mingled; both types of fibers also contain NPh. The zona externa, however, exhibits a regional pattern of distribution for different hormones. In both the rat and guinea pig, LRH fibers are more heavily concentrated in the lateral portions of the external zone, whereas somatostatin fibers are more heavily concentrated in the medial portion. A similar pattern of distribution has been reported for these two hormones in the rat by KING et al. (1975). In the rat, AVP and NPh fibers can be found light microscopically, scattered throughout the medial portion of the external zone (Fig. 1d,e). The discrete localization of the hormones in various parts of the median eminence, with no overlap in certain areas, is evidence of the specificity of the immunohistochemical procedure for localizing individual hormones.

The perikarya of origin of the various peptide-containing fibers are distributed over a wide area of the hypothalamus. While AVP and OT producing perikarya in the SON are intermingled, there is a special pattern of distribution for magnocellular perikarya in the PVN. In the rat, a cluster of AVP-positive perikarya is located in the center of this nucleus. OT-positive perikarya occur primarily rostrally and dorsally to this cluster, and some are located more dorsally and caudally to it (Figs. 1b,d,e, and 2). The PVN of the guinea pig shows two distinct divisions of magnocellular perikarya. OT perikarya extend rostrocaudally in a periventricular layer, while AVP perikarya form a compact cluster corresponding to the PVN proper (SOFRONIEW et al., 1978). We find somatostatin-positive perikarya close to the third ventricle in the area of the anterior hypothalamic nucleus. This nucleus has been described by CHRIST (1969), based on conventional staining methods, to consist of medium-sized, loosely clustered perikarya ventral and slightly rostral to the PVN, which correlates well with the size and distribution of the somatostatin perikarya (Figs. 1, 2). Electrophysiologic stimulation of the anterior hypothalamus has been reported to inhibit growth hormone secretion (see MARTIN, 1976). ALPERT et al. (1976) have also described somatostatin perikarya in the anterior hypothalamic nucleus. There also appears to be a slight overlap of magnocellular perikarya with smaller somatostatin perikarya in the PVN. This is not unusual, since perikarya of several sizes are found in the PVN (see CHRIST, 1969). This finding may also explain the effect of electrophysiologic stimulation of the PVN on growth-hormone secretion (see MARTIN, 1976). The somatostatin perikarya (diameter 14-18 µm; Fig. 1g) are smaller than magnocellular perikarya (diameter 22-28 µm; Fig. 1f), yet larger than the parvocellular perikarya of the SCN (diameter 10-14 µm; Fig. 1h) containing vasopressin. This suggests that there are more than two different sizes of peptide producing perikarya in the hypothalamus. BARRY et al. (1973) also defined LRH-positive perikarya in the guinea pig as mediocellular.

Within the parvocellular SCN of the rat (Fig. 1d,e) and guinea pig (WEINDL and SOFRONIEW, 1976) a distinct group of perikarya located medially and dorsally react with AVP and NPh, but not with OT antiserum. Finely beaded AVP- and NPh-positive fibers leaving these perikarya are directed dorsally in both rat (Fig. 1d,e) and guinea pig; they do not descend to the median eminence as suggested by others (VANDESANDE et al., 1974). Within a separate central portion of the SCN we find finely beaded fibers stained with somatostatin antiserum (Figs. 1c, 2).

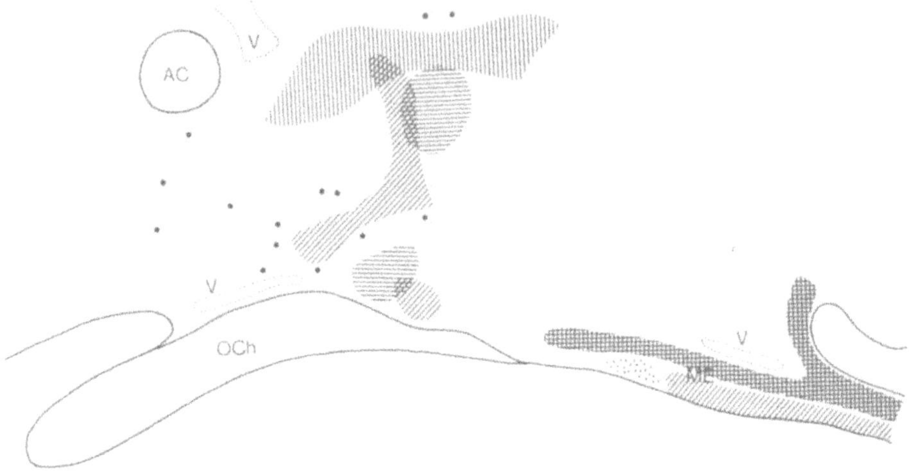

Fig. 2. Different locations of perikarya and fibers containing LRH (░░░), somatostatin (//////), vasopressin (≡≡≡), and oxytocin (||||||) are compared. *AC* - anterior commissure; *ME* - median eminence, *OCh* - optic chiasm; *V* - third ventricle. × 38

We find perikarya immunoreactive for LRH widely dispersed in the preoptic anterior hypothalamic region of castrated rats (Figs. 1a, 2). Some are located above the PVN. LRH perikarya appear not to be confined to a distinct nuclear group. Our staining of LRH perikarya, however, is not as intense as that found for other hormones, nor are there as many perikarya stained. The location of LRH-containing perikarya remains controversial, our data supporting the distribution of the perikarya in the preoptic anterior hypothalamic area originally described by BARRY et al. (1973). Some somatostatin-containing perikarya are located in the vicinity of the organum vasculosum of the lamina terminalis (OVLT). In the guinea pig, AVP- and OT-containing perikarya immediately surround the OVLT (SOFRONIEW and WEINDL, 1978). In the rat and guinea pig, LRH fibers are located around the vascular plexus of the OVLT. Within the OVLT, we find LRH fibers, in agreement with BARRY et al. (1973), as well as somatostatin fibers. The OVLT is a neurohemal zone where the blood-brain barrier does not exist. It has a possible neuroendocrine function (WEINDL, 1973).

Outside of the hypothalamus we have observed AVP- and NPh-containing neurons in several different areas of the guinea pig (Figs. 3, 4) and rat brain. Perikarya containing NPh, but not AVP are found in the triangular nucleus of the septum in the guinea pig (WEINDL and SOFRONIEW, 1976) and rat. We have also found two types of fibers containing AVP and NPh outside the hypothalamus (WEINDL and SOFRONIEW, 1976). Large-caliber fibers positive for AVP and NPh ascend from the magnocellular nuclei and join the stria terminalis. These fibers can be traced within the stria terminalis to the central amygdala, where a cluster of large-caliber fibers containing both AVP and NPh is found in the guinea pig (Fig. 3) (WEINDL and SOFRONIEW, 1976), as well as in the rat.

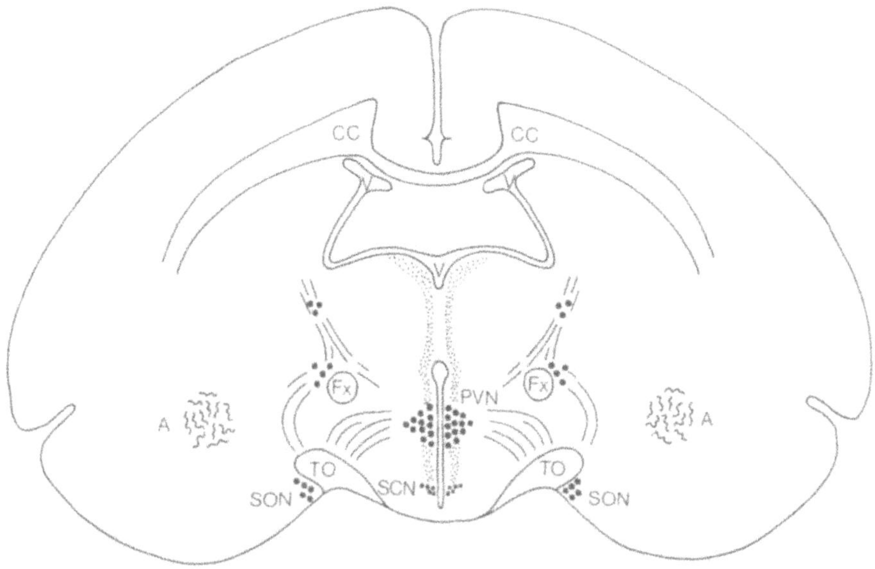

Fig. 3. Distribution of neurophysin- and vasopressin-containing perikarya and fibers in a frontal section of guinea-pig brain. Large-caliber fibers descend to neurohypophysis from magnocellular perikarya of supraoptic (*SON*) and paraventricular nuclei (*PVN*), and of perifornical region. Extrahypothalamic fibers from magnocellular perikarya ascend to stria terminalis, and appear to project to the central amygdala (*A*). Finely beaded small fibers found in medial and dorsal parts of thalamus ascend from parvocellular perikarya of the suprachiasmatic nucleus (*SCN*). *CC* - corpus callosum, *Fx* - fornix, *V* - ventricle, *TO* - optic tract. × 5

A smaller type of finely beaded NPh- and AVP-immunoreactive fibers has been described ascending from medial parts of the hypothalamus along the ventricle to the thalamus (WEINDL and SOFRONIEW, 1976). These fibers arise from the SCN, and can be traced to the lateral septum and to the lateral habenulae (Figs. 3, 4), in both the rat and guinea pig. In the guinea pig, fine fibers appear to descend to the lower brainstem (Fig. 4).

In the rat, large-caliber NPh and OT fibers descend from hypothalamic magnocellular nuclei to the lower brainstem and spinal cord, where they lie adjacent to the central canal and in the region of the anterior horn. These fibers are present in Brattleboro rats with a hereditary inability to produce AVP and its associated NPh. At present, large-caliber OT and NPh fibers do not appear to exist in the brainstem and spinal cord of the guinea pig.

The morphologic demonstration of fibers containing specific peptide hormones outside the hypothalamus may be related to the neurotropic effects of peptide hormones discussed by BARKER (1976).

Summary: Closely neighboring sections of normal guinea pig, normal rat, or castrated rat brains were stained alternately for arginine vasopressin (AVP), oxytocin (OT), neurophysin (NPh), somatostatin, and LRH, using antisera to these peptides and the

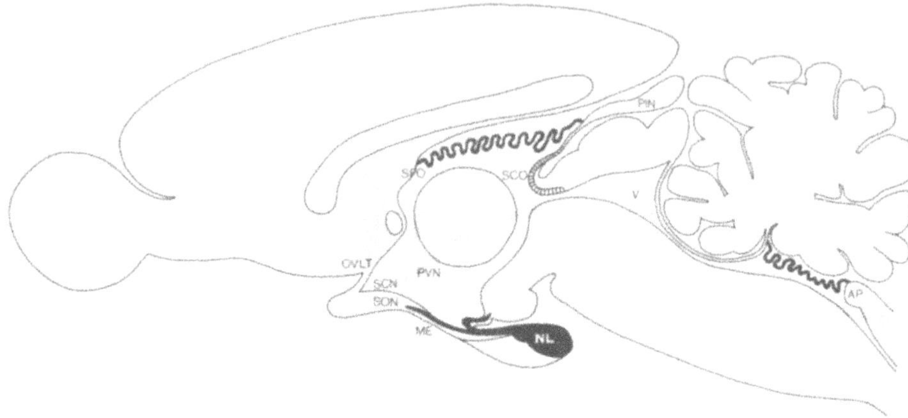

Fig. 4. Diagram of sagittally sectioned guinea pig brain. Lightly shaded regions represent extrahypothalamic areas where finely beaded small fibers, positive for neurophysin, have been found. These include the lateral septum, mediodorsal thalamus, and areas beneath the floor of the aqueduct and fourth ventricle. Fibers in the lateral septum and mediodorsal thalamus also contain AVP, and can be traced from the SCN. *AP* - area postrema, *ME* - median eminence, *NL* - neural lobe, *OVLT* - organum vasculosum of the lamina terminalis, *PIN* - pineal organ, *PVN* - paraventricular nucleus, *SCN* - suprachiasmatic nucleus, *SCO* - subcommissural organ, *SON* - supraoptic nucleus, *V* - ventricle. × 3

immunoperoxidase technique. AVP, OT, and NPh were found in the magnocellular components of both nuclei of the classic hypothalamo-neurohypophyseal system. In addition, AVP and NPh were found within a portion of the parvocellular perikarya of the suprachiasmatic nucleus (SCN) in both species. Somatostatin and LRH were found within fibers in discrete areas of the external zone of the median eminence in patterns similar to those described by others. Furthermore, a distinct cluster of somatostatin-containing perikarya was detected close to the third ventricle in the anterior hypothalamus, slightly ventro-rostral to the magnocellular neurons of the paraventricular nucleus containing AVP, OT, or NPh. Fibers containing somatostatin were also found in the SCN. Scattered individual perikarya containing LRH were seen at periventricular sites in the preoptic anterior hypothalamic area of castrated rats. In addition, AVP, OT, and NPh, as well as somatostatin-containing perikarya were found in the vicinity of the OVLT in the guinea pig; numerous fibers containing LRH were also found in the area around the OVLT, and small amounts of LRH and somatostatin were found within the organ itself in both species. The OVLT is a highly vascular area similar to the median eminence, where the blood-brain barrier does not exist. With increasing information, its hitherto unknown function seems to be involved in neuroendocrine activity. Numerous AVP, OT, and NPh fibers are found outside the hypothalamus. Large-caliber fibers, probably deriving from hypothalamic magnocellular perikarya ascend to and join the stria terminalis; they can be traced to the central amygdala in both species. In the rat, large-caliber OT and NPh fibers can be traced from the hypothalamus to the brainstem and spinal cord. Small-caliber AVP and NPh fibers, probably deriving from the parvocellular SCN, are found in the lateral septum and dorsal thalamus in both species.

References

ALPERT, L.C., BRAWER, J.R., PATEL, Y.C., REICHLIN, S.: Somatostatinergic neurons in anterior hypothalamus: immunohistochemical localization. Endocrinology 98, 255-259 (1976)

BARKER, J.L.: Peptides: Roles in neuronal excitability. Physiol. Rev. 56, 435-452 (1976)

BARRY, J., DUBOIS, M.P., POULAIN, P.: LRF producing cells of the mammalian hypothalamus. A fluorescent antibody study. Z. Zellforsch. Mikrosk. Anat. 146, 351-366 (1973)

BURLET, A., MARCHETTI, J., DUHEILLE, J.: Immunohistochemistry of vasopressin: Study of the hypothalamo-neurohypophyseal system of normal, dehydrated and hypophysectomized rats. In: Neurosecretion - The Final Neuroendocrine Pathway. KNOWLES, F., VOLLRATH, L. (eds.). Berlin-Heidelberg-New York: Springer-Verlag 1974, pp. 24-30

CHRIST, J.F.: Derivation and boundaries of the hypothalamus, with atlas. In: The Hypothalamus. HAYMAKER, W., ANDERSON, W., NAUTA, W.J.H. (eds.). Springfield: C. Thomas 1969, pp. 13-60

KING, J.C., GERALL, A.A., FISHBACK, J.B., ELKIND, K.E., ARIMURA, A.: Growth hormone-release inhibiting hormone (GH-RIH) pathway of rat hypothalamus revealed by the unlabeled antibody peroxidase-antiperoxidase method. Cell Tissue Res. 160, 423-430 (1975)

MARTIN, J.B.: Brain regulation of growth hormone secretion. In: Frontiers in Neuroendocrinology. MARTINI, L., GANONG, W.F. (eds.). New York: Raven Press 1976, Vol. IV, pp. 129-168

SOFRONIEW, M.V., WEINDL, A., SCHINKO, I., WETZSTEIN, R.: The distribution of vasopressin, oxytocin and neurophysin producing neurones in the guinea pig brain. I. The classical hypothalamo-neurohypophyseal system. Cell Tissue Res. (1978) (in preparation)

SOFRONIEW, M.V., WEINDL, A.: The distribution of vasopressin, oxytocin and neurophysin producing neurones in the guinea pig brain. II. Cell groups within the hypothalamus distinct from the supraoptic and paraventricular nuclei. Cell Tissue Res. (1978) (in preparation)

VANDESANDE, F., DE MAY, J., DIERICKX, K.: Identification of neurophysin producing cells. I. The origin of the neurophysin-like substance-containing nerve fibers of the external region of the median eminence of the rat. Cell Tissue Res. 151, 187-200 (1974)

VANDESANDE, F., DIERICKX, K., DE MEY, J.: Identification of the vasopressin-neurophysin II and the oxytocin-neurophysin I producing neurons in the bovine hypothalamus. Cell Tissue Res. 156, 189-200 (1975)

WEINDL, A.: Neuroendocrine aspects of circumventricular organs. In: Frontiers in Neuroendocrinology. GANONG, W.F., MARTINI, L. (eds.). New York: Oxford University Press 1973, pp. 3-32

WEINDL, A., SOFRONIEW, M.V.: Demonstration of extrahypothalamic peptide secreting neurons. A morphological contribution to the investigation of psychotropic effects of neurohormones. Pharmakopsychiatrie 5, 226-234 (1976)

ZIMMERMAN, E.A.: Localization of hypothalamic hormones by immunocytochemical techniques. In: Frontiers in Neuroendocrinology. MARTINI, L., GANONG, W.F. (eds.). New York: Raven Press 1976, Vol. IV, pp. 25-62

Immunohistologic Identification of Vertebrate Neurophysins

G. WOLF
Section of Biosciences, Karl Marx University, Leipzig, GDR

A. Introduction

According to WUU et al. (for review, see WALTER, 1975), there is a striking similarity in the molecular structure of different types of mammalian neurophysins (NP), associated with an extensive immunologic cross-reactivity. The cross-reactivity has been utilized very successfully by many authors in radioimmunoassays and immunohistologic investigations of the mammalian neurosecretory system. Moreover, the staining and histochemical properties of NP of all vertebrates are very similar. Thus, we decided to search for an immunologic relationship between NP within the vertebrate subphylum. The special aim of our work was to find a convenient immunohistologic method for the identification of NP and NP-like substances that would be applicable to all vertebrates; only one type of anti-NP antisera would be used, based on the principle of heterology. WATKINS (1975) started to investigate species-dependent cross-reactivity. In order to study the range limits of this cross-reactivity, we examined immunohistologically the reaction between the antiserum to porcine NP and, on the other hand, NP and NP-like substances inside and outside the hypothalamus in representatives of different vertebrate classes (see also WOLF, 1976).

B. Materials and Methods

New Zealand rabbits were used to produce an extensive cross-reacting antiserum against purified porcine NP. The antiserum was employed for the three-layer immunoperoxidase technique according to STERNBERGER (1972) (for details see WOLF, 1976). The following species were used: Mammalia: man (female, aged 82 years), Wistar rats (during and after day 15 of intrauterine life, newborns and adults); Aves: Japanese quail, pigeon; Reptilia: tortoise (*Testudo horsfieldii*); Amphibia: frog (*Rana temporaria*); Teleostei: crucian (*Carassius carassius*), bream (*Abramis brama*), carp (*Cyprinus carpio*); Chondrostei: sturgeon (*Acipenser güldenstaedti*)[2]; Cyclostomata: lamprey (*Lampetra planeri*); Insecta: cockroach (*Periplaneta americana*). The animals were killed by decapitation. Nerve tissues were fixed by immersion in Bouin's fluid, according to the technique of Bouin-Hollande (see VANDESANDE et al., 1975). Embedding in paraffin, serial sections, 5 µm thick.

---

[1] This study was supported by the Ministerium für Wissenschaft und Technik der DDR.

[2] Kindly supplied by Prof. Polenov of Leningrad.

C. Results and Discussion

In each of the vertebrate species studied, the magnocellular neurosecretory system was immunoreactive in all of its parts (Figs. 1 and 2); these were the same parts known to give a specific reaction for neurosecretory material by appropriate staining and histochemical methods. It appears that on an immunologic basis there is a close relationship between the NP-types in the whole vertebrate subphylum. This is true also for the fetal NP in rats. NP were seen in cells of the supraoptic nucleus of 16-day fetal rats, i.e., some days earlier than by staining methods.

Moreover, we showed the existence of immunoreactive material outside the classic magnocellular system. In all of these cases there was no clear evidence to establish the identity of the reacting material. However, it does seem to be closely related to NP. In the rat brain, we found NP or NP-like material in neurons of the parvicellular part of the paraventricular nucleus and in the suprachiasmatic nucleus, as well as in fibers of the external zone of the median eminence. These immunoreactive fibers were

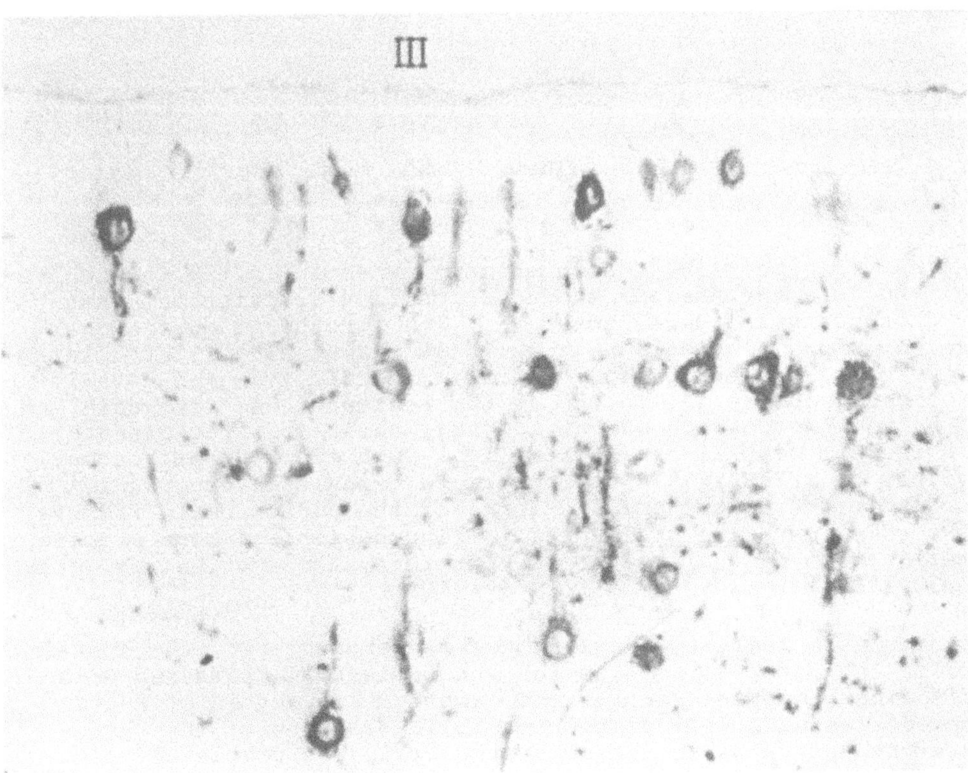

Fig. 1. Immunoperoxidase labeling of neurophysin-containing neurons of tortoise paraventricular nucleus. Frontal section; *III* - third ventricle

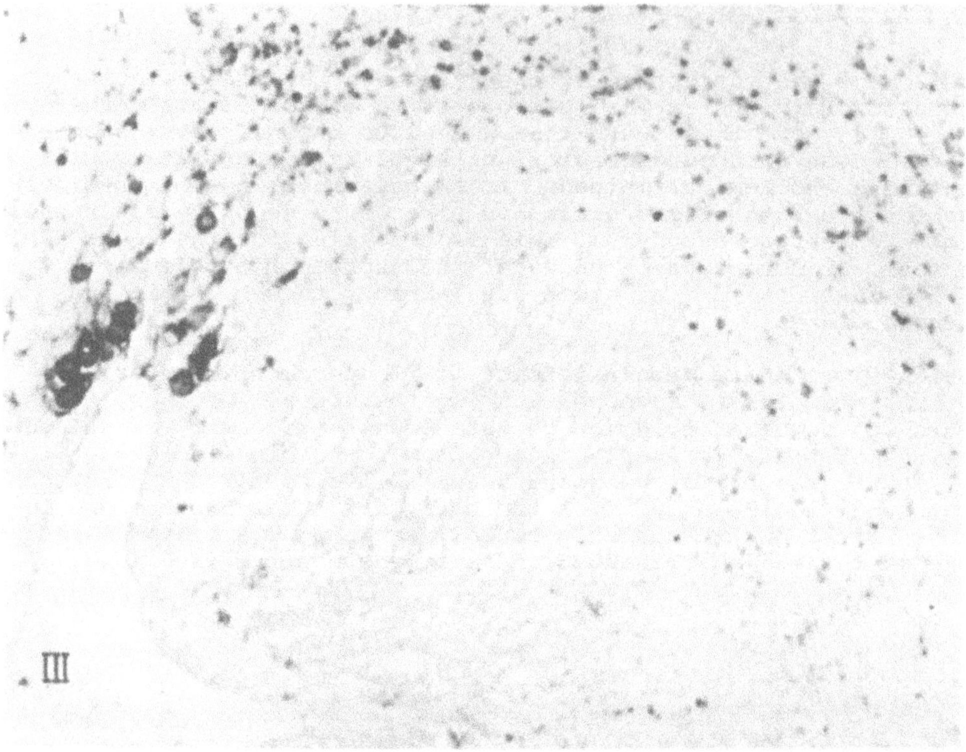

Fig. 2. Neurosecretory cells and fibers of adult female lamprey. Sagittal section, immunoperoxidase reaction for neurophysin; *III* - third ventricle

the last to appear in newborn animals, whereas in the suprachiasmatic nucleus the neurons showed a positive reaction only after day 3 of postnatal development (cf. the hypothesis on the character of suprachiasmatic neurons (DIERICKX et al., 1976)). In preliminary studies we showed that immunoreactive exohypothalamic fibers were, e.g., in the septum region of the rat brain and in the rhombencephalon of the lamprey; these observations are in agreement with findings from light- and electron microscopy, reviewed by STERBA (1974). Furthermore, single mesencephalic neurons in the torus semicircularis of the adult female lamprey showed NP or NP-like substances, making possible a more precise determination of the cystine-rich protein, as described by STERBA et al. (1973).

The urophysis and the caudal neurosecretory cells in the spinal cord of the carp, as well as the subcommissural organ and Reissner's fiber, examined in rat and lamprey, are devoid of any immunoreactive material. Immunohistologic staining of the neurosecretory apparatus in the cockroach brain was completely negative. Evidently, the secretory materials of the latter structures are characterized by substances unlike NP.

References

DIERICKX, K., VANDESANDE, F., MEY, J. DE: Identification, in the external region of the rat median eminence, of separate neurophysin-vasopressin and neurophysin-oxytocin containing nerve fibres. Cell Tissue Res. 168, 141-151 (1976)

STERBA, G.: Das oxytocinerge neurosekretorische System der Wirbeltiere. Beitrag zu einem erweiterten Konzept. Zool. Jb. Physiol. 78, 409-423 (1974)

STERBA, G., HOHEISEL, G., RÜHLE, H.-J., ENGELMANN, E.: Extrahypothalamische peptiderge Neurosekretion. I. Neurosekretion im Mittelhirn der Neunaugen. Z. Zellforsch. 142, 329-345 (1973)

STERNBERGER, L.A.: The unlabelled antibody-peroxidase and the quantitative immunouranium methods in light and electron immunohistochemistry. In: Techniques of Biophysical and Biochemical Morphology. GLICK, D., ROSENBAUM, R.M. (eds.). New York: Wiley Interscience 1972, Vol. I, pp. 67-88

VANDESANDE, F., DIERICKX, K., MEY, J. DE: Identification of the vasopressin-neurophysin II and the oxytocin-neurophysin I producing neurons in the bovine hypothalamus. Cell Tissue Res. 156, 189-200 (1975)

WALTER, R. (ed.): Neurophysins: carriers of peptide hormones. Ann. N.Y. Acad. Sci. 248 (1975)

WATKINS, W.B.: Immunocytochemical identification of neurophysin-secreting neurons in the hypothalamo-neurohypophysial system of some non-mammalian vertebrates. Cell Tissue Res. 162, 511-521 (1975)

WOLF, G.: Immunohistological identification of neurophysin and neurophysin-like substances in different vertebrates. Endokrinologie 68, 288-299 (1976)

Hypothalamic Neurosecretion in Mink (*Mustela vison* Schreb.) Kept Under Various Photoperiodic Conditions

M. N. YURISOVA and D. V. KLOTCHKOV
Institute of Cytology and Genetics, USSR Academy of Sciences Sibirian Department, Novosibirsk, USSR

The hypothalamo-hypophyseal neurosecretory system (HHNS) of male standard mink were studied cytomorphologically in November. The control (group I) was kept under natural photoperiodic conditions. For group II, daylight was prolonged from November 10-25 by 17 h. Group III was exposed to conditions simulating a halving of the natural light year; the day's length was gradually decreased from July to September up to 7.30 h and then increased by the end of November up to 17.00 h. In mink of groups II and III, the numbers of nuclei and nucleoli of the neurosecretory cells of the supraoptic nucleus were increased. The neurosecretion content in the cells and fibers of the supraoptic, postoptic, and paraventricular nuclei and of the median eminence (ME) was reduced twofold. The glial and vascular elements of these areas were activated. A twofold reduction of neurosecretory material in the posterior pituitary (PP) was observed in mink of group II only. The cells of the arcuate nucleus demonstrated increases in the size of nuclei (insignificant) and nucleoli (significant) in mink of group III. In these mink, the glial elements of the ME were markedly hyperplastic (by 107%) and hypertrophic (by 139%). The glial cells of the ME of group II were slightly activated (by 28% and 36%, respectively). The proliferative processes in gonads of mink of group III were much more advanced than those of group II. It is possible that the regulatory effect of the peptidergic HHNS is exerted through the PP in mink of group II. This effect is exerted in mink of group III by the complex comprising the magnocellular and arcuate nuclei acting, largely, through the adenohypophysis.

Annual Dynamics of Activity of the Hypothalamo-Hypophyseal Neurosecretory System in Ground Squirrels, *Citellus erythrogenys* Brandt and *C. undulatus* Pallas

M. N. YURISOVA, A. L. POLENOV, and A. D. SLONIM
Institute of Cytology and Genetics, Novosibirsk and Sechenov Institute of Evolutionary Physiology and Biochemistry, Leningrad, USSR

An important role of the neurosecretory mechanisms in the regulation of hibernation is well known. However, the role of the "Gomori-positive" hypothalamo-hypophyseal neurosecretory system (HHNS) in hibernation is far from clear. The results and interpretations are rather contradictory (see YURISOVA, 1970; POLENOV and YURISOVA, 1976).

Morphology of all parts of the HHNS in 120 hibernating ground squirrels of two species characterized by different ecology was studied monthly. In *C. undulatus* hibernation is shorter and awakenings are more frequent than in *C. erythrogenys*. Cytometry (Gomori-Gabe's paraldehyde fuchsin (PAF) + Azan preparations) and spectrophotometry (evaluation of the relative amount of neurosecretory material (NSM) in the posterior pituitary (PP)) were used.

Changes found in the neurosecretory centers show unidirectional character, and those in the nucleus supraopticus (NSO) are more profound. In *C. erythrogenys* the volume of nuclei and nucleoli in the neurosecretory cells decreases gradually during hibernation, up to its minimal size in December (Fig. 1). At the same time the NSM is progressively accumulated in the perikarya (Table 1). Glial nuclei are very small, and the capillaries are collapsed. The content of the NSM increases sharply in the neurosecretory fibers of the hypothalamic regions and in the median eminence (ME), up to the height of hibernation. Concentration of NSM in the PP rises from the beginning of torpidity (262.6 ± 3.9 arbitrary units (AU)) up to December (336.1 ± 1.26 AU). Small nuclei of pituicytes and collapsed capillaries are hardly seen, due to the abundant content of NSM. Synthesis and transport of the NSM in the HHNS are reduced to a minimum in December.

Beginning in January some indications of activation of the HHNS are evident. The size of the neurosecretory cells (NSC) and of the nuclei and nucleoli increases. Up to the end of March the NSM content decreases progressively in the perikarya and in the PP (up to 162.2 ± 10.4 AU). Vacuoles occur more frequently in the cytoplasm. Hyperemia increases in all parts of the HHNS. In February, transport of the NSM along the fibers to the ME where it is accumulated becomes apparent. Capillaries of the Mantelplexus are hyperemized; neurosecretory endings often make contact with them.

A decrease of the amount of NSM in the HHNS that takes place in hibernating animals is most active in arousing ground squirrels in April and leads to almost complete devastation of the HHNS. The maximum nuclear and nucleolar volume of the NSC, almost complete

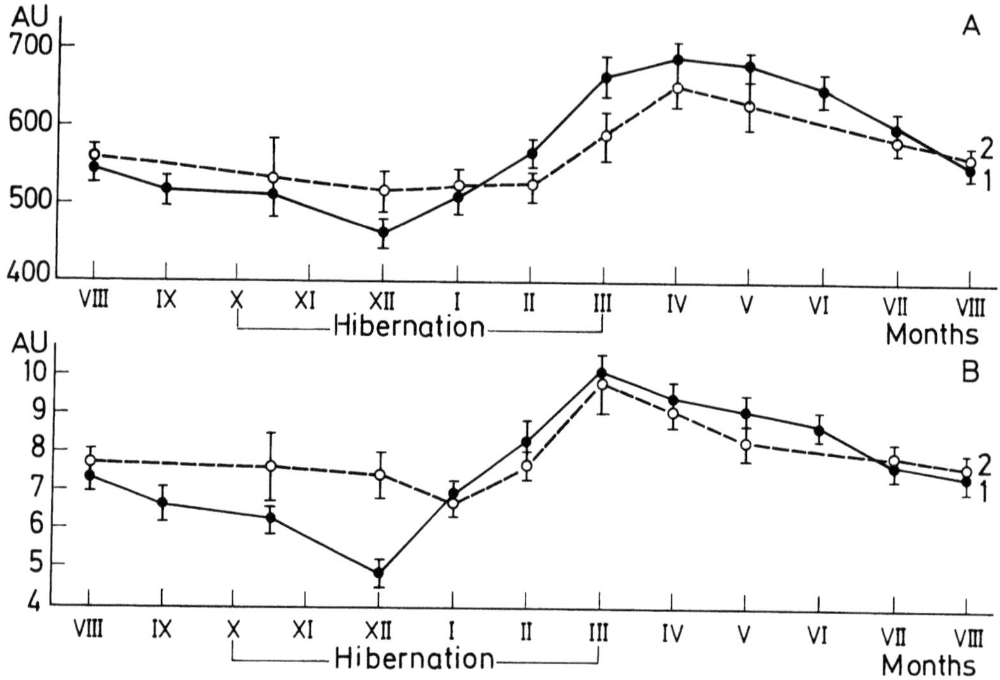

Fig. 1. Seasonal dynamics of volume (AU) of (A) nuclei and (B) nucleoli of neurosecretory cells of NSO in *C. erythrogenys* Brandt (*1*) and *C. undulatus* Pallas (*2*). *AU* - arbitrary units

absence of NSM in their perikarya and in the PP up to beginning of May, and the appearance of a large number of pyknomorphous cells (up to 47%) speak for a high activity of the NSC. All regions of the HHNS show hyperemia, their glial elements a maximum activity. In June and during the summer-autumn months, progressive accumulations of NSM in the NSC and in the PP, a decrease of the nuclear and nucleolar volume of the neurosecretory and glial cells are observed. Hyperemia of all parts of the HHNS decreases. In September, the state of the HHNS is similar to that at the beginning of hibernation.

In *C. undulatus* the same seasonal changes of the HHNS are seen, but they are not so clearly expressed as in *C. erythrogenys*. The amplitude of fluctuations of the karyometric index is smaller (Fig. 1). Accumulations of NSM during hibernation and its reduction in the HHNS in the spring are less prominent than in *C. erythrogenys*.

These data demonstrate changes of the functional state of the HHNS not only in the period of active life of ground squirrels but also during their hibernation. It is interesting to note that changes in the HHNS precede corresponding changes of some important physiologic processes. The revealed peculiarities of the HHNS during seasonal changes are in accordance with the ecological specificity of the ground squirrels.

Table 1. Amount of NSM (arbitrary 5-unit scale) in different parts of the HHNS

Months	Nucleus supraopticus		Nucleus postopticus		Nucleus paraventricularis		Neurohypophysis	
	Perikarya	Processes	Perikarya	Processes	Perikarya	Processes	Median eminence	Posterior pituitary
	Hibernation							
October-November	4.2	1.0	3.8	0.8	4.0	0.7	3.7	3.9
December	4.8	1.1	4.7	0.6	4.6	1.2	2.6	5.0
January	4.9	0.2	4.8	0.3	5.0	0.3	0.6	5.0
February	3.8	0.5	4.5	0.8	4.6	1.3	2.0	4.2
March	2.8	1.5	3.3	0.9	4.2	1.0	2.8	3.5
	Active Period							
March	2.7	0.8	2.8	1.1	3.6	1.0	3.0	3.0
April	2.3	1.0	2.6	1.5	2.8	1.0	2.5	2.2
May 1	0.3	0.1	1.2	0.7	2.0	0.3	1.3	1.5
May 20	1.5	1.3	1.5	0.9	2.5	1.2	1.1	2.3
June	2.1	1.1	2.1	1.5	3.0	1.4	1.5	2.5
July	2.9	1.0	2.5	1.0	3.3	1.0	2.3	3.0
August	3.5	1.3	3.2	1.8	3.6	1.3	2.9	3.7
September	3.8	3.8	3.5	2.0	3.8	2.0	3.3	3.8

References

POLENOV, A.L., YURISOVA, M.N.: The hypothalamo-hypophysial system in the ground squirrels, *Citellus erythrogenys* Brandt and *Citellus undulatus* Pallas. I. Microanatomy and cytomorphology of the Gomori-positive neurosecretory system with special reference to its state during hibernation. Z. mikrosk.-anat. Forsch., Leipzig (in press)

YURISOVA, M.N.: Ecological histophysiology of the hypothalamo-hypophysial neurosecretory system in the red-cheeked (*Citellus erythrogenys* Brandt) and long-tailed (*Citellus undulatus* Pallas) ground squirrels. Thesis. Novosibirsk 1970 (in Russian)

Morphofunctional Basis of Involutional Changes in the Neuroendocrine System

T. B. ZHURAVLEVA, R. A. PROCHUKHANOV, V. A. GRANTYN, G. V. IVANOVA, G. B. KOVALSKY, T. I. ROSTOVTSEVA-BAIDACHENKO, L. I. PLINER, and I. A. RAVKIN
Department of Pathologic Anatomy, Leningrad I.P.Pavlov Medical Institute, USSR

A. Introduction

It is generally accepted in modern endocrinology and gerontology that changes in the neuroendocrine system (NES) play a decisive role in the involution processes of an organism (BENDER et al., 1970; DILMAN, 1968; GITMAN, 1967; ROBERTSON et al., 1972). The contribution of the neurosecretory apparatus of the hypothalamus is considered of particular importance (DILMAN et al., 1975; EVERITT, 1973; FROLKIS et al., 1972). There are numerous works in the literature that deal with functional characteristics of different components of the NES at different ages. However, there are no data on functional morphology based on quantitative cytochemical methods at initial stages of aging.

The purpose of the present investigation is to analyze the initial manifestation of the changes connected with aging in the main components of the NES. We attempted to elucidate the structural and metabolic substrates responsible for such changes.

B. Materials and Methods

Two hundred female albino rats (from a mixed line) were used in this study. They comprised two age groups: (1) young mature rats (4-5 months old) with a 5-day estrous cycle (EC), and (2) aging animals (12 months old). We observed that rats from our breeding colony displayed a prolonged EC up to 6-9 days (due to the prolonged diestrus) by the end of the first year of life. Biochemical analysis of rats of this age revealed some signs of disintegration of the endocrine system, e.g., the disturbance of synchronization between the major endocrine glands (ovarian, adrenal, thyroid) (LEDOVSKAYA and PROCHUKHANOV, 1976). Morphofunctional analysis in the present research included a complex cytochemical investigation with subsequent cytophotometry and mathematical calculations, applying a specialized computer program (PROCHUKHANOV, 1975). Calculations were performed on an ES-1020 computer.

C. Organs Subjected to Analysis and Methods

(1) Hypothalamus: paraventricular (PVN) and arcuate (AN) nuclei, median eminence (ME), posterior lobe of pituitary (PH), nucleic acids (gallocyanin), monoamines (MA), NAD and NADP-diaphorase (NAD, NADP), acid and alkaline phosphatase (ASP, ALP), monoaminoxidase (MAO), proteins and karyometry, (2) adeno-

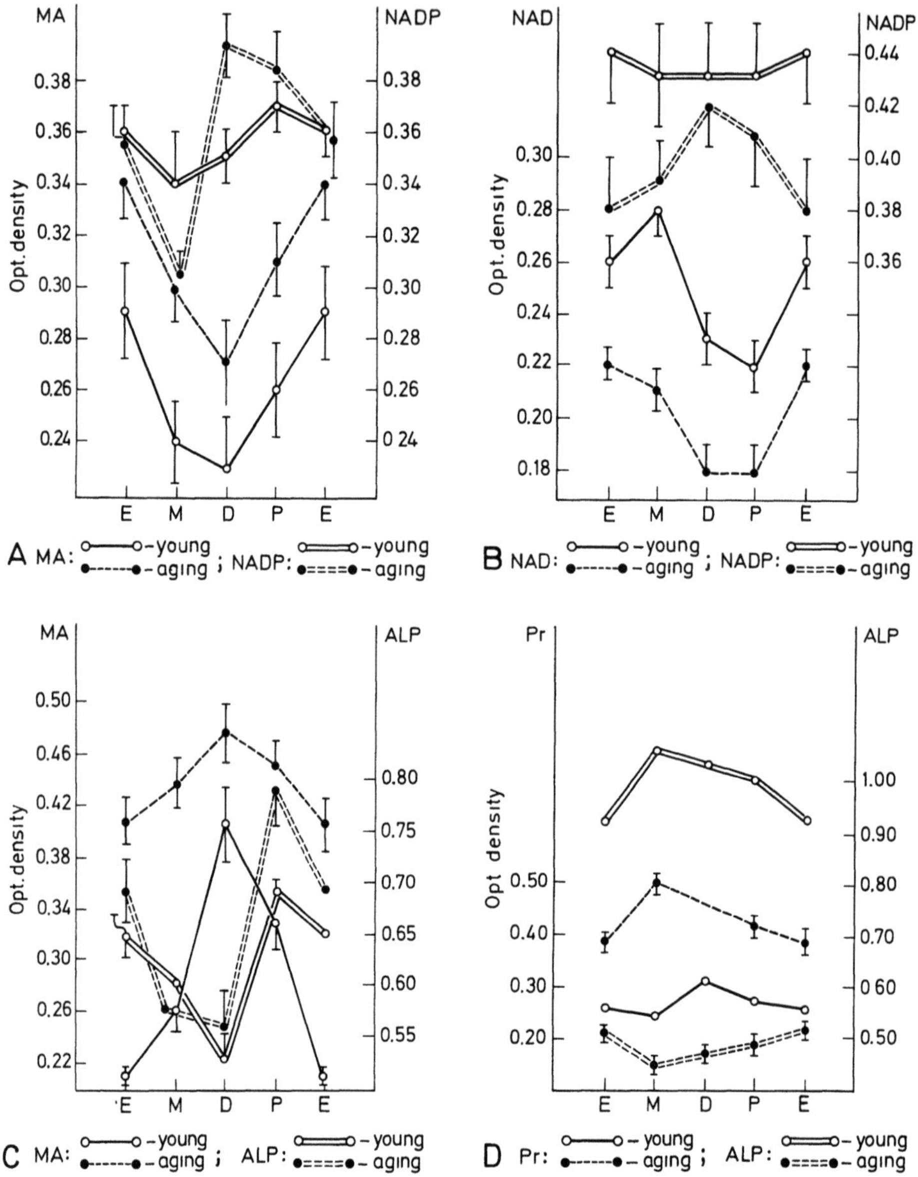

Fig. 1. (A) Content of monoamines (*MA*) and activity of NADP-diaphorase (*NADP*) in AN of hypothalamus during EC. (B) Activity of NAD and NADP-diaphorase (*NAD, NADP*) in PVN of hypothalamus during EC. (C) Content of MA and activity of alkaline phosphatase (*ALP*) in ME of hypothalamus during EC. (D) Content of proteins (*Pr.*). and activity of ALP in PH during EC. *E* - estrous, *M* - metestrous, *D* - diestrous, *P* - proestrous

hypophysis: common proteins, nucleic acids, NAD, NADP, ASP, ALP, and karyometry, (3) adrenal cortex: NAD, NADP, glucose-6-phosphate-dehydrogenase (G-6-PD), 3β-OH steroiddehydrogenase (3β-OH-SD), and 11-hydroxysteroiddehydrogenase (11-β-OH), (4) ovary: NAD, NADP, ALP, 3β-OH-SD, G-6-PD, 17β-OH-SD, 20α-OH-SD, esterase, and stereometry.

D. Results

I. Arcuate Nucleus (AN)

Compared to young animals, the AN in rats from the "aging" group displayed an increased content of MA, combined with a reduction of MAO activity. There was some activation of NAD and NADP (Fig. 1A). The cyclic dynamics of these indexes remained unchanged, but the degree of the cyclic changes and the number of cells displaying fluctuations of enzyme activity and the MA content in the course of the EC were increased. The nucleic acid "activity" (nuclear and cytoplasmic DNA and RNA) was slightly reduced. The character of the cyclic changes was modified, but the degree of modulation remained unchanged.

The MA content of the ME of aging rats was markedly increased when compared to that of young animals. In contrast to the observation of the AN, the amplitude of fluctuations of the MA concentration of the ME in the course of the EC was greatly diminished. At the same time, no changes in the activity or the dynamic pattern of the ALP in the capillary plexus of the portal system could be found. Moreover, the degree of proestrous activation of this enzyme was even greater than in young animals (Fig. 1C).

These data testify to the increased functional activity of the AN in aging animals, which is reflected by a rise in MA content and activation of oxidation-reduction enzymes. The susceptibility of the AN neurons to peripheral hormonal influences is still preserved at this age, as is seen from the absence of any reduction in the amplitude of the cyclic modulation both with respect to the histochemical indices mentioned above, and to the number of cells displaying functional changes correlated with the EC.

The constant and relatively high content of MA in the ME at all stages of the EC indicates a disturbance of transport functions at the level of the ME in aging animals. The results of the experiment correspond to data in the literature (BARANOV et al., 1970).

II. Paraventricular Nucleus (PVN)

PVN in aging rats is characterized by a decrease (compared to young control animals) in the activity of NAD and NADP (Fig. 1B). At the same time, the fluctuations in AP and ALP occur more slowly though the level of their activity is unchanged. Changes of activity of the nucleic acid in the PVN of aging animals consisted of an increase of DNA activity and deviations from the normal cyclic changes in DNA and RNA. Furthermore, the synchrony of the dynamic changes of nuclear and cytoplasmic RNA, which is typical of young animals, is markedly disturbed in the aging animals. Analysis of the posterior hypophyseal lobe showed a marked decrease in the ALP activity of the vascular walls during aging. These changes develop parallel to the accumulation of protein in this organ (Fig. 1D). The data show a depression of transport processes at the level of the PH, as well as a decrease in the metabolism of the PVN neurons. In summary, we conclude that the initital stage of functional-morphologic changes associated with aging can be revealed in the arcuate and paraventricular hypothalamic nuclei. Desynchronization between parvi- and magnocellular nuclei is observed in the hypothalamus during aging, while the level of metabolism is preserved.

III. Adenohypophysis

The analysis of DNA and RNA of aging animals shows a marked reduction of the amplitude of DNA oscillations in all the zones of adenohypophysis, while nuclear and cytoplasmic RNA oscillations were changed only in shape. Contrary to the changes seen in young animals, the RNA level decreases in proestrus in all the zones, regardless of the cell contacts with active vessels. The greatest modifications are observed in the dorsal zone, where the ACTH cells are accumulated. These changes in DNA and RNA are reflected in the dynamics of the other morphofunctional patterns. Thus, the analysis of simple proteins reveals a real increase in their concentration and in the amplitude of their oscillations in the cells of aging animals. The analysis of histograms proved that the increased level of simple proteins in aging animals is maintained by the same number of cells as within the young animals. Hence, the amplification of protein metabolism or some changes in transport processes is marked. The study of enzymes of the mitochondria, endoplasmic reticulum, and lysosomes showed a diminishing level of hydrolysis and energy supply (Fig. 2). The increase in the average content of proteins is probably due to the suppression of transport of proteins from the cells. This is confirmed by the simultaneous analysis of the nucleic-acid system and of the activity of oxidation-reduction and and hydrolytic enzymes.

Thus, during the first stages of involution, the stabilization of synthesis and transport processes takes place in the cells of all parts of the adenohypophysis, regardless of the cellular contacts with the vessels. These changes are most vividly expressed in the dorsal zone of the adenohypophysis, the zone of accumulation of the adrenocroticotrophic cells.

IV. Adrenal Cortex

The involutional peculiarities were expressed in a sharp leveling of the cyclic dynamics of enzyme activity (G-6-PD, NAD, NADP). Though the average level of activity of these enzymes did not differ from that in young animals, the character of mor-

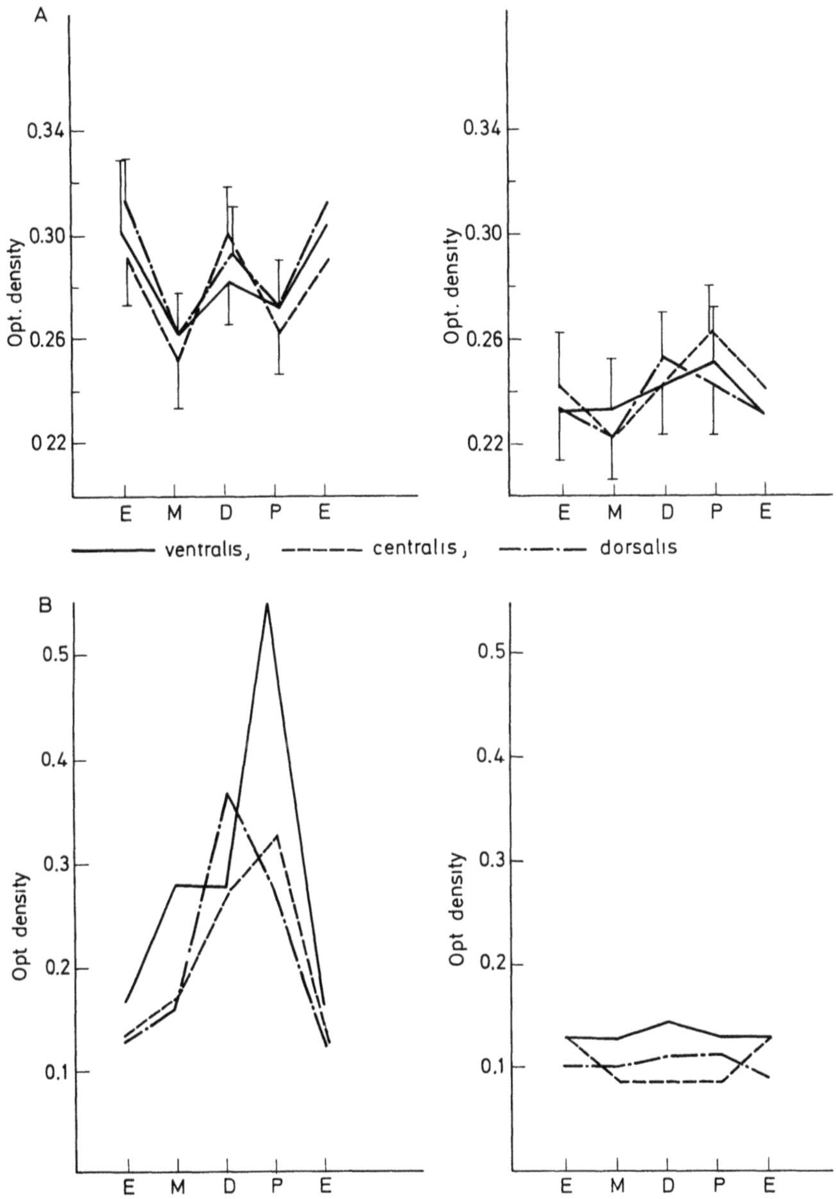

Fig. 2. (A) Activity of NADP-diaphorase in adenohypophysis during EC. (B) Activity of alkaline phosphatase in adenohypophysis during EC. *1* - young, *2* - aging. *E* - estrous, *m* - metestrous, *D* - diestrous, *P* - proestrous

phofunctional relations between different parts of the cortex was altered. The activity of oxidation-reduction enzymes was relatively higher in the zona reticularis, but the changes in the specific enzymes of steroid synthesis that took place in aging were different. The cyclic dynamics not only did not decrease, but tended to intensify. The average level of activity of these enzymes was approximately equal in young and aging animals. Nevertheless, there appeared to be a lack of integration between different zones of the cortex. For 3β-OH this was expressed by a relative increase of activity in the zona reticularis, and for the 11β-OH by a threefold increase in the amplitude of oscillations in the inner part of the cortex.

Thus, the activity of all the enzymes studied in the cells of the adrenal cortex was similar in both the young and the aging animals. The enzymes of steroid synthesis, however, preserve cyclic oscillations. At the same time, a strong depression in the cyclic dynamics of enzymes providing initial stages of steroid synthesis (G-6-PD, NADP) points to a reduction of central stimulation of steroidogenesis. A lack of integration between the function of energetic and specific enzymes was reflected in the changing level of corticosteroid secretion. The age-specific features of adrenalcortical function are marked by a changing of the mechanisms of structural integration, i.e., in the amplification of activity of the zona reticularis compared to the zona fasciculata.

V. Ovary

According to histologic and stereometric data, there is a depression of follicle development and a decrease in the mass of interstitial tissue in the ovaries of aging rats and in the corpus luteum in the organ. Our data point to a slight decrease in hormonal function of the follicles. The initial level of activity of 3β-OH-SD and of esterase in follicle walls is reduced, but in the preovulatory period the decrease of energy supply (NAD, NADP) occurs there as well. The general index of steroidogenesis in interstitial tissue (3β-OH-SD) is lowered. The levels of oscillations of (17β-OH-SD, 20α-OH-SD, G-6-PD) and of esterase are preserved. The quantitative analysis of ALP activity in vascular walls revealed diminishing levels of reaction, with a decrease in the amplitude of oscillations in the interna of follicles, old old corpora lutea, and in interstitial glands without cavities.

In summary, a decreased integration of the morphofunctional system of the follicle-interstitial gland and the corpus luteum occurs in the ovaries of aging rats. It is seen in the relative disconnection of energy supply and hormonal synthesis as well as in the decrease of vascular transport processes in some types of ovarian structures.

E. Conclusion

In this investigation, a complex approach has been applied to evaluate the development of the initial stages of involution. The analysis was based on the cytophotometric assay of proteins, monoamines, and nucleic acids as well as the enzyme activity in energy supply, synthesis, metabolism, and transport within the main subdivisions of the neuroendocrine system (NES). The results indicate that the initial disintegration of NES functions is characterized by two features: on one hand, the structural and metabolic patterns are maintained at a level close to optimal, and on the other hand, the amplitude of their cyclic modulations is reduced. At the same time, there is an accumulation of the products of synthesis (monoamines, proteins) in the neurohemal organs and hypophysis. These results, combined with observations on the state of the blood vessels within the main NES subdivisions, show that the development of the aging processes is determined, not by a primary impairment of specific functions of certain NES structures, but rather by the disturbance of interactions between them. It is defined by the initial changes in vascular transport first in the hypothalamic-portal system and adenohypophysis. The development of all the alterations of the microcirculatory system is probably a result of chronic interference by the so-called "ballast" reactions, which accompany any compensatory reaction in all kind of disturbance (stress) and are known to affect primarily the microcirculation. The presence of such "ballast" reactions is determined in its turn by the structural-metabolic "attachment" within each endocrine organ, as has been illustrated by our previous investigations of each separate link of the NES (II).

References

BARANOV, V.G., PROPP, M.V., SAVTCHENKO, O.N., STEPANOV, G.S.: Physiological changes of the hypothalamic-hypophyseal control of the ovarian function in ageing rats. Physiol. J. USSR 56 (7), 1013-1019 (1970)

BENDER, A.D., KORMENDY, C.G., POWELL, R.: Pharmacological control of aging. Exp. Gerontol. 5 (2), 97-129 (1970)

DILMAN, V.M.: Ageing, Clima and Cancer. Leningrad 1968

DILMAN, V.M.: Elevationary mechanism of development, ageing and age-related pathology. Comm. 1. Elevation of the hypothalamic threshold to feedback suppression in ageing. Physiol. Man 1 (2), 336-343 (1975)

EVERITT, A.V.: The hypothalamic-pituitary control of ageing and age-related pathology. Exp. Gerontol. 8 (5), 265-277 (1973)

FROLKIS, V.V., BEZRUKOV, V.V., DUPLENKO, Y.K., GENIS, E.D.: The hypothalamus in Ageing. Exp. Gerontol. 7 (3), 169-184 (1972)

GITMAN, L.: Endocrines and Ageing. Springfield (Illinois): Charles C. Thomas 1967

LEDOVSKAYA, S.M., PROCHUKHANOV, R.A.: On the character of functional links in the endocrine system of female albino rats and its age specific changes. Probl. Endocrinol. 22 (3), 103-107 (1976)

PROCHUKHANOV, R.A.: Objectives and prospects of quantitative histochemistry. Arch. Pathol. 37, (2), 77-84 (1975)

ROBERTSON, O.H., BREZNOCK, E.M., RIEGLE, G.D.: Endocrines and Ageing. New York: MSS Information Corporation 1972

ZHURAVLEVA, T.B., PROCHUKHANOV, R.A.: Functional Morphology of Neuroendocrine System. Leningrad: 1976

Interrelationship of the Hypothalamus and the Gonads in the Fish *Aspro zindel* L.

M. ŽORIĆ
Institute of Biology, Medical Faculty, Niš, Yugoslavia

In the course of the investigation of the sexual cycle of the fish Asproon (*Aspro zindel* L.), variation of the microstructure of the preoptic nucleus (NPO and NLT) and β-cells of the meso-adenohypophysis related to morphodynamics of the ovary and testis was observed.

During the analysis of the preoptic nucleus according to POLENOV's classification (1965), three stages in the development of the neurosecretory cells were noted: multiplication, migration from the ependyma, and a storage stage. The period of degeneration was noted in most cases before spawning. With the exceptions of the preoptico-hypophyseal and tubero-hypophyseal tracts, hydro-encephalocrinia was noted within the recess of the infundibulum and in the preoptic recess in most cases. β-cells display marked basophilia before and during spawning, while they are hypobasophilic in the period after spawning. The cells of the preoptic nucleus and the β-cells show signs of activity before and during spawning, while immediately after spawning they are in an involutive condition. It can be concluded that correlative relations exist between these organs and the maturation of the ovary and testis.

Reference

POLENOV, A.L.: Functional Morphology of Diencephalic Neurosecretory Elements in Several Vertebrates. (In Russsian). Leningrad: Academy of Science of USSR (Institute of Physiology) 1965, p. 57

Effects of Low-Molecular-Weight Substances on Synthesis and Release of Prolactin in Rat

O. N. ZRYAKOV and N. P. KORNYUSHENKO
Institute of Endocrinology and Metabolism, Kiev, USSR

Hypothalamic low-molecular-weight biogenic substances take part in the control of anterior-pituitary function (KAMBERI et al., 1971). The effects of various concentrations of some of them on prolactin synthesis and release were investigated in vitro (ZRYAKOV, 1975). It has been shown that serotonin and tryptamine had no effect on prolactin synthesis and release. Dopamine and noradrenaline (7×10^{-6} *M*–2.8×10^{-5} *M*) inhibited these processes, whereas the same concentrations of γ-aminobutyric acid and acetylcholine stimulated them. These actions were realized via hypothalamic factors, as the actions mentioned disappeared in the absence of hypothalamic tissue in the incubation system. Histamine (1.4×10^{-5} *M*–2.8×10^{-5} *M*), cyclic 2.3-AMP, and cyclic 3.5-AMP (5×10^{-6} *M*) depressed prolactin release and probably also synthesis at the pituitary level. As an experimental model in vivo, a sharp rise in prolactin synthesis was produced by estradiol injection into 30-day-old female and male rats (VOOGT et al., 1970). The results of the experiments in vivo confirmed the data gained in vitro, i.e., that catecholamines are specific inhibitors and acetylcholine a specific stimulator of prolactin synthesis and release, their action being mediated by hypothalamic factors.

References

KAMBERI, I.A., MICAL, R.S., PORTER, J.C.: Endocrinology 88, 1021-1020 (1971)
VOOGT, J.L., CHEN, C.L., MEITES, J.: Am. J. Physiol. 218, 396-399 (1970)
ZRYAKOV, O.N., DOPOVIDI: Acad. Sci. Ukr. SSR 12, 1106-1108 (1975)

Caudal Neurosecretory System of Fishes

Caudal Neurosecretory System of Fishes in 1976

H. A. BERN[1] and K. LEDERIS[2]
[1]Department of Zoology and Cancer Research Laboratory, University of California, Berkeley, California 94720, USA, and [2] Division of Pharmacology and Therapeutics Faculty of Medicine, University of Calgary, Alberta, Canada

A. Introduction

The nature of the caudal neurosecretory system and its products has been surveyed frequently in the past, despite the small number of laboratories actively concerned with its functional attributes. At the last International Symposium on Neurosecretion in London, we presented several aspects of our interest in this challenging neuroendocrine complex (LEDERIS et al., 1974). Since then our laboratories have surveyed the properties of the urotensins (LEDERIS, 1976) and the possible functional duality of the caudal system (CHAN and BERN, 1976).

The present report summarizes our recent observations on the nature of the urophysial peptides, the putative neurohormones of this system, and of the urophysial proteins and the putative carriers of these neurohormones.

B. Status of the Active Principles

Although the two generally recognized putative neurohormones from the caudal system are urotensins I and II, there remains evidence for the existence of three other active principles in urophysial tissues.

Urotensin I is hypotensive in mammals (and apparently in some amphibian species, in reptiles, and in birds; CHAN and KONG, unpublished; cf. CHAN and BERN, 1976). In the rat it also has a transient antidiuretic effect, which is not seen after chronic administration. In the eel it is hypertensive and diuretic. No physiologically significant effect has yet been demonstrated in fishes.

Urotensin II is a potent, and diuretic agent in the eel. The principle appears to stimulate all piscine smooth muscle. Particular attention has been paid to the urinary bladder, the genital ducts, intestine, and caudal lymph hearts (cf. CHAN and BERN, 1976).

Urotensin III, a stimulant of branchial sodium influx, according to MAETZ et al. (1964), has not been investigated further. However, in *Catastomus commersoni* urophysectomy leads to a significant decrease in plasma Na^+, without a corresponding increase in urinary Na^+ excretion. This would point to elimination of a factor like urotensin III (GILL and LEDERIS, unpublished).

Urotensin IV, which is indistinguishable from arginine vasotocin (LACANILAO, 1972), is present in the urophyses of only some teleostean species. Whereas it is present in *Gillichthys*, it is absent from *Catastomus*.

Acetylcholine is present in large quantities in the urophysis of the carp and other species (ICHIKAWA and KOBAYASHI, personal communication). Its occurrence has been discussed by Professor KOBAYASHI at this symposium.

C. Pharmacologic Properties of Urotensins I and II

I. Urotensin I

The effects of pharmacologic amounts of urotensin I in the eel *Anguilla rostrata* have been recorded in Calgary by Dr. D.K.O. Chan (CHAN, 1975). These observations can be summarized as follows: (1) Urotensin I increases the systemic blood pressure (dorsal and ventral aorta) in the eel, but is only approximately one-tenth as potent as urotensin II when related to the Urophysial Standard Unit (BERN and LEDERIS, 1969), (2) Urotensin I induces diuresis with a concomitant increase in renal excretion of divalent ions (Ca^{++}, Mg^{++}), (3) Urotensin I, unlike urotensin II, does not affect the lymph-heart rate or the caudal-vein pressure.

In mammalian species (rat, sheep, dog, monkey) urotensin I exerts a uniquely longlasting depression of systemic blood pressure, accompanied by a variable degree of reflex tachycardia (cf. LEDERIS, 1976). These effects of urotensin I have been shown to be due to a direct vasodilatory action on various vascular beds of the rat (MEDAKOVIC et al., 1975), but a highly selective vasodilatation in the mesenteric region only has been observed in the dog (MACCANNELL and LEDERIS, 1976).

In contrast to the highly selective and localized systemic effects of urotensin I, there appears to be a nonselective vasodilatation of isolated blood vessels from different regions of the dog, sheep, rabbit, and rat (GERRITSEN and LEDERIS, unpublished observations). Moreover, preliminary studies of the molecular mechanisms of action in isolated blood vessels indicate a dose-dependent accumulation of cAMP and cGMP, thus suggesting a participation of the cyclic nucleotides in the vasodilatory action. An antagonistic interaction between prostaglandins of the B, G, E, and F series and urotensin I is indicated in experiments using such prostaglandins and the prostaglandin synthetase inhibitors indomethocin or acetylsalicylate; both of the latter substances potentiate the effects of urotensin I on the isolated rat tail artery.

II. Urotensin II

The original observation of potent pressor activity of crude urophysial extracts in the eel (BERN et al., 1967) led to the chromatographic separation of urotensin I and II peptides and the finding that the pressor effects were due to urotensin II (ZELNIK and LEDERIS, 1973). The spectrum of activities of urotensin II in fishes has now been studied in some detail (cf. CHAN, 1975; LEDERIS, 1976). In addition to the pressor effects, glomerular diuresis, stimulation of the caudal-lymph heart (eel), and contractile action on all smooth muscles of fish (vascular, intestinal, urogenital) have been demonstrated. It is noteworthy that the amounts of urotensin II required to produce all these effects strongly suggest a hormonal nature for this peptide; only picogram quantities are needed in all cases (thus paralleling urotensin II effects in fish systems, with the effects of similar quantities of neurohypophysial peptides on appropriate mammalian smooth muscle). Whatever the physiologic role of urotensin II in fishes, the stimulatory effects of various smooth muscle systems are likely to prove to be of some importance.

Urotensin II does not cause significant effects in mammalian systems or on isolated mammalian tissues, other than weak contractile response in guinea-pig ileum and rat uterus when very high doses are administered (MEDAKOVIC and LEDERIS, unpublished observations). An interesting analogy can be drawn with reference to receptor recognition of urotensin II and the neurohypophyseal peptides: To produce comparable contractile responses in a fish system (*Lebistes* oviduct; LEDERIS, 1970), amounts of arginine vasotocin or isotocin at least three orders of magnitude greater than those of urotensin II are required (LEDERIS, 1976). Conversely, amounts of urotensin II from four to five orders of magnitude greater than those of oxytocin are required to induce comparable contractile responses in the isolated rat uterus (MEDAKOVIC and LEDERIS, unpublished observations).

D. Chemistry of Urotensins I and II

I. Urotensin I

The original observation of KOBAYASHI et al. (1968) that acidic extracts of carp urophyses induce hypotensive responses in the rat, has led to the isolation of urotensin I as a peptide responsible for such pharmacologic effects (ZELNIK and LEDERIS, 1973).

The isolated urotensin I of *C. commersoni* has now been purified employing gel-filtration chromatography, isoelectric focusing and ion-exchange chromatography (see LEDERIS, 1976). Three urotensin I fractions, similar in amino acid composition and in pharmacologic effects, are usually found. The main peptide peak, which accounts for > 85% of total biologic activity, was found to contain the following amino acids: Asp_5, Thr, Ser_2, Glu_5, Pro_2, Gly, Ala_2, Val, Met_2, $Ileu_2$, Leu_5, Tyr, Phe, His, Lys_2, Arg_3 (LETTER, MOORE, MCMASTER and LEDERIS, unpublished observations).

The following interesting structural aspects of the urotensin I peptide are now apparent: (1) Urotensin I is a straight-chain peptide with two methionine residues in positions 15 and 18, (2) Cleavage of urotensin I at Met with cyanogen bromide does not cause a diminution of the rat-hypotensive activity. Until such time that a suitably sensitive (and specific) piscine target organ is discovered, it cannot be predicted whether or not the entire peptide or the cleaved partial sequence represent the "hormonal" urotensin I in fishes. The relatively low eel-pressor potency of urotensin I is unlikely to indicate a hormonal function of this peptide in cardiovascular regulation of fishes; as much as 15 times more urotensin I is needed to induce a pressor response in the eel than will induce a measurable hypotensive effect in the rat (LEDERIS and MEDAKOVIC, 1974).

II. Urotensin II

The chemical nature of urotensin II has been investigated in a number of laboratories. Even the information on the size of this peptide has resulted in divergent conclusions. Urotensin II activity in *A. anguilla* was reported to reside in a peptide as small as a few hundred daltons (CHAN and HO, 1969; CHAN, in discussion of LEDERIS, 1976). GESCHWIND et al. (1968) and LEDERIS et al. (1971) found that urotensin II from *G. mirabilis* behaved in chromatographic and ultrafiltration procedures as a peptide of about 1000 daltons. The purification of urotensin II from *C. commersoni* by gel filtration on Bio-Gel and ion-exchange columns, followed by an estimation and comparison of molecular weights with SDS-8M urea polyacrylamide gel electrophoresis, have indicated the likely presence of two peptides, one of 1100-1400 daltons and another of 2000-2400 daltons (MOORE et al., 1975).

Whether these not inconsiderable differences in conclusions about the molecular size of urotensin II are real, and thus represent significant interspecific variation, or whether combination of different starting material with different experimental approach has led to these differing findings, cannot be resolved until the structural analyses of urotensin II peptide(s) have been completed and sequence and molecular configurations have been confirmed by subsequent synthesis and pharmacologic evaluation.

Extensive purification of *Catastomus* urotensin II by ion-exchange chromatography on SP-Sephadex, followed by rechromatography and thin-layer chromatography, has yielded a highly purified peptide with a specific activity of > 1920 units/mg amino acid nitrogen. Amino acid analysis of the hydrolysate of this peptide showed the following composition: Asx_2, Thr, Ser_2, Glx, $\frac{1}{2}Cys_4$, Gly_3, Ala_2, Val_2, Tyr_2, Phe_2, Lys_2 (LETTER and LEDERIS, unpublished observations). Subject to sequence determination and structural confirmation by synthesis, the possibility of two S-S linkages or of a dimerization of a smaller peptide cannot be excluded. Therefore, the divergence in size of urotensin II by a factor of two in different teleostean species remains a definite possibility.

E. Status of Urophysial Proteins (Urophysins)

Urophysis-specific proteins are possible intracellular carrier proteins (urophysins) for urophysial active principles, analogous to the relationship between neurophysins and neurohypophysial peptides. Evidence for urophysins in teleosts is substantial; differences in numbers (1-4) and in mobility in polyacrylamide gel electrophoresis characterize different species (LEDERIS et al., 1974). However, no conclusion as to their true carrier status can be drawn until these proteins have been isolated and purified and their specific binding of urotensins has been demonstrated.

A true urophysin must form an essential part of the elementary neurosecretory granule, which also contains the neurohormone. Using discontinuous sucrose gradients on *Gillichthys* urophysial homogenates, a high concentration of unique urophysial proteins was found at the interface between the 35% and the 40% sucrose layers. One of these proteins, with an R_f of 0.43 in 10.5% acrylamide gel at pH 8.3, was associated with a high level of urotensin II activity. Electron microscopy of the 35%-40% interface revealed large numbers of neurosecretory granules. This preliminary study, then, associates urotensin II activity, a specific protein, and neurosecretory granules, and supports the concept of a urophysin for urotensin II in the caudal neurosecretory system of *Gillichthys* (NISHIOKA, GUNTHER and BERN, unpublished).

The one neuron-one hormone concept may apply to the caudal neurosecretory system, analogous to a similar duality claimed for the hypothalamo-neurohypophyseal complex (HELLER, 1961). In another series of density gradient centrifugation experiments, a partial separation of urotensin I- and urotensin II-containing subcellular particles (elementary granules?) was reported by us in the previous Symposium in London (LEDERIS et al., 1974). Such experiments, if extended to include the localization of the urophysin-specific proteins (urophysins), may strengthen the duality (two neuron-two hormone) hypothesis discussed by CHAN and BERN (1976).

Urotensin II is clearly present in the caudal neurosecretory system of elasmobranchs (BERN et al., 1973). Attempts were made (NISHIOKA and GUNTHER, unpublished) to determine if one or more binding proteins are present in the area of the caudal neurosecretory perikarya, inasmuch as a urophysis is absent from non-teleostean fishes. In the shark *Squalus acanthias*, a unique band was detected with a R_f of 0.59-0.61 on 7% acid polyacrylamide gel; in the ray *Raja binoculata*, a band occurred with a R_f of 0.51-0.52 on 10% basic gel. Both of these are possible urophysins. In the ratfish *Hydrolagus colliei*, a band similar to that in the ray was encountered. Since evidence for urotensin II activity in the ratfish has been somewhat questionable (BERN, 1972; BERN et al., 1973), the finding of a band in encouraging.

It was initially disconcerting to find slight evidence for these unique proteins in spinal cord areas where caudal neurosecretory perikarya are completely lacking. However, in view of the close relationship between ependyma and caudal neurosecretory neurons (cf. FRIDBERG et al., 1966), it may not be surprising that a carrier protein would prove to be related to an ependymal secretory protein.

Four specific proteins have been demonstrated in the urophysis of *Catostomus* by polyacrylamide gel electrophoresis (MOORE et al., 1975). Equilibrium dialysis, followed by bioassays of urotensins I and II, showed that a mixture of these proteins bound both urophysial peptides. Maximum binding of urotensin I occurred over a relatively broad pH range (5-8), but maximum binding of urotensin II was found at pH 4-5. Depending on methodology employed for the separation of the urophysins, as few as two proteins and as many as five protein bands can be demonstrated with isoelectric points ranging from 5.0 to 6.2.

In order to establish which of these proteins are definitive urophysins and what their specific peptide-binding properties are, procedures to separate the individual proteins were devised (MASUR et al., 1976) for subsequent characterization of these peptide-binding properties. Partial purification of the proteins and their separation from urotensins I and II were achieved by gel filtration in columns of either Bio-Gel P_6 or Sephadex G-75. Further purification and isolation of the individual proteins, designated as urophysins A, B, C, and D, were effected by chromatography on diethylaminoethane (DEAE)-Sephadex columns over a pH gradient to pH 3.0 in citric acid-phosphate buffer. At all purification steps, the proteins were localized and the different components identified by analytic polyacrylamide gel electrophoresis and correlated with ultraviolet absorption spectra (using a LKB Uvicord).

Aliquots of all four urophysial proteins were taken for amino acid analysis. Proteins A, B, C, and D were lyophilized, and hydrolyzed in 6N HCl containing 0.1% β-mercaptoethanol and 0.1% phenol to protect any cysteine and tyrosine residues, respectively, from oxidation during hydrolysis. Amino acid analyses were done using an automated Beckman M-121 analyser. The amino-acid analyses indicated an estimated total of 150-179 amino-acid residues for the individual proteins, all sharing two unique characteristics: (1) absence of cysteine and tyrosine, and (2) presence of the amino acid ornithine, which is usually only found in avian proteins.

F. Control of the Caudal Neurosecretory System

SWANSON et al. (1975) have established an important aminergic innervation of the caudal neurosecretory systen in *Gillichthys*. What the physiologic import of this input may be is still conjectural. For this reason and others, a collaborative research program with David Pearson and Irving Geschwind at the University of California, Davis, was established that will allow examination of possible controlling factors, using the isolated caudal system maintained in organ culture.

To date, it has become evident that the caudal neurosecretory system can be maintained in organ culture for at least 7 days and probably longer. Electron microscopy reveals that many axon endings in the urophysis retain their in situ characteristics, while others have obviously degenerated. Perikarya of neurons projecting to the urophysis are often degenerate, but others can be found with considerable evidence of cellular activity. The rough endoplasmic reticulum is prominent, but less well organized than in situ. Interestingly enough, the neuronal cytoplasm may contain many more elementary granules in vitro than are ordinarily encountered in vivo. It is possible that the surviving neurosecretory neurons (and endings) may be removed from inhibitory control by the cord transection prior to explantation, whereas the dead and dying cells (and endings) are dependent on a neural input no longer available. Preliminary assay results indicate that the explanted systems continue to synthesize and release urotensin II.

It should become possible to test various agents (amines, acetylcholine, hormones, ions, etc.) for their effects on synthesis, transport, and release of neurohormones and also of urophysial proteins. These studies are being pursued actively at the present time (PEARSON, NISHIOKA, GUNTHER, DEWEY, GESCHWIND and BERN, unpublished).

G. Conclusion

The caudal neurosecretory system with its urophysis is becoming increasingly recognized as an important endocrine structure in fishes. Its morphology has been carefully analyzed in a variety of species of elasmobranch and actinopterygian fishes. Its neural connections are being elucidated. The chemistry and pharmacology of its products, presumably neurohormones, are increasingly well understood, at least in the few species of fishes from which adequate amounts of material can be collected. Parallelism of structural and subcellular features between the caudal system and the cranial (hypothalamo-neurohypophyseal) system is underlined by the recognition of probable carrier proteins (urophysins) in the former analogous to those (neurophysins) found in the latter. Despite all this increase in functionally oriented information (which still regrettably comes from too few laboratories), we can only reiterate what we have stated in the past: the functions of the caudal system - its contributions to the biology of the organism - continue to elude us. Indications, indeed strong indications, exist for a contribution of urotensins to osmoregulation, to cardiovascular function, and to reproduction (cf. CHAN and BERN, 1976). Nevertheless, the challenge to the physiologist of neurosecretory systems, to the comparative physiologist generally, remains. Hopefully, the next International Symposium on Neurosecretion will reveal the true functions(s) of this prominent piscine neuroendocrine apparatus.

Acknowledgments. The research reported herein was supported by U.S. National Science Foundation grant MBS-16345 and by the Medical Research Council of Canada. We are grateful to many colleagues for their recent contributions to the studies surveyed herein, including G. Burford, D.K.O. Chan, R. Dewey, M.E. Gerritsen, I.I. Geschwind, V. Gill, R. Gunther, B.L. Horne, A. Letter, K.L. MacCannell, L. Masur, D. McMaster, M. Medakovic, G. Moore, R.S. Nishioka, and D. Pearson. We are indebted to Ms. Mollie Field for her help in preparing the manuscript and to Hugo Lee for technical assistance.

References

BERN, H.A.: Some questions on the nature and function of cranial and caudal neurosecretory systems. Prog. Brain Res. 38, 85-96 (1972)

BERN, H.A., GUNTHER, R., JOHNSON, D.W., NISHIOKA, R.S.: Occurrence of urotensin II (bladder-contracting activity) in the caudal spinal cord of anamniote vertebrates. Acta Zool. (Stockh.) 54, 15-19 (1973)

BERN, H.A., LEDERIS, K.: A reference preparation for the study of active substances in the caudal neurosecretory system of teleosts. J. Endocrinol. 45, xi-xii (1969)

BERN, H.A., NISHIOKA, R.S., CHESTER JONES, I., CHAN, D.K.O., RANKIN, J.C., PONNIAH, S.: The urophysis of teleost fish. J. Endocrinol. 37, xl-xli (1967) (abstract)

CHAN, D.K.O.: Cardiovascular and renal effects of urotensins I and II in the eel, *Anguilla rostrata*. Gen. Comp. Endocrinol. 27, 52-61 (1975)

CHAN, D.K.O., BERN, H.A.: The caudal neurosecretory system - a critical evaluation of the two-hormone hypothesis. Cell Tissue Res. (1976) (in press)

CHAN, D.K.O., HO, M.W.: Pressor substances in the caudal neurosecretory system of teleost and elasmobranch fishes. Gen. Comp. Endocrinol. 13, 498 (1969)

FRIDBERG, G., NISHIOKA, R.S., BERN, H.A., FLEMING, W.R.: Regeneration of the caudal neurosecretory system in the cichlid teleost *Tilapia mossambica*. J. Exp. Zool. 162, 311-336 (1966)

GESCHWIND, I.I., LEDERIS, K., BERN, H.A., NISHIOKA, R.S.: Purification of bladder-contracting principle from the urophysis of the teleost, *Gillichthys mirabilis*. Am. Zool. 8, 758 (1968) (abstract)

HELLER, H.: Occurrence storage and metabolism of oxytocin. In: Oxytocin. CALDERYO-BARCIA, R., HELLER, H. (eds.). London: Pergamon 1961, p. 3-23

KOBAYASHI, H., MATSUI, T., HIRANO, T., IWATA, T., ISHII, S.: Vasodepressor substance in fish urophyses. Annot. Zool. J. 41, 154-158 (1968)

LACANILAO, F.: The urophysial hydrosmotic factor of fishes: II. Chromatographic and pharmacologic indications of similarity to arginine vasotocin. Gen. Comp. Endocrinol. 19, 413-420 (1972)

LEDERIS, K.: Active substances in the caudal neurosecretory system of bony fishes. Mem. Soc. Endocrinol. 18, 465-484 (1970)

LEDERIS, K.: Chemical properties and the physiological and pharmacological actions of urophysial peptides. Am. Zool. (1976) (in press)

LEDERIS, K., BERN, H.A., MEDAKOVIC, M., CHAN, D.K.O., NISHIOKA, R.S., LETTER, A., SWANSON, D., GUNTHER, R., TESANOVIC, M., HORNE, B.: Recent functional studies on the caudal neurosecretory system of teleost fishes. In: Neurosecretion - The Final Neuroendocrine Pathway. VI Int. Symp. on Neurosecretion, London. KNOWLES, F., VOLLRATH, L. (eds.). Berlin-Heidelberg-New York: Springer-Verlag 1974, p. 94-103

LEDERIS, K., BERN, H.A., NISHIOKA, R.S., GESCHWIND, I.I.: Some observations on biological and chemical properties and subcellular localization of urophysial active principles. Mem. Soc. Endocrinol. 19, 413-433 (1971)

LEDERIS, K., MEDAKOVIC, M.: Effects and assay of urotensin I on the perfused hind limb of the rat. Gen. Comp. Endocrinol. 24, 10-16 (1974)

MACCANNELL, K.L., LEDERIS, K.: Selective dilatation of the mesenteric vascular bed. Proc. Can. Fed. Biol. Soc. 19, 554 (1976) (abstract)

MAETZ, J., BOURGUET, J., LAHLOU, B.: Urophyse et osmorégulation chez *Carassius auratus*. Gen. Comp. Endocrinol. 4, 401-414 (1964)

MASUR, L., BURFORD, G., MOORE, G., LEDERIS, K.: Isolation of urophysial hormone-binding proteins. Proc. Can. Fed. Soc. 19, 95 (1976) (abstract)

MEDAKOVIC, M., CHAN, D.K.O., LEDERIS, K.: Pharmocological effects of urotensins. I. Regional vascular effects of urotensins I and II in the rat. Pharmacology 13, 409-418 (1975)

MOORE, G., BURFORD, G., LEDERIS, K.: Properties of urophysial proteins (urophysins) from the white sucker, *Catostomus commersoni*. Mol. Cell. Endocrinol. 3, 297-307 (1975)

SWANSON, D.D., NISHIOKA, R.S., BERN, H.A.: Aminergic innervation of the cranial and caudal neurosecretory systems in the teleost *Gillichthys mirabilis*. Acta Zool. (Stockh.) 56, 225-237 (1975)

ZELNIK, P.R., LEDERIS, K.: Chromatographic separation of urotensins. Gen. Comp. Endocrinol. 20, 392-400 (1973)

Acetylcholine in the Urophysis and Release of Urophysial Hormones by Neurotransmitters in Vitro

T. ICHIKAWA and H. KOBAYASHI
Misaki Marine Biological Station, University of Tokyo, Misaki, Kanagawa-ken 238-02, Japan

In 1963, KOBAYASHI et al. demonstrated a high concentration of a substance similar to acetylcholine (ACh) in the urophyses of several species of fish, by bioassay using a bivalve-heart preparation (Table 1). In the present study, this substance was identified as ACh by pyrolysis-gas chromatography combined with mass spectrometry (Figs. 1 and 2). The concentration of ACh in the urophysis of freshwater fish was at least 6 times higher than that in seawater fish (Table 1), and the concentration was higher than that in any other tissues or organs.

Differential centrifugation (500, 4000, 8500, 70,000, and 100,000 *xg*) of carp urophysial homogenates in 0.4 *M* sucrose solution revealed that ACh was concentrated in the sediment fraction "A" at 70,000 *xg*. When examined with an electron microscope, this fraction "A" mainly consisted of granules (~ 150 nm) and vesicles (~ 50 nm). Following subsequent ultracentrifugation of fraction "A" in a density gradient (0.60-2.00 *M* sucrose, 100,000 *xg* for 1 h), one distinct layer was obtained between 1.34 and 1.45 *M*. This layer consisted mostly of large granules (150-200 nm) and vesicles (50-80 nm), and showed the highest concentration of ACh of all the fractions. The large granules are the carriers of urophysial hormones (LEDERIS et al., 1974; and unpublished observations). Consequently, the small vesicles must be the carrier of ACh.

Table 1. Acetylcholine in the urophysis

Species	Body length (cm)	Assay method	ACh (nmol/ urophysis)	ACh (μmol/ g tissue)
Freshwater fish				
Cyprinus carpio	30-35	B[a]	1.87 ± 0.32[b]	1.49 ± 0.32
	34-46	GC[c]	1.60 ± 0.07	0.63 ± 0.03
	38-45	GC	2.02 ± 0.03	0.71 ± 0.01
Carassius carassius	12-20	B	0.32 ± 0.07	0.94 ± 0.18
	24-35	GC	0.56 ± 0.01	0.86 ± 0.01
Tribolodon hakonensis	23-30	GC	1.03 ± 0.02	1.37 ± 0.02
Seawater fish				
Lateolabrax japonicus	29-33	B	0.16	0.18
Acanthopagrus schlegelii	22-28	B	0.07	0.10
Hexagrammos otakii	21-33	B	0.06	0.12
Laphiomus setigerus	79-95	GC	2.50 ± 0.27	0.16 ± 0.004

[a] Bioassay with bivalve heart (KOBAYASHI et al., 1963)

[b] Mean ± SE

[c] Gas chromatography

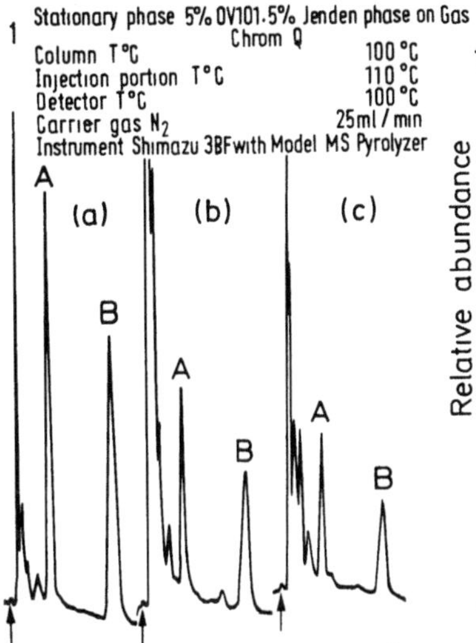

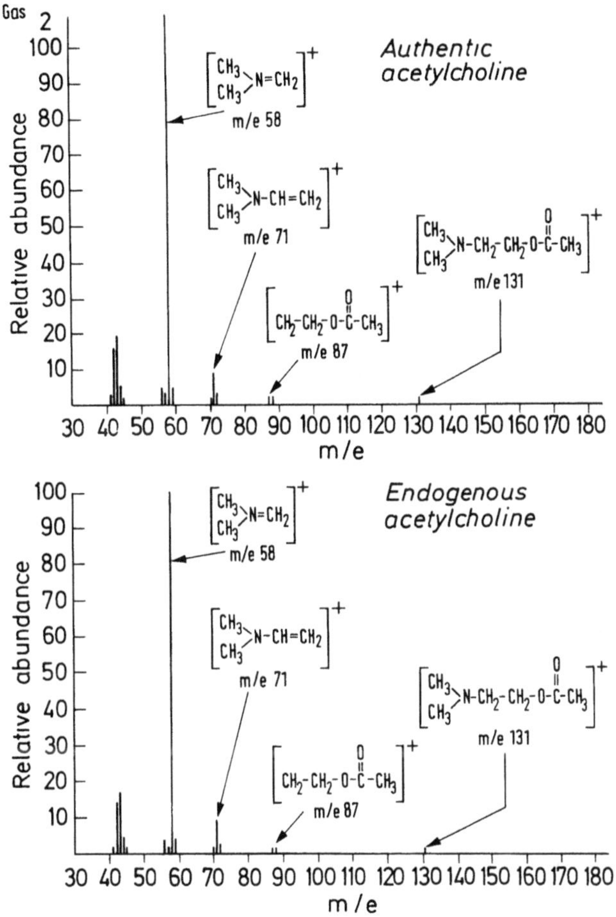

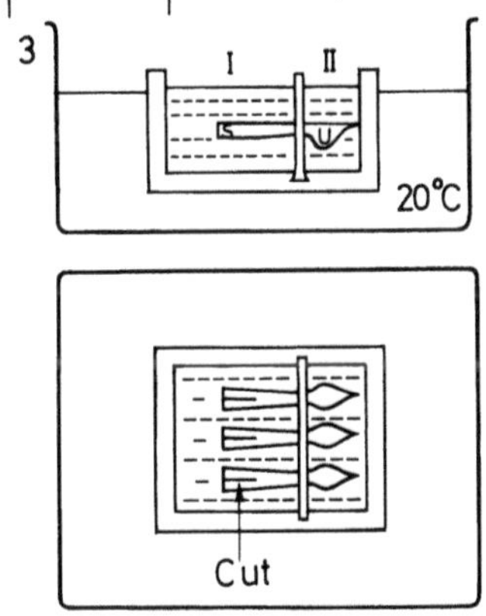

Fig. 1. Gas chromatograms of pyrolytic products of (a) authentic AChI (*A*) and BChI (*B*) as an internal standard, (b) authentic AChI and BChI subjected to entire extraction procedure, and (c) ACh (*A*) and BChI (*B*) fractions from carp urophysis

Fig. 2. Mass spectra of authentic ACh and ACh extracted from carp urophysis. Upper spectrum was obtained from peak *A* of chromatogram in Fig. 1a; lower spectrum was obtained from peak *A* of chromatogram in Fig. 1c

Fig. 3. Diagram of culture aquarium (3 cm in length, 1 cm in width, 1.5 cm in depth). *s* - spinal cord, *u* - urophysis

Since electron microscopy of the carp urophysis showed that the small vesicles always coexist with the granules in neurosecretory nerve endings, and that nerve endings containing only small vesicles were not found, it was concluded that ACh must be associated with small vesicles in the neurosecretory nerve endings.

In the next experiment, neural regulation of caudal neurosecretory activity was investigated in the carp. Innervation of the Dahlgren cells has been shown in fishes by several investigators using electrophysiological, histochemical, and electron microscopic methods (see FRIDBERG and BERN, 1968); LEDERIS et al., 1974). We have also confirmed the presence of acetylcholinesterase in the cytoplasm of Dahlgren cells and monoamine oxidase around the cells in the caudal neurosecretory system of carp. Further, synapses and possible monoaminergic neurons were found between the Dahlgren cells. Based on these data, the effects of neurotransmitters on the release of urophysial hormones were examined. Three spinal-cord-urophysial preparations were cultured in a small aquarium with a partition wall, as shown in Figure 3; both chambers (I and II) of the aquarium contained fish Ringer solution. When adrenaline, noradrenaline (NA), or ACh were introduced into chamber I, rat antidiuretic substance(s) (probably urotensin I) were released in chamber II (Table 2). The amount of the substance(s) released by ACh seems to be dose-dependent. Serotonin and dopamine had no effect. The stimulation by NA was inhibited by phenoxybenzamine (PBA), but not by propranolol and atropine. The effect of ACh was blocked by atropine, but not by hexamethonium and PBA. These results show that (1) both adrenergic and cholinergic mechanisms seem to be involved independently in the control of release of urophysial hormones, (2) the monoaminergic stimulative effect is mediated by an α-adrenergic receptor, and (3) the action of ACh is of a muscarinic nature.

Table 2. Neurotransmitters and release of antidiuretic substance

Neurotransmitters	Antidiuretic activity[a] (m units/gland)		
Adrenaline (10^{-4} *M*)	21.5 ± 2.21,[b]	26.4 ± 2.55,	31.6 ± 2.68
Noradrenaline (10^{-4} *M*)	23.5 ± 2.99,	34.8 ± 1.98,	36.8 ± 2.95
Dopamine (10^{-4} *M*)	<8.3		
5-Hydroxytryptamine (10^{-4} *M*)	<8.3		
Acetylcholine (10^{-4} *M*)	33.7 ± 2.30,	37.2 ± 2.45,	39.2 ± 3.02
(10^{-6} *M*)	32.6 ± 2.68,	35.3 ± 1.98	
(10^{-8} *M*)	23.9 ± 2.00,	26.8 ± 2.57	
Control	<8.3		

[a]Activity induced by 1 mg acetone-dried carp urophysis is defined as one unit

[b]Mean ± SE

References

FRIDBERG, G., BERN, H.A.: The urophysis and the caudal neurosecretory system of fishes. Biol. Rev. 43, 175-199 (1968)

KOBAYASHI, H., UEMURA, H., OOTA, Y., ISHII, S.: Cholinergic substance in the caudal neurosecretory storage organ of fish. Science 141, 714-716 (1963)

LEDERIS, K., BERN, H.A., MEDAKOVIC, M., CHAN, D.K.O., NISHIOKA, R.S., LETTER, A., SWANSON, D., GUNTHER, R., TESANOVIC, M., HORNE, B.: Recent functional studies on the caudal neurosecretory system of teleost fishes. In: Neurosecretion: The Final Neuroendocrine Pathway. KNOWLES, F., VOLLRATH, L. (eds.). Berlin-Heidelberg-New York: Springer-Verlag 1974, pp. 94-114

Caudal Neurosecretory System in Acipenseridae and Some Aspects of Its Evolution

I. I. SAENKO
Leningrad State University, Leningrad, USSR

The study of the evolutionary aspect of the caudal neurosecretory system (CaNS) in fish is of great interest because the origin and function of this formation are as yet unknown. For this reason, we have undertaken research on the Acipenseridae, an ancient and primitive family of fish. Light- and electron-microscopic investigation of the spinal cord of sturgeons established the existence of a CaNS (SAENKO, 1970), which has some peculiar characters in comparison with that of teleosts. While in the latter the CaNS is distributed in the terminal part of the spinal cord, corresponding to several of the caudal vertebrae, in Acipenseridae the CaNS occupies a large region corresponding to 20-25 segments of the body (from the end of the dorsal fin to the middle of the upper tail blade). The cells of the CaNS in these fishes are not concentrated in a conspicuous group, as in teleosts, but are scattered throughout the medulla (Fig. 1). The CaNS is composed of cells with noticeable cytological features of secretory activity (Fig. 2). As in teleosts, these cells are often large in size, frequently more than 100 µm in maximum diameter, and polygonal in shape with intensively staining cytoplasm. They have large polymorphic nuclei with several nucleoli. While the nuclei of these cells in teleosts often have many lobes or projections, the nuclei of caudal cells in Acipenseridae are characterized by cytoplasmic invaginations of spherical shape and of 6-10 µm in diameter. This difference does not seem to be critical because both forms increase the nuclear surface and are characteristic of secreting cells. Different inclusions are occasionally observed in the perikarya of neurosecretory cells. These take the form of single acidophilic droplets 2-6 µm in diameter and basophilic globules 4-13 µm in diameter. Optically lucent vacuoles of up to 34 µm in maximum diameter are observed more frequently in the caudal neurosecretory cells of Acipenseridae. The abundance of vacuoles is also a characteristic of the cells of the hypothalamo-hypophyseal system in these fish. The processes, 8-17 µm in diameter, extend from the cells to form the unmyelinated neurosecretory fibers. Their enlargements, filled by secretion, give rise to Herring bodies. Acidophilic granules that are occasionally observed along the neurosecretory tract in teleosts, are lacking in sturgeons. The neurosecretory fibers end with the dilated bulbous terminals 3-34 µm in diameter at the meninx of the spinal cord (Figs. 1 and 3). There are some differences in the intensity of staining, both among and within the terminals, while small vacuoles are rarely present. The terminals occupy a large region of the ventrolateral surface of the spinal cord, somewhat more caudal to the neurosecretory cells. The meninx in this area is richly vascularized. Similar contact is also found in the brain of Acipenseridae, where the proximal contact area has been described by POLENOV (1966). The lack of the urophysis is the main difference in the

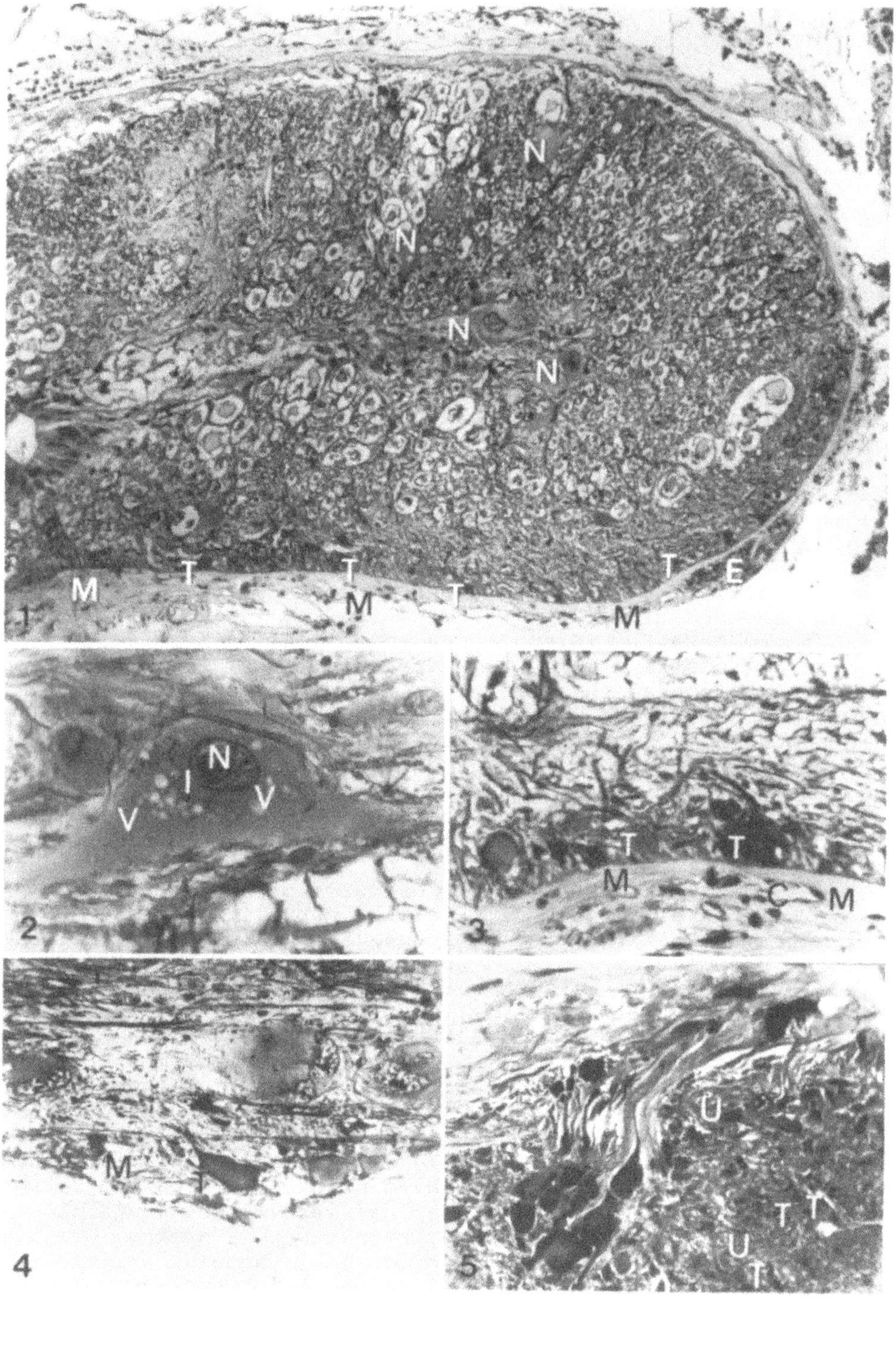
N
N
N
N
M
T
T
M
T
T
E
M
1
N
I
V
V
2
T
T
M
C
M
3
M
4
U
T
T
U
T
5

structure of the CaNS in Chondrostei in comparison with Teleostei. A urophysis is also lacking in the CaNS in Elasmobranchs (FRIDBERG, 1962). At the same time, in the ontogeny of CaNS in teleosts, there are stages when the urophysis is absent and the neurosecretory terminals are situated at the meninx. On the other hand, there are accessory neurohemal areas in the definitive caudal system of some primitive teleosts (Fig. 4). In some cases (5 fish out of 50) in Acipenseridae the single terminals were situated within the meninx in close proximity to its vessels (Fig. 4). Such formations lack a certain form, size, and distribution. Probably they are the material from which a special neurohemal organ is derived in evolution. In summary, it may be concluded that lack of the urophysis and the presence of neurosecretory terminals at the meninx are primitive features in the organization of the CaNS in general, and of CaNS in Acipenseridae in particular. It may be proposed that in the course of evolution the isolation of neurosecretory terminals from the spinal cord occurs. It is possible to observe three stages in this process (Fig. 6): (1) Terminals are situated within the spinal cord at the meninx (CaNS of Acipenseridae, some elasmobranchs, early stages in ontogeny of CaNS in teleosts; Figs. 3 and 6a). (2) Terminals penetrate the meninx of some elasmobranchs: intermediate stages in the ontogeny of the CaNS in teleosts; accessory neurohemal organs in primitive teleosts; Figs. 4 and 6b). (3) Terminals are situated outside the spinal cord in the urophysis (definitive CaNS of teleosts; Figs. 5, 6c). Besides the above-mentioned features, the CaNS of Acipenseridae differs from that of teleosts by a more diffuse distribution of its elements. This involves both the cells and the terminals. A similar peculiarity was also noticed in the CaNS of elasmobranchs (FRIDBERG, 1962). Comparison of the CaNS in primitive fish with that in more advanced families of teleosts (Salmonidae, Cyprinidae, and Percidae), leads to a similar conclusion. Thus the second tendency revealed in the evolution of the CaNS is an increasing concentration of its elements with advanced organization. This is in agreement with the hypothesis (STERBA and NAUMANN, 1970) that cranial and caudal neurosecretory systems can be understood as differentiated parts of an original segmentally organized neurosecretory system extending throughout the central nervous system. In any event, the CaNS of Acipenseridae represents the more primitive type, and is possibly near to the initial type of caudal neurosecretory system.

◄

Figs. 1-3. Illustration of caudal neurosecretory system (CaNS) in *Acipenser güldenstädti* Brand

Fig. 1. Cross section of the spinal cord at the level of the caudal neurosecretory system. *N* - neurosecretory cells, *T*, *E* - neurosecretory terminals (*T* - at the meninx, *E* - inside the meninx), *C* - central canal, *M* - meninx of the spinal cord. × 150

Fig. 2. Neurosecretory cell: *N* - nucleus, *I* - intranuclear cytoplasmic invagination, *V* - vacuoles. × 490

Fig. 3. Neurosecretory terminals (*T*) at the meninx (*M*): *C* - capillary. × 351

Figs. 4 and 5. Illustration of neurosecretory terminals from the CaNS of *Salmo salar* L.

Fig. 4. Neurosecretory terminals (*T*) in the meninx (*M*) from accessory neurohemal organ. × 300

Fig. 5. Neurosecretory terminals (*T*) in the urophysis (*U*). × 370

Figs. 1-5. Fixation in Bouin's fluid; staining with Heidenhain's iron hematoxylin

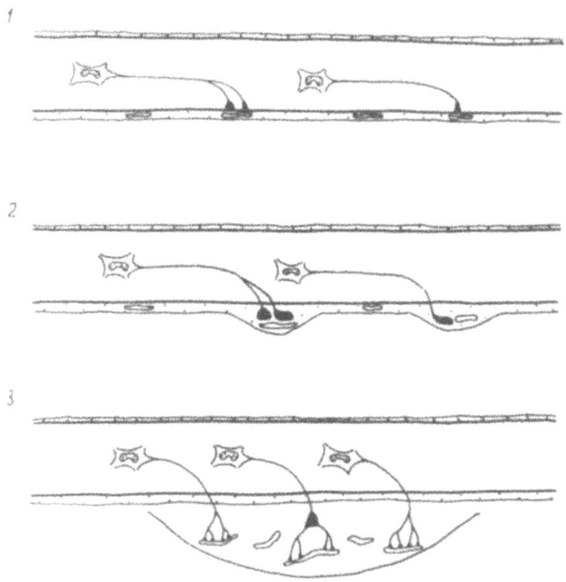

Fig. 6. Diagrams represent sagittal sections through caudal spinal cord of fish to show possible evolution of neurosecretory terminals. Explanation in text

References

FRIDBERG, G.: The caudal neurosecretory system in some elasmobranchs. Gen. Comp. Endocrinol. 2, 249-265 (1962)

POLENOV, A.L.: Concerning the proximal neurosecretory contact region of the preoptic-hypophysial system in Acipenseridae. (In Russian). Dokl. Acad. Sci. USSR 169, 1467-1470 (1966)

SAENKO, I.I.: Concerning the caudal neurosecretory system in Acipenseridae. (In Russian). Dokl. Acad. Sci. USSR 194, 218-221 (1970)

STERBA, G., NAUMANN, W.: Neural and glial secretion in the spinal cord. Acta Zool. 51, 159-168 (1970)

Ultrastructure of the Caudal Neurosecretory System in Acipenseridae

I. I. SAENKO and N. A. EFIMOVA
Leningrad State University, Leningrad, USSR

The fine structure of the cells of the caudal neurosecretory system in Acipenseridae exhibits all characteristic neurosecretory features. They have large, polymorphic nuclei rich in chromatin, with numerous nucleoli. The nuclear envelope has many pores. Numerous intranuclear cytoplasmic invaginations are observed; these are characteristic of the nuclei of caudal cells in Acipenseridae. At the cross section they are round in form and 900 nm - 20 μm in diameter. Granular endoplasmic reticulum is well developed, especially at the periphery of the perikaryon. The reticulum in nuclear invaginations differs from that in the rest of the cell by a more regular distribution of dilated canaliculi. Conspicuous aggregations of polysomes and free ribosomes are also observed here. Neurosecretory granules 100-250 nm in diameter are scattered over the whole cytoplasm and their structure corresponds almost exactly to that described for other neurosecretory systems. Golgi complexes are located in the perinuclear region, and consist of long and narrow cisterns, vacuoles, and vesicles. Numerous mitochondria of a different form, microtubules, microfilaments, and random lysosomes are also evident in the cells. The unmyelinated neurosecretory fibers contain elongated mitochondria, microtubules, and numerous neurosecretory granules. At the meninx they form dilated neurosecretory endings of various size. There are many electron-lucent vesicles 40-100 nm in diameter within these terminals: some of them contact the axolemma contiguous to the meninx. Neurosecretory granules are also present in the terminals in varying amounts. The granules vary in electron density and the grainy ones predominate.

Structure and Function of Neurosecretory Systems in Invertebrates

Neurosecretion in the Frontal Ganglion of the Stick Insect, *Carausius morosus*

A. DORN
Institut für Zoologie, Johannes Gutenberg-Universität, 6500 Mainz, FRG

The presence of neurosecretory cells in the frontal ganglion (FG) has been demonstrated only in the Lepidoptera *Bombyx* (BOUNHIOL et al., 1953), *Manduca* (BORG et al., 1973; BELL et al., 1974), and *Diatraea* (YIN and CHIPPENDALE, 1975). In *Manduca* and *Diatraea* the neurosecretory material of the FG is apparently involved in the regulation of diapause.

In several representatives of other orders, for example *Leptinotarsa* (SCHOONEVELD, 1970), *Schistocerca* (DELPHIN, 1965), and *Locusta* (CLARKE and LANGLEY, 1963a) no substances that stain with the paraldehyde fuchsin method (PAF) were found in the FG. In *Locusta*, however, electron microscopy revealed neurosecretory fibers in the neuropil of the FG. This report deals with neurosecretory fibers identified by light and electron microscope in the FG of *C. morosus*.

No positive reaction was obtained with PAF. After staining with azan, however, red-staining granules were observed in the neuropil of the anterior and medial parts of the ganglion, whereas the posterior part was almost devoid of them. Relatively large amounts of red granules were also found in the frontal connectives. The perikarya of the FG apparently contain no azan-positive material.

Electron-microscopic examination shows that in the anterior part of the ganglion numerous axons in the neuropil carry neurosecretory granules. Three types of neurosecretory fibers can be differentiated (Fig. 3). Most frequent are type-I fibers, with granules of high electron density and an average diameter of 1000 Å, and type-II fibers, with granules of moderate density and an average diameter of 900 Å, which give an impression of fragility. Type-III fibers are rare; the granules are completely electron lucent and have a diameter of about 1500 Å. In the medial part of the FG the neurosecretory fibers of types I and II form synaptoid structures facing intercellular spaces, glial elements, nerve fibers of the conventional type, or other neurosecretory fibers (Figs. 4, 5). Such release sites are very frequent; in a given axonal profile as many as eight synaptoids can be observed. It should be pointed out that the synaptoid-forming nerve endings are located within the neuropil and consequently are separated from the hemocoelom by perineurium, neural lamella, and fat body (Fig. 1). Cross sections through the posterior part of the FG show only very few profiles of neurosecretory fibers.

It is now uncertain whether the FG has a neurohemal function as was suggested by CHANUSSOT et al. (1969) and CHANUSSOT (1972)) for the hypocerebral ganglion of *Blabera*, or whether the neurons

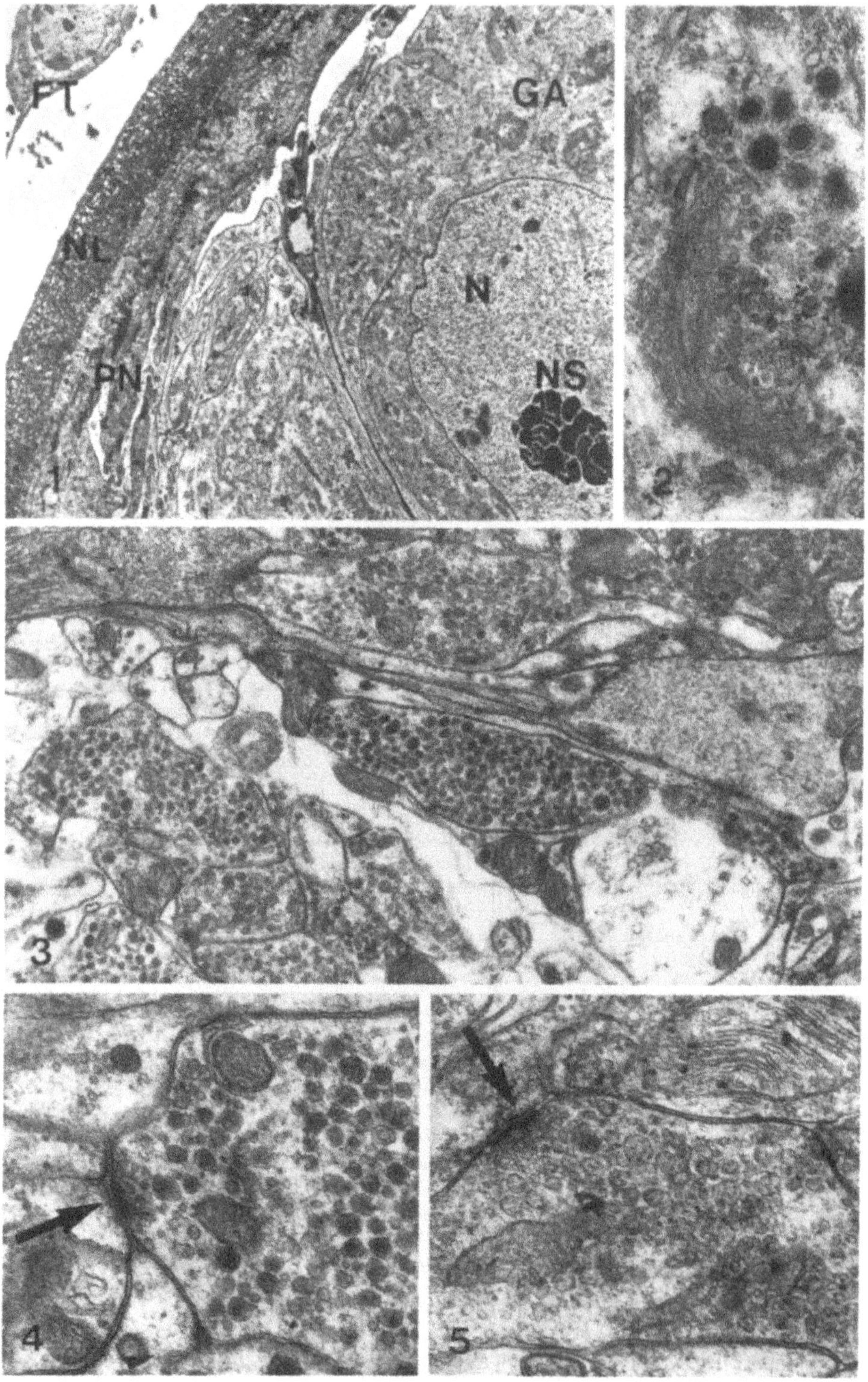
FT
GA
NL
N
PN
NS
1
2
3
4
5

Fig. 1. Dorsal, peripheral part of FG. *FT* - fat tissue, *NL* - neural lamella, *PN* - perineurium, *GA* - Golgi apparatus, *N* - nucleus of ganglion cell; *NS* - nucleolus. × 3400
Fig. 2. Golgi apparatus of ganglion cell with dense-core vesicles in its vicinity. × 34,000
Fig. 3. Numerous axons with different types of neurosecretory granules in anterior part of neuropil. × 18,000
Fig. 4. Synaptoid formation of type-I neurosecretory axon in medial part of FG (*arrow*). × 38,000
Fig. 5. Synaptoid formation of type-II neurosecretory axon in medial part of FG (*arrow*). × 38,000

of the FG are the effector sites of the released neurosecretory material. The latter hypothesis is favored since it is doubtful that neurohormones can penetrate the perineurium. However, the functional significance of this phenomenon remains obscure. Extirpation experiments on the FG in several other species indicated an important neuroendocrine role of this ganglion (CLARKE and LANGLEY, 1963a,b; CLARKE and GILLOT, 1965; PENZLIN and STÖLZNER, 1971).

The site of origin of the neurosecretory granules in the neuropil of the FG is uncertain. Electron-dense granules produced by the Golgi complexes of the intrinsic ganglion cells (Figs. 1,2) are of a different size and appearance than the axonal neurosecretory granules, and are apparently not identical with them. They never accumulate in the cell bodies, and are not considered neurosecretory products. The light-microscopic observations seem to indicate that the neurosecretory granules observed in the FG neuropil might stem from perikarya within the brain.

Summary. The neuropil of the frontal ganglion of *C. morosus* contains numerous neurosecretory axons; the cells of origin of these axons apparently lie outside the ganglion. Three types of neurosecretory fibers can be differentiated. Most of the neurosecretory granules are released within the ganglion. The functional meaning of these phenomena is unknown.

Acknowledgments. This paper was supported by grants of the Deutsche Forschungsgesellschaft. I wish to thank Miss J. Tröster and Mrs. M. Ullmann for technical assistance.

References

BELL, R.A., BORG, T.K., ITTYCHERIAH, P.I.: Neurosecretory cells in the frontal ganglion of the tobacco hornworm *Manduca sexta* (L). J. Insect. Physiol. 20, 669-678 (1974)
BORG, T.K., BELL, R.A., PICARD, D.J.: Ultrastructure of neurosecretory cells in the frontal ganglion of the tobacco hornworm, *Manduca sexta* (L). Tissue Cell 5, 259-267 (1973)
BOUNHIOL, J.J., GABE, M., ARVY, L.: Données histophysiologiques sur la neurosécrétion chez *Bombyx mori* L., et sur ses rapports avec les glandes endocrines. Bull. Biol. Fr. Belg. 87, 323-333 (1953)

CHANUSSOT, B.: Étude histologique et ultrastructurale du ganglion ingluvial de *Blabera craniifer* Burm. (Insects, Dictyoptère). Tisse Cell 4, 85-97 (1972)

CHANUSSOT, B., DANDO, J., MOULINS, M., LAVERACK, M.S.: Mise en évidence d'une amine biogène dans le système nerveux stomatogastrique des insectes: étude histochimique et ultrastructurale. C. R. Acad. Sc. (D) (Paris) 268, 2101-2104 (1969)

CLARKE, K.U., GILLOTT, C.: Relationship between the removal of the frontal ganglion and protein starvation in *Locusta migratoria* L. Nature 208, 808-809 (1965)

CLARKE, K.U., LANGLEY, P.: Studies on the initiation of growth and moulting in *Locusta migratoria migratorioides* R & F - II. The role of the stomatogastric nervous system. J. Insect Physiol. 9, 363-373 (1963a)

CLARKE, K.U., LANGLEY, P.: Studies on the initiation of growth and moulting in *Locusta migratoria migratorioides* R & F - III. The role of the frontal ganglion. J. Insect Physiol. 9, 411-421 (1963b)

DELPHIN, F.: The histology and possible functions of neurosecretory cells in the ventral ganglia of *Schistocerca gregaria* Forskål (Orthoptera: Acrididae). Trans. R. Entomol. Soc. Lond. 117, 167-214 (1965)

PENZLIN, H., STÖLZNER, W.: Frontal ganglion and water balance in *Periplaneta americana* L. Experientia 27, 390-391 (1971)

SCHOONEVELD, H.: Structural aspects of neurosecretory and corpus allatum activity in the adult Colorado beetle, *Leptinotarsa decemlineata* (Say) as a function of day-length. Neth. J. Zool. 20, 151-237 (1970)

YIN, C.-M., CHIPPENDALE, G.M.: Insect frontal ganglion: fine structure of its neurosecretory cells in diapause and non-diapause larvae of *Diatraea grandiosella*. Can. J. Zool. 53, 1093-1100 (1975)

Immunochemical Investigations on the Neuroendocrine System of the Cockroach, *Periplaneta americana* L.

M. ECKERT and M. GERSCH
Sektion Biologie, Tierphysiologie der Universität Jena, GDR

The morphological appearance of the neurosecretion in the brain of most insects is very uniform after staining with classical techniques. In contrast to this, a physiological diversity of neurohormones exists. Therefore attempts have been made to characterize neurosecretory cell groups by means of histochemical and experimental methods (see: MADDRELL, 1973). PRENTÖ (1972) reported that A- and B-cells of the pars intercerebralis of the locust *Schistocerca gregaria* produce chemically different peptides. Assuming the peptide or protein nature of the neurosecretory material, we have tried to determine a selective morphological and chemical distinction of the neurosecretion in the brain, using immunological techniques. The investigations indicated that immunological techniques are very useful in the analysis of this problem, because high sensitivity and specificity are typical for immunological reactions. A sufficient amount of neurosecretory material can be obtained by extraction of the retrocerebral complex of the cockroach, *P. americana*. The crude retrocerebral complex extract was fractionated by means of gel chromatography, ion-exchange chromatography and preparative polyacrylamide electrophoresis according to the following scheme:

Retrocerebral complex extract (0.01 *N* NH_4OH)

Sephadex G-200 (0.01 *N* NH_4OH)	Sephadex G-100 (0.01 *N* NH_4OH)	
	Preparative polyacrylamide electrophoresis after MAURER (gel system No. 1a, pH 8.9 -15%)	DEAE sephadex A-50 (0.1 *M* Tris-HCl, pH 8.3, gradient: 0.0-0.5 NaCl)
Polyvalent antineurosecretion sera	Monovalent anticardiaca secretion serum	Monovalent antineurosecretion serum

Antisera were prepared by immunization of rabbits with fractionated neurosecretions of the retrocerebral complex. From 3000 to 5000 retrocerebral complexes are necessary as starting material for the preparation of one antiserum.

After immunochemical staining of brain sections of *P. americana* the aldehyde fuchsin(AF)-positive neurons of the pars intercerebralis and the AF-negative lateral neurosecretory cells are selectively marked by polyvalent antineurosecretion sera (ECKERT, 1973). The immunohistochemical neurosecretion staining is not species-specific. Cross-species reactivity was demonstrated in cockroaches and locusts using enzyme-labeled anti-Periplaneta antibodies (Fig. 1). In Lepidoptera the reation of the neuro-

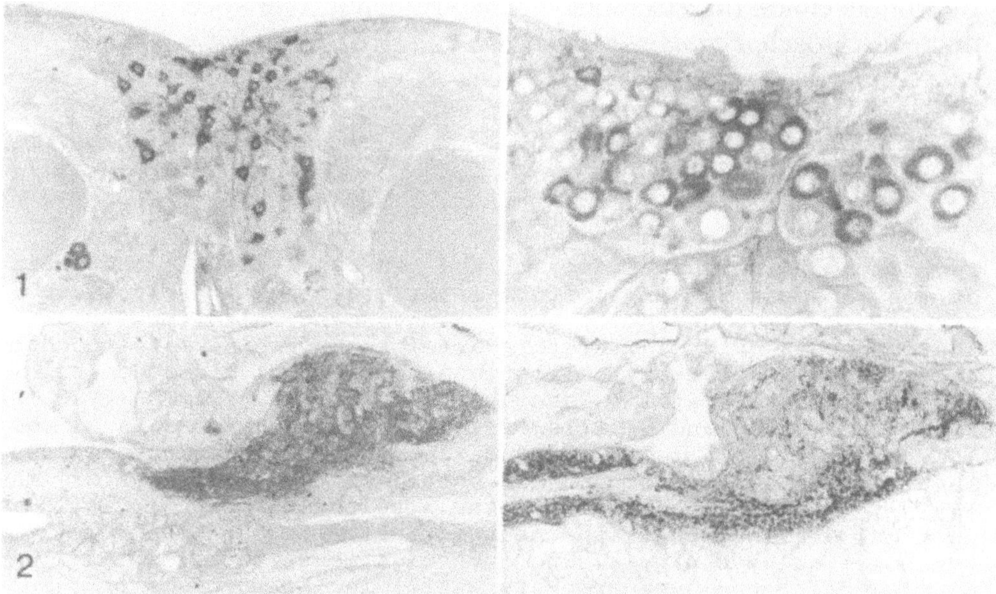

Fig. 1. Immunohistochemical staining of the pars intercerebralis of *Blaberus craniifer* (*left*) and *Locusta migratoria* (*right*). Typical neurosecretory cells react with antibodies of polyvalent antiserum to *Periplaneta* neurosecretion
Fig. 2. Sagittal sections of the corpora cardiaca of *P. americana* stained immunohistochemically for two separate antigens. Corpora-cardiaca secretion is located caudal of parenchyma cells (*left*). Nerve terminals containing neurosecretory material are demonstrated by the antigen-antibody reaction in the periphery of the gland (*right*)

secretory material of the pars intercerebralis is either weak (*Galleria mellonella*) or negative (*Mamestra brassicae*), with the polyvalent antineurosecretion sera against *Periplaneta* neurosecretion. However, the neurosecretory material of the lateral neurosecretory cells still exhibits an intensive cross-reaction. These results demonstrate on the one hand the chemical similarity of the neurosecretions of various insects, and on the other hand the distinct differences in the structure of neurosecretions between different species of insects. The combination of the immunohistochemical technique with the AF-staining of histological slides allows us to demonstrate three neurosecretory cell types besides the lateral neurosecretory cells. An adequate number of precipitation lines will be obtained after immunoelectrophoresis of the retrocerebral-complex extract.

For selective immunohistochemical staining of neurosecretory elements, monovalent antisera to the neurosecretory material of the corpora cardiaca must be prepared. The production of monovalent antisera is described in detail by ECKERT (1976). In this way, it was demonstrated that the AF-positive neurosecretory cells of the pars intercerebralis produce different neurosecretions. Whereas the large AF-positive neurosecretory cells in a rostral posi-

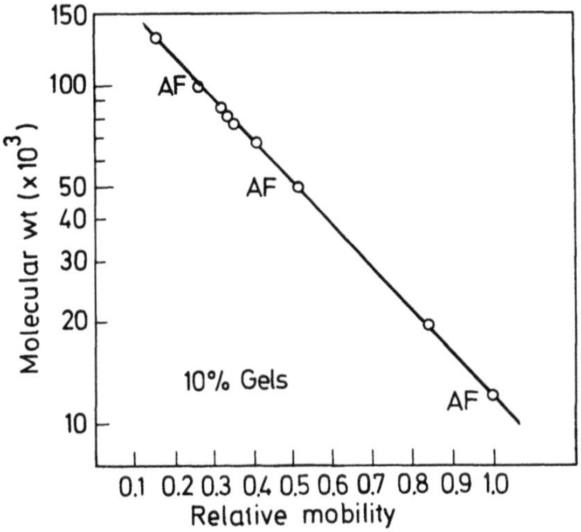

Fig. 3. Molecular-wt. estimation of immunochemically isolated neurosecretions by means of disc electrophoresis in SDS on 10% gels (gel system according to GAINER, and buffer system according to PAGE et al.). Migration distances of proteins were converted to relative mobilities by dividing each migration distance by that of cytochrome "c". *AF*-positive neurosecretion band with relative mobility 1.0 consists of two components with molecular sizes 9000 and 7000 daltons, estimated on 15% gels

tion can be stained by antibodies of the monovalent antineurosecretion serum, the smaller and also AF-positive cells in a median position are not stainable. This is direct chemical evidence for the production of different neurosecretions by the pars intercerebralis. Staining of the corpora cardiaca with two monovalent antisera indicates different storage sites for the neurosecretory material descending from the brain and for the secretion of parenchymal cells of the corpora cardiaca (Fig. 2).

In further experiments, the antigenic neurosecretions were characterized chemically. The neurosecretory materials were quantitatively precipitated by incubation of a retrocerebral-complex extract with polyvalent antineurosecretion serum. The washed neurosecretion-antibody complexes were dissolved in sodium dodecyl sulfate (SDS) containing sample solution for molecular wt. estimation by polyacrylamide-gel electrophoresis. The results of these investigations are presented in Figure 3. Of the nine protein bands detected by amino black staining, only four bands react with AF and periodic acid-Schiff reagent (PAS). The molecular sizes of the AF- and PAF-positive proteins are 100,000, 48,000, 9000, and 7000 daltons, respectively. Using immunoelectronmicroscopical techniques, antibodies against the isolated proteins stain the electron-dense content of the neurosecretory elementary granules selectively. At present it is not possible to decide whether the immunoreactive materials are the neurohormones themselves, carrier proteins, or other components of the elementary granules.

A direct relationship between the biologically active material (or factors) and the immunohistochemically detected neurosecretory material was only demonstrated in relation to activation-factor II. This factor is a fraction of the so-called "brain hormone," active in the development of insects. It causes changes in the permeability of the cell membranes of the molting gland in the wax moth *G. mellonella* (GERSCH et al., 1973). Activation-factor II, isolated by immunoabsorbance, produces a concentration-dependent biphasic modification of the membrane po-

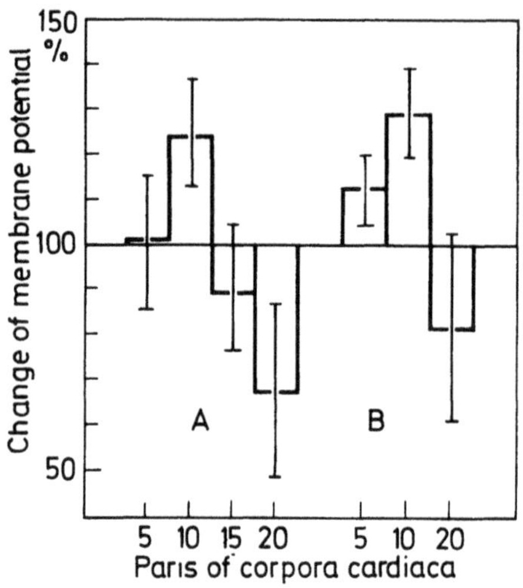

Fig. 4. Influence of activation-factor II isolated by sephadex G-100 gel filtration *A* and by immunoabsorption *B* on membrane potential of prothoracic-gland cells of *G. mellonella* in vitro

tential of the prothoracic gland cells (GERSCH et al., in press). This agrees with earlier results using chemically prepared activation-factor II. We believe that activation-factor II is a component of cardiaca secretion, which was demonstrated immunohistochemically by monovalent anticardiaca-secretion serum.

This study also demonstrates the possibility of correlating the physiological diversity of neurosecretion on a morphological level.

References

ECKERT, M.: Immunologische Untersuchungen des neuroendokrinen Systems von Insekten. III. Immunhistochemische Markierung des neuroendokrinen Systems von *Periplaneta americana* mit durch Fraktionierung von Retrocerebralkomplexextrakten gewonnenen Anti-Seren. Zool. Jb. Physiol. 76, 29-35 (1973)

ECKERT, M.: Immunologische Untersuchungen des neuroendokrinen Systems von Insekten. IV. Differenzierte immunhistochemische Darstellung von Neurosekreten des Gehirns und der Corpora cardiaca bei der Schabe *Periplaneta americana*. Zool. Jb. Physiol. 80 (1976) (in press)

GAINER, H.: Micro-disc electrophoresis in sodium dodecyl sulfate: an application to the study of protein synthesis in individual, identified neurons. Annal. Biochem. 44, 589-605 (1971)

GERSCH, M., BRÄUER, R., BIRKENBEIL, H.: Experimentelle Untersuchungen zum Wirkungsmechanismus der beiden entwicklungsphysiologisch aktiven Fraktionen des "Gehirnhormons" der Insekten (Aktivationsfaktor I und II) auf die Prothorakaldrüse. Experientia 29, 425-427 (1973)

GERSCH, M., ECKERT, M., BAUMANN, E., BIRKENBEIL, H.: Immunologische Untersuchungen des neuroendokrinen Systems von Insekten. V. Zur Kennzeichnung des Aktivationsfaktors II mit immunologischen, biochemischen und physiologischen Methoden. Zool. Jb. Physiol. (1973) (in press)

MADDRELL, S.H.P.: Neurosecretion. In: Frontiers of Biology. XXXV. Insect Neu Neurobiology. NEUBERGER, A., TATUM, E.C. (eds.). Amsterdam-Oxford: 1974, pp. 307-357

PACE, J.L., KEMPER, D.L., RAGLAND, W.L.: The relationship of molecular weight to electrophoretic mobility of fluorescamine-labeled proteins. Biochem. Biophys. Res. Commun. 57, 482-487 (1974)

PRENTÖ, P.: Histochemistry of neurosecretion in the pars intercerebralis-corpus cardiacum system of the desert locust *Schistocerca gregaria*. Gen. Comp. Endocrinol. 18, 482-500 (1972)

Neural and Neurohormonal Control of the Circadian Rhythm of Blood Trehalose in the Cockroach *Periplaneta americana* (Insecta)

M. GERSCH
Sektion Biologie der Universität Jena, GDR

The question of whether neurosecretions and/or neurohormones control rhythmic events, and if, accordingly, neurosecretory cells have an autonomous rhythmicity, is of general importance in neuroendocrinology. There exist numerous observations on circadian rhythms in insects, but the data concerning their control by neurohormones are quite contradictory (BRADY, 1974). On the one hand, neurosecretory cells of single ganglia (e.g., the subesophageal ganglion serving the control of locomotor activity) are thought to be directly responsible for certain circadian rhythms. On the other hand, the role of neurosecretory centers (e.g., pars intercerebralis of the brain) in the control of rhythms is still open to discussion. Arhythmic states occurring in some cases after the extirpation of neurosecretory areas do not necessarily mean that these areas are involved in the control of biologic rhythms. Considering the contradictory results and conclusions, it seems impossible to present a general scheme that could serve to explain all functional states. Therefore, one should refer only to well-analyzed data and avoid generalizations. A suitable system for this type of analysis is the circadian rhythm of the blood sugar content in *Periplaneta americana* and its neurohormonal control.

Some data concerning the blood sugar concentrations in *P. americana* and its circadian rhythm should first be considered. The content of trehalose in its hemolymph is known to be controlled by a hyperglycemic neurohormone from the corpora cardiaca (STEELE, 1961). In previous investigations we demonstrated the release of the hyperglycemic neurohormone in vitro, after stimulation of the corpora cardiaca via Nervus corporis cardiaci II (Ncc II) (GERSCH et al., 1970).

Furthermore, it is known that the blood sugar content of *P. americana* shows a circadian rhythm with a minimum at 5 p.m. and a maximum at 5 a.m. (HILLIARD and BUTZ, 1969; GERSCH, 1976). It was essential for the elucidation of the control of this circadian rhythm that the content of blood sugar could be influenced experimentally under in vivo conditions (GERSCH, 1974). These statements represent the experimental starting point for the investigation of regulation of the circadian rhythmicity of the trehalose content in the hemolymph of *P. americana*.

It had to be clarified whether or not the circadian rhythm of blood sugar in this insect is directly controlled by the corpora cardiaca and is accordingly under direct neurosecretory influence. The other possibility to be discussed is that nervous centers are responsible for the control mechanism that regulates the rhythmic release of the neurohormone from the corpora cardiaca.

To examine this question experimentally, the Ncc II of male imagines 6 days after molting were sectioned on both sides. Four days later, the trehalose level in the hemolymph of these animals was estimated at 5 p.m. (minimum in normal animals) and 5 a.m. (maximum in normal animals). The result was very strikking: the circadian rhythm was abolished. The sectioning of the Ncc II had prevented the release of the hyperglycemic hormone. With respect to the circadian rhythmicity the transection of the Ncc I is of particular significance. From previous experiments it is known that in this case the content of trehalose in the hemolymph would not show any change.

The Ncc I of male imagines 6 days after molting were transected and the hemolymph trehalose was measured 4 days later, at minimum and maximum times in two experimental groups. In both groups the results were identical: the circadian rhythm had ceased. In the sham-operated controls, however, the rhythm remained unchanged. From the loss of the rhythm after sectioning of the Ncc I it was concluded that in *P. americana* the neurohormonal regulation of the blood sugar rhythm is under the control of nervous centers. This is further supported by the fact that the rhythm ceased, although the transection of the Ncc I per se did not influence the release of the hyperglycemic hormone from the corpora cardiaca.

No exact information is yet available about the precise location of the superimposed centers. It could be shown that the circadian rhythm is abolished after elimination of the cerebral ganglion, the subesophageal ganglion or the 2nd thoracic ganglion, whereas elimination of the 2nd abdominal ganglion has no influence on the rhythm. Therefore the brain does not seem to be the only master center. The results obtained after the elimination of some ganglia of the ventral chain speak in favor of the participation of certain parts of the nerve cord in control of the rhythm.

The regulation of the blood sugar content in the cockroach *P. americana* and its circadian rhythm cannot be considered an isolated phenomenon. Particularly, the question arises whether other functions neurohormonally dependent on the corpora cardiaca are controlled in a similar manner. A number of different functions in cockroaches are regulated by neurohormones of the corpora cardiaca.

Therefore we can assume that with respect to (1) the control of the circadian rhythm of blood sugar, and (2) the diversity of the control mechanisms exerted by the neurohormones from the corpora cardiaca, the regulatory pattern of the corpora cardiaca is much more complex than has previously been suggested.

Although in the CNS of *P. americana* the precise location of the center controlling the circadian level of blood sugar through the corpora cardiaca is unknown, the fundamental functional relationship between the nervous system and the neuroendocrine system is evident. However, in this particular case, neurosecretion per se is not responsible for the maintenance of circadian rhythm.

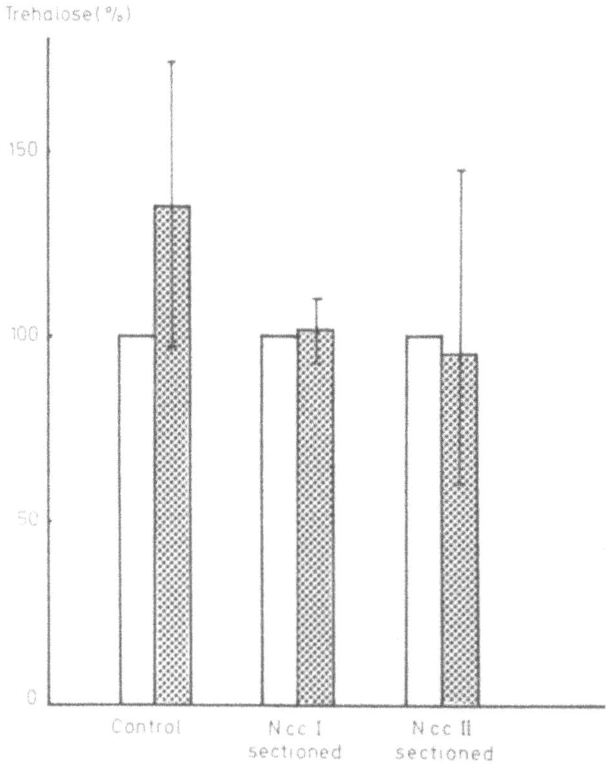

Fig. 1. Effect of sectioning Ncc on circadian rhythm of blood sugar in *P. americana*. Note that transection of Ncc I abolishes circadian rhythm although hormonal control of trehalose content of hemolymph is not directly influenced via Ncc I. Contrary to this, sectioning of Ncc II influences trehalose level of blood as well as circadian rhythm. Therefore it may be concluded that circadian rhythm of blood sugar level depends on action of nervous centers and cannot be considered an autonomous neurosecretory function. □ blood trehalose level at 5 p.m. (min.), ▨ blood trehalose level at 5 a.m. (max.)

References

BRADY, J.: The physiology of insect circadian rhythms. Adv. Insect Physiol. 10, 1-115 (1974)

GERSCH, M.: Experimentelle Untersuchungen zum Freisetzungsmechanismus von Neurohormonen nach elektrischer Reizung der corpora cardiaca von *Periplaneta americana* in vitro. J. Insect Physiol. 18, 2425-2439 (1972)

GERSCH, M.: Selektive Freisetzung des hyperglykaemischen Faktors aus den corpora cardiaca von *Periplaneta americana* in vivo. Experientia 30, 767 (1974)

GERSCH, M.: Kontrolle der circadianen Rhythmik des Trehalosegehaltes der Haemolymphe von *Periplaneta americana*. Zool. Jb. Physiol. 80, 1-15 (1976)

GERSCH, M., RICHTER, K., BÖHM, G.-A., STÜRZEBECHER, J.: Selektive Ausschüttung von Neurohormonen nach elektrischer Reizung der Corpora cardiaca von *Periplaneta americana* in vitro. J. Insect Physiol. 16, 1991-2013 (1970)

HILLIARD, S.D., BUTZ, H.: Daily fluctuation in the concentrations of total sugar and uric acid in the haemolymph of *Periplaneta americana*. Ann. Ent. Soc. Am. 62, 71-74 (1969)

STEELE, J.E.: Occurrence of a hyperglycaemic factor in the corpus cardiacum of an insect. Nature 192, 680-681 (1961)

Midgut of Coleopteran Larvae, the Possible Target Organ for the Action of Neurohormones

J. IVANOVIĆ, M. JANKOVIĆ-HLADNI, V. STANIĆ, V. NENADOVIĆ, and M. MILANOVIĆ
Laboratory of Physiologic Ecology of Insects, Institute for Biologic Research, 29 November 142, Belgrade, Yugoslavia

A. Introduction

Detailed knowledge concerning the role of neurohormones in the regulation of metabolic processes in the larvae of insects is still lacking. In our previous studies, a functional relationship between the physiologic state of the neurosecretory cells of brain and midgut proteolytic activity in larvae of *Tenebrio molitor* and *Morimus funereus* was reported. Moreover, prolonged exposure of the larvae to certain temperatures resulted in reversible inactivation of the neurosecretory system (APPLEBAUM et al., 1964; IVANOVIĆ et al., 1975a; IVANOVIĆ et al., 1975b; JANKOVIĆ-HLADNI and GROZDANOVIĆ, 1969). This work studies the role of neurohormones in regulation of midgut proteolytic and amylolytic activities in phytophagous larvae of two coleopteran species of very different phylogenetic age: *T. molitor* (Tenebrionidae) and *M. funereus* (Cerambycidae).

B. Materials and Methods

The larvae of *T. molitor* (100 mg) and *M. funereus* (600-1200 mg) were used in the experiments. The reversible inactivation of the neurosecretory system by use of prolonged exposure to certain temperatures is a novel technique in this field and, in combination with the ligature and injection techniques, it was employed in the course of this work. *Morimus* larvae were ligated proximally to the metathoracic region; fed and unfed intact larvae served as controls. After 4 days the isolated abdomina were injected with cerebral-complex extract (CCE) or saline. The larvae were sacrificed 20 h after injection. In order to inactivate the neurosecretory system, *Tenebrio* larvae were kept at 31 °C for one week, and *Morimus* larvae at 23 °C for 2 weeks. After that period the larvae were injected with CCE or saline and sacrificed 20 h after treatment. The extract was prepared (without c. allata in *Morimus*) in saline solution, from donors with high-enzyme activity (24 heads/ml). Each recipient (low-enzyme activity) received 0.2 µl/mg body wt of the extract or saline. Proteolytic and amylolytic activities, and the amount of proteins were determined spectrophotometrically in crude midgut extracts.

Fig. 1A-F. Regulation of midgut proteolytic and amylolytic activities in larvae of *T. molitor* and *M. funereus*. (A,B) The effect of ligation on *M. funereus*; C_f - control (untreated, fed); C_U - control (untreated, unfed); *L* - ligated; *L* + *S* - saline-injection into ligated larvae; *L* + *E* - extract-injection into ligated larvae. (C,E) The effect of temperature on *T. molitor*; C_{23} - control (grown at 23°C); T_{31} - kept at 31°C for 1 week; *S* - group of T_{31} larvae injected with saline; *E* - group of T_{31} larvae injected with extract. (D,F) The effect of temperature on *M. funereus*; C_N - control (from natural habitat); T_{23} - kept at 23°C for 2 weeks; *S* - group of T_{23} larvae injected with saline; *E* - group of T_{23} larvae injected with extract

C. Results

I. Proteolytic Activity of the Midgut

(1) The effect of ligation and temperature: Figure 1A,D shows that in larvae of *M. funereus*, both ligation and exposure to 23°C decrease the proteolytic activity to a negligible level, while in *T. molitor* (Fig. 1C) the enzyme activity was significantly lowered at 31°C. (2) The effect of the extract: from Figure 1A,D one can conclude that the extract injected into ligated and temperature-treated larvae of *M. funereus* exerts a significant stimulatory effect on the proteolytic activity. The same holds true for *T. molitor* (Fig. 1C).

II. Amylolytic Activity of the Midgut

(1) The effect of ligation and temperature: the results shown in Figure 1B,F indicate that ligation and exposure to a temperature of 23°C significantly decreased the amylolytic activity in *M. funereus*, whereas in *T. molitor* (Fig. 1E) the amylolytic activity was increased at 31°C. (2) The effect of the extract: it is evident from Figure 1B, E, F that the extract evokes a significant increase of the amylolytic activity in both species.

D. Discussion

Our discussion is based on data reported in the literature, i.e., the existence of a correlation between the cytologic changes in the neurosecretory cells and changes in brain-hormone titer (MARKS et al., 1973), the control of synthesis and release of the brain hormone (HIGHNAM, 1967), and on our results concerning cytologic analysis of the cephalic neurosecretory system and the midgut epithelial cells of the larvae (unpublished data). Our results show that ligation, exposure to different temperatures, and starvation decrease the proteolytic and amylolytic activities of both species, while CCR prepared from active donors and injected into inactive recipients stimulates them. Stimulation of protease by CCE is more pronounced in ligated recipients (with cephalic neurosecretory system and prothoracic gland irreversibly

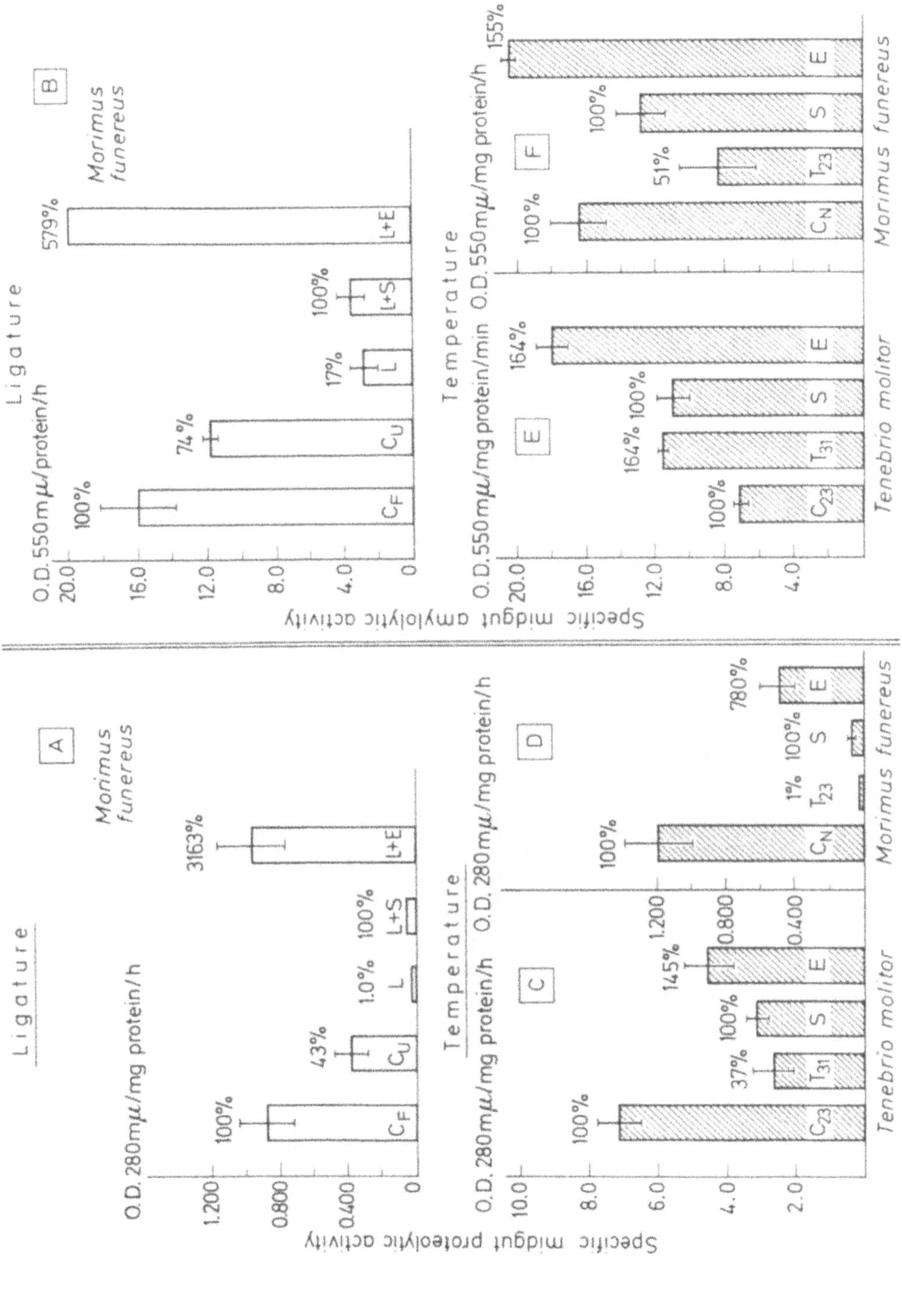
Ligature
A
Morimus funereus
O.D. 280mμ/mg protein/h
Specific midgut proteolytic activity
1.200
0.800
0.400
0
100%
43%
1.0%
100%
3163%
C_F
C_U
L
L+S
L+E
B
Ligature
Morimus funereus
O.D. 550mμ/protein/h
Specific midgut amylolytic activity
20.0
16.0
12.0
8.0
4.0
0
100%
74%
17%
100%
579%
Temperature
C
D
O.D. 280mμ/mg protein/h
10.0
8.0
6.0
4.0
2.0
100%
37%
100%
145%
C_{23}
T_{31}
S
E
Tenebrio molitor
1.200
0.800
0.400
100%
1%
100%
780%
C_N
T_{23}
S
E
Morimus funereus
Temperature
E
F
O.D. 550mμ/mg protein/min
O.D. 550mμ/mg protein/h
20.0
16.0
12.0
8.0
4.0
100%
164%
100%
164%
C_{23}
T_{31}
S
E
Tenebrio molitor
100%
51%
100%
155%
C_N
T_{23}
S
E
Morimus funereus

isolated) than in temperature-treated recipients (with reversibly inactivated neurosecretory systems), in which overdosage of the hormone might exert inhibitory influence on the enzyme activity. Such larvae show decreased amount of the neurosecretory material in c. cardiaca (unpublished data); this is perhaps due to the presence in the extract of activating-factor II, which alters the permeability of the cell membranes of the prothoracic gland (GERSCH and BIRKENBEIL, 1973). Differences in the activity of the two enzymes under identical conditions may depend upon different regulatory centers and/or specific enzyme properties (half life of enzyme, stability, isozymes). Our cytologic study of the midgut of temperature-treated larvae showed that changes occur in the cytoplasm and the nucleus of the enterocytes and regenerative cells, correlated with changes in the cephalic neurosecretory system (unpublished data). It was suggested (HRUBEŠOVA and SLÁMA, 1967) that in adult *Pyrrhocoris apterus* the midgut is the target organ of the activating hormone. The above results suggest that the cells of the midgut in *T. molitor* and *M. funereus* larvae are target cells of the brain hormone.

Acknowledgment. The authors wish to thank Mr. M. Božidarac for his skilfull technical assistance.

References

APPLEBAUM, S.W., JANKOVIĆ, M., GROZDANOVIĆ, J., MARINKOVIĆ, D.: Compensation for temperature in digestive metabolism of *Tenebrio molitor* larvae. Physiol. Zool. 37, 90-95 (1964)

GERSCH, M., BIRKENBEIL, H.: Das Membranpotential der Prothoracaldrüsenzellen von *Galleria mellonella* in Beziehung zum Entwicklungsstadium und nach Einwirkung von Neurohormonen. Zool. Jb. (Physiol.) 77, 1-24 (1973)

HIGHNAM, K.C.: Insect hormones. J. Endocrinol. 39, 123-150 (1967)

HRUBEŠOVA, H., SLÁMA, K.: The effect of hormones on the intestinal proteinase activity of adult *Pyrrhocoris apterus* L. (Hemimptera). Acta Ent. Bohemoslov. 64, 175-183 (1967)

IVANOVIĆ, J., JANKOVIĆ-HLADNI, M., MILANOVIĆ, M.: Effect of constant temperature on survival rate, neurosecretion and endocrine cells, and digestive enzymes in *Morimus funereus* larvae (cerambycidae:Coleoptera). Comp. Biochem. Physiol. 50A, 125-130 (1975a)

IVANOVIĆ, J., JANKOVIĆ-HLADNI, M., MILNOVIĆ, M.: Possible role of neurosecretory cells: type A in response of *Morimus funereus* larvae to the effect of temperature. J. Thermal Biol. 1, 53-57 (1975b)

JANKOVIĆ-HLADNI, M., GROZDANOVIĆ, J.: The effect of temperature on medial neurosecretory cells of *Tenebrio molitor* larvae. Gen. Comp. Endocrinol. 13, 68 (1969)

MARKS, E., HOLMAN, G., BORH, T.: Synthesis and storage of neurohormone in insect brains in vitro. J. Insect Physiol. 19, 471-479 (1973)

Regulation of Midgut Amylolytic Activity in *Tenebrio molitor* Adults

M. JANKOVIĆ-HLADNI, J. IVANCOVIĆ, V. STANIĆ, V. NENADOVIĆ, and M. MILANOVIĆ
Laboratory of Physiologic Ecology of Insects, Institute for Biologic Research, 29 November 142, Belgrade, Yugoslavia

MORDUE has stated (Gen. Comp. Endocrinol. 9, 406-415, 1967) that in *T. molitor* females, midgut proteolytic activity is regulated via the median neurosecretory cells of the protocerebrum. The aim of this work was: (1) to study whether or not the amylolytic activity of *T. molitor* adults is regulated in a similar way, and (2) to find out if there is some relationship between cytodifferentiation of midgut epithelium and the amylolytic activity. Comparative studies of amylolytic activity, midgut epithelium, and the neuroendocrine system were undertaken. Adults 0-2 h and 18-20 h after emergence were ligated around the head, and others (0-6 h and 18-20 h after emergence) were injected with crude head extract, 10 µl/individual prepared in saline solution from 4-5 day-old, fed adults. Following this treatment, ligated insects were sacrificed after 18 h and 72 h, and the injected ones after 18 h. The results show that in ligated adults the amylolytic activity was decreased, while in recipients of head extract it was significantly increased. The ligature was more effective in older adults, the injection of extract was more effective in newly emerged ones. In older (18 h) insects the old epithelium was replaced by a new one, the number of epithelial cells was significantly increased, and the neuroendocrine system was in a more active physiologic state. In ligated adults (72 h) a decreased number of epithelial cells, their incomplete differentiation, and degenerative changes were observed.

The results suggest that hormones are involved in regulation of midgut amylolytic activity in *T. molitor* adults, and that this regulation is probably closely related to the cytodifferentiation of the midgut epithelium.

Neurosecretory Cells of the Brain of *Mamestra brassicae* (Lepidoptera, Noctuidae) During Metamorphosis and Diapause Development

T. W. KIND
Laboratory of Entomology, Biologic Institute, Leningrad State University, Leningrad, USSR

Activation of the prothoracic glands is due to the brain prothoracotropic hormone. The source of this hormone is the medial neurosecretory cells (NSC) of the protocerebrum (WILLIAMS, 1969) and, in *Lepidoptera*, the major part of prothoracotropic hormone biosynthesis most likely occurs in the A'-NSC of M_1-group (PANOW, 1969). The inactivation of the brain endocrine centers that occurs during the onset of diapause is usually accompanied by a cessation of hormone release and hence the accumulation of a great quantity of secretory material in the NSC perikarya (HIGHNAM, 1965; KIND, 1968; KONO, 1973). Renewal of brain-endocrine activity takes place after a long period of diapause development in low-temperature conditions.

There are two types of pupal diapause in the armyworm *M. brassicae*: a winter diapause, which is determined by the influence of short-day photoperiods, and a summer diapause (estivation). In the pupae with the summer diapause, development is delayed for about a month and is restored without a reactivation by cold.

The NSC of the pupal brain were studied in active and diapause pupae, during diapause development (at 5°C), and subsequent incubation. A'-NSC of *M. brassicae* can be divided into two subtypes: A_1'- and A_2'-NSC, the first containing much more stainable material (Fig. 2). There are four cells of each subtype in the brain. Both in active and diapause pupae the quantity of neurosecretory material in the A_1'-cells undergoes negligible changes during metamorphosis and the early stages of diapause. A_2'-cells do not →

Fig. 1. Amount of neurosecretory material in A'-NSC of active and diapause *M. brassicae* pupae. o——o - A_1'-NSC of active pupae; ●——● - A_1'-NSC of diapause pupae, □---□ - A_2'-NSC of active pupae, ■---■ - A_2'-NSC of diapause pupae; ◪---◪ - A_2'-NSC of estivating pupae; *ordinate* - amount of material in conventional units, *abscissa* - days after pupation

Fig. 2. Young pupa. First and second medial groups of NSC. Note difference between A_1'- and A_2'-cells and absence of stainable material in NSC of M_2-group

Fig. 3. A'-cell of a diapause pupa, 16 days after pupation

Fig. 4. A'-cell of a diapause pupa, 2 months of chilling

Fig. 5. A'-cell of a diapause pupa, 3 months of chilling. Vacuoles are observed in blocks of secretory material

Fig. 6. A'-cell of a diapause pupa, 6 months of chilling. Cell is highly vacuolated

Fig. 7. A'-cell of a postdiapause pupa, 3 months of chilling and 2 days of incubation

Fig. 8. M_2-cell of an active pupa, 5 days after pupation

Fig. 9. M_2-cell of an active pupa, 16 days after pupation

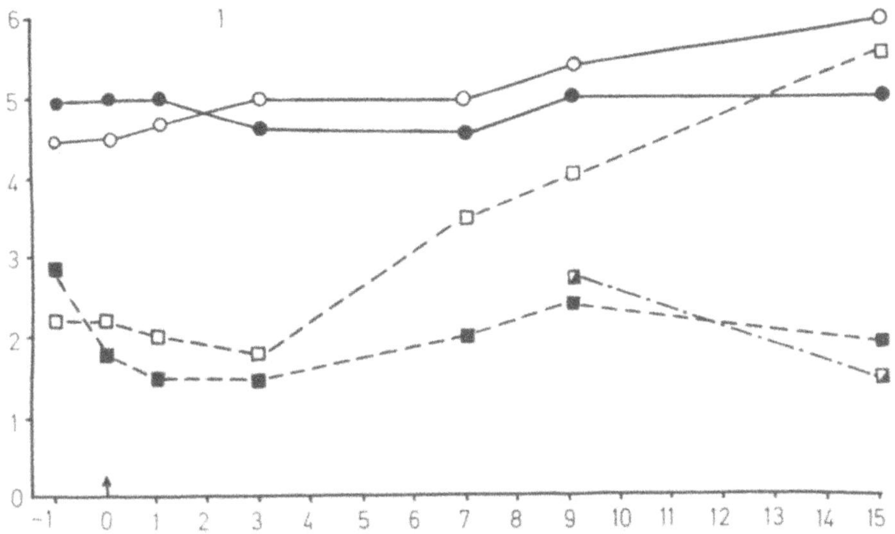
1
0
1
2
3
4
5
6
-1
0
1
2
3
4
5
6
7
8
9
10
11
12
13
14
15

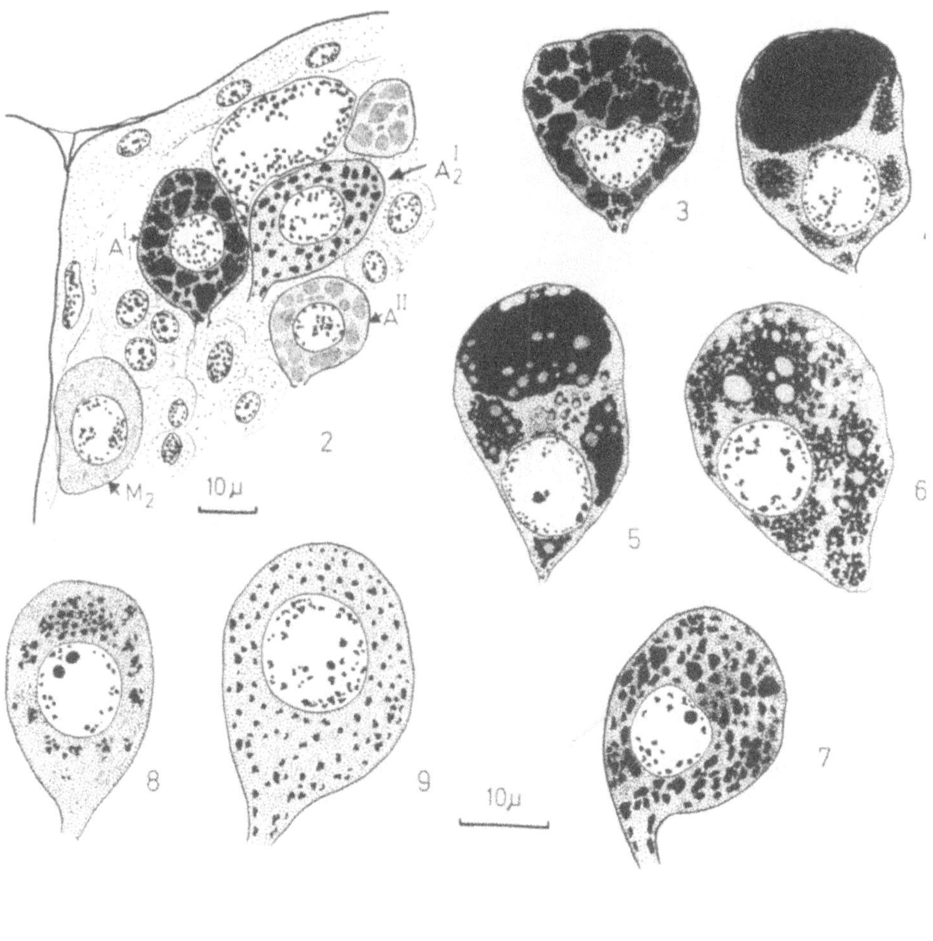
A_2^I
A_1^I
A^{II}
M_2
10μ
2
3
5
6
8
9
10μ
7

change their activity in the course of adult development, but in the diapause specimens they gradually become filled with secretory material (Fig. 1). After pupation for 15-20 days A_2'-NSC cannot be distinguished from the A_1'-NSC of the same group (Fig. 3). Extirpation experiments show that the brain-hormone threshold titer was reached on the third day of pupal life. After that time the brain may be extirpated without any effect on imaginal differentiation. Yet the differences between the A_2'-cells of active and diapause pupae can be observed only at the seventh day after pupation. It is very likely that the synthesis of the brain hormone in *M. brassicae* pupae is very low, and if its release is blocked, neurosecretory material accumulates gradually in diapause pupae NSC.

Only scanty information concerning NSC patterns during estivation was obtained. A'-cells of such pupae do not differ in their content of secretion from the same NSC of active pupae (Fig. 1). It is quite possible that during estivation the rate of hormone release falls insignificantly, but enough to delay the activation of the prothoracic glands.

A_1'- and A_2'-NSC of old diapause pupae are undistinguishable and can be united into one A'-type. After 3 months at 5°C (the minimal period of chilling for reactivation) the first change is that vacuoles can be discerned in the colloidal blocks of secretion in these NSC (Figs. 3, 4, 5); they increase sharply in numbers after 1 month of further reactivation. In pupae maintained for 5-6 months in low temperature conditions, blocks of the secretion in A'-cells break up into granules (Fig. 6). This indicates the renewal of NSC endocrine activity, but the prothoracotropic-hormone titer does not reach the threshold since brain extirpation during this period leads to the state of permanent diapause.

Activity of A'-cells in the early stages varies after different periods of chilling but, on the second day of incubation in all samples, the neurosecretory material becomes granulated and is distributed uniformly throughout the cell body (Fig. 7). In the postdiapause pupae the threshold titer of the brain hormone is reached at 1.5-2 days after the onset of incubation. Thus, in the postdiapause pupae activity of the brain NSC is higher than in the active pupae.

The second group of NSC that change their activity during imaginal development are the M_2-groups of cells of the pars intercerebralis. There is a lack of secretory material in the young active and diapause pupal M_2-cells (Fig. 2); it can be recognized only after 4-5 days of pupal life. Both in active and postdiapause pupae a great increase in the size of M_2-cells may be observed shortly before imaginal ecdysis (Figs. 8, 9). They became filled with faint granules of secretory material. In the young imago this disappears from the cells once more. Such cycles of cell activity have also been observed in some silkworms (PANOW, 1968). It may be supposed that these NSC are the source of eclosion hormone (TRUMAN and RIDDIFORD, 1970). The probability of this supposition is confirmed by the fact that, when brain extirpation is performed after the critical period, imagines cannot ecdyze, and die within the pupal sheath.

References

KIND, T.W.: Functional morphology of the insect neurosecretory systems during active development and different types of diapause. In: Photoperiodic Adaptations in Insects and Acari. (In Russian). Leningrad: State Univ. 1968, pp. 153-191

KONO, Y.: Light and electron microscopic studies on the neurosecretory control of diapause incidence in *Pieris rapae crucivora*. J. Ins. Physiol. 19 (2), 255-272 (1973)

PANOW, A.A.: Neurosecretory processes in the brain of some silkworms. In: The Aspects of Functional Morphology and Embryology of Insects. (In Russian). Moscow: Nauka 1968, pp. 93-132

PANOW, A.A.: A'-neurosecretory cells of same *Lepidoptera* as a possible source of the activation hormone. (In Russian). J. Gen. Biol. 30 (1), 87-93 (1969)

TRUMAN, J.W., RIDDIFORD, L.M.: Neuroendocrine control of ecdysis in silkmoths. Science 167 (3925), 1624-1626 (1970)

WILLIAMS, C.M.: Photoperiodism and the endocrine aspects of insect diapause. Symp. Soc. Exp. Biol. 23, 285-300 (1969)

Neurosecretory System of the Polychaete *Nephthys minuta* Theel (Annelida, Polychaeta) and Its Possible Function in Salinity Acclimatization

E. E. KULAKOVSKI and T. G. L'VOVA
Zoologic Institute, Academy of Sciences, USSR, Leningrad, USSR

The neurosecretory system of the supraesophageal ganglion of the polychaete *Nephthys minuta* is represented by diffusely localized neurosecretory cells (NSC), among which two types may be distinguished by cytomorphologic features. The cerebrovascular complex, which is present in other, more highly organized polychaetes, is absent here. The NSC function in an asynchronous way, and due to this a definite quantity of neurohormones constantly enters the blood. When the salinity of the environment is changed, neurosecretory material is removed from the NSC and a disturbance of the normal secretory cycle occurs. Formation of a new rhythm of the function, which corresponds to the changed circumstances, takes place 9-11 days later. This period of time is similar to that of the completion of the animals' acclimatization to the new salinity conditions. The dynamics of the polychaetes' acclimatization to lower salinity (measured by O_2 consumption) represents a regular modification of that value in relation to the control level and its further stabilization after 11-12 days. Extracts prepared from supraesophageal ganglia of animals acclimated to 10% and 40% saline were introduced to the environment of control animals (26%). This resulted in a considerable increase in the level of O_2 consumption. Daily measurements of respiration revealed that addition of the extract caused a change of the functional states of the animals that was similar to the natural process of acclimatization to a direct lowering of salinity. The results suggest an initial neurohormonal stimulation and regulation of the processes that form the foundation of phenotypic adaptations.

Evolution of the Composition of the Brain Medial Neurosecretory Cells Within Neuropteroid and Mecopteroid Insects

A. A. PANOV and E. D. DAVYDOVA
A.N. Severtzov Institute of Evolutionary Morphology and Ecology of Animals, Academy of Sciences of the USSR, Moscow, USSR

The neurosecretory system (NSS) of the insect brain controls numerous processes of life activity. At present it is already known to produce at least six different hormonal substances: hyperglycemic, diuretic, prothoracotropic, as well as neurohormone D, bursicon, and eclosion hormone. This has produced a great interest in the complexity of the cell composition of the brain NSS and in the elucidation of its origin during onto- and phylogenesis. However, in spite of an intense study of brain NSS during the last 25 years, these problems still remain inadequately investigated. The qualitative composition of the brain neurosecretory cells (NSC) has not yet been studied in about a half the orders of insects.

To ascertain the manner of development of the brain NSS, the medial NSC composition was studied in a large range of holometabolous insects. The latter include four superorders: Neuropteroidea, Coleopteroidea, Hymenopteroidea, and Mecopteroidea. Coleopteroidea and Hymenopteroidea are each characterized by a particular direction of their evolution, and their origin is not yet sufficiently clear. By contrast, a close relationship between Neuropteroidea and Mecopteroidea is generally accepted, the former being considered as deriving from the latter (ROHDENDORF, 1962). The members of these two superorders were the subject of our present study. The medial NSC were investigated in about 70 insect species.

The general organization of the medial NSS was found to be very similar in all insects studied. In members of both superorders, the medial NSC are gathered in three paired groups (M1, M2, and M3). Such an organization of medial NSC is apparently a very ancient feature, in so far as the origin of the most ancient Mecopteriodea dates from the Devonian period. In the majority of species studied, groups M2 and M3 are characterized by their stable composition and each includes two identical NSC. Only in some Diptera does group M3 consist of a single NSC. Composition of groups M2 and M3 does not change in the course of ontogenesis.

By contrast, the composition of group M1, which corresponds to the medial NSC of the pars intercerebralis of other authors, is highly variable. Among Neuropteroid and Mecopteroid insects, a tendency to reduce the number of NSC of group M1 is observed, and is accompanied by ontogenetically early stabilization of its composition. The lowest degree in this process occurs in Neuropteroidea, whereas the highest occurs in cyclorhaphous Diptera and some Lepidoptera.

In most Neuropteroidea, a "larval" and "imaginal" set of the NSC can be distinguished in group M1, including at least three cell types: A1, A2, and B. The A1-NSC stain intensely with PTh and PF, whereas the A2-cells stain more strongly with PF than with PTh. The B-NSC are phloxinophil. In Neuroptera larvae, group M1 includes four A1, 16 A2- and from three to five B-cells. Besides, neuroblasts and small undifferentiated cells also occur in the medial part of the brain. In adult insects, the number of the A2-NSC does not generally change. By contrast, the A1- and B-cells increase significantly in number, apparently on account of differentiation of the above-mentioned small cells and of division of neuroblasts.

In scorpion flies, the most archaic among Mecopteroid insects, the same three cell types occur in group M1. In *Panorpa*, the NSC are numerous, and composition of the A-cells (approximately 23 A1- and 42 A2-cells for each pars intercerebralis) is the same already in the second instar larvae as in adults. The number of B-cells rises during the pupal stage on account of neuroblast divisions. However, in *Boreus*, another member of Mecoptera, only eight A1- and 24 A2-cells were found in imaginal pars intercerebralis: these were similar to the larval set of the NSC of Neuroptera.

The subdivision of the A-NSC into A1- and A2-cells apparently also occurs in Diptera. At least, it is the case in *Calliphora* and *Lucilia* (PANOV, 1976). But in contrast to the insects described above, the A1-, A2-, and B-cells are less numerous in higher Diptera, and their number is the same in mature larvae and in adults.

Lepidoptera and Trichoptera form a particular branch among Mecopteroid insects. Apparently, they lack the A2-cells. However, in Lepidoptera, there are eight A1-cells in each group M1, which are subdivided into two subtypes: A' and A". Moreover, in several Lepidoptera, further differentiation of the A'-cells takes place. As for higher Diptera, early ontogenetic stabilization of the composition of A1-NSC is characteristic of Lepidoptera. It is possible, however, that in some Lepidoptera, as in *Panorpa*, multiplication of the B-cells occurs during metamorphosis.

Finally, in Trichoptera, a more primitive insect order than Lepidoptera, composition of the group M1 is the simplest. There are neither A2- nor B-cells, and the number of the A1-NSC varies from between 2 and 3 up to nine in larval brains of different members of this order. Among these cells, one A_b-NSC can be singled out by its strong affinity to PTh and PF. Apparently, it has no homologs among the NSC of other Mecopteroid insects. The remaining A-cells seem to belong to a single cell type and correspond in general to A'- and A"-cells of Lepidoptera.

In so far as high stability of chemical properties is generally characteristic of the nerve cells (SAKHAROV, 1970), the establishment of homology of NSC types and of their groups in large insect axons allows us to suppose a similarity or identity in chemical composition of the hormones elaborated and released by these NSC types. However, it is less probable that these homologous types of the NSC control the same processes of life activity in the members of different insect groups.

References

PANOV, A.A.: The composition of the medial neurosecretory cells of the pars intercerebralis in *Calliphora* and *Lucilia* adults. Zool. Anz. 196, 23-27 (1976)

ROHDENDORF, B.B.: Holometabola. Coleopteroidea. Hymenopteroidea. In: Principles of Paleontology. ORLOV, J.A. (ed.). Moscow: Acad. Sci. USSR 1962, Vol. IX, pp. 239-241, 345 (in Russian)

SAKHAROV, D.A.: Grounds for construction of the nerve cell system. Zhurn. Obsh. Biol. 31, 449-457 (1970) (in Russian)

Ultrastructure of the Dorsal Neurohemal Area of the Snail *Theba pisana* L. (Stylommatophora, Gastropoda)

A. NOLTE
Zoologisches Institut, Abteilung Histophysiologie, Hüfferstraße 1, 4400 Münster, FRG

In most species of Stylommatophora that have been investigated, two or rarely three small nerves extend from the cerebral commissure and branch out within the dispersed dorsal body (DB). This dorsal neurohemal area and two lateral neurohemal areas belong to the peptidergic system of the cerebral ganglia (KUHLMANN, 1963, 1966; NOTTE, 1965, 1968; VAN MOL, 1967). No electronmicroscopic investigations of this dorsal area in Stylommatophora have been published until now (see MARTOJA, 1972; BOER and JOOSSE, 1975). *Theba pisana*, a hermaphroditic xerophilous landsnail, seems adequate for an ultrastructural examination of the supposed morphologic connection between the neurosecretory nerves and the dorsal body (NOLTE, 1965). This species has well-developed PAF-positive cerebral commissure nerves (CCNs) and a DB lying at a clear distance from the cerebral commissure so that the close contact of these two tissues (CCNs and DB) cannot only be due to chance.

By using serial semithin sections and montages of electron micrographs of cerebral ganglia of 21 adult specimens sacrificed during 4 different months of a year (including the reproductive phase) we tried to trace the branches of the CCNs to the axon terminals (fixation: 2% glutaraldehyde in 0.05 *M* cacodylate buffer; 2% OsO_4). *

The CCNs (Fig. 1) and their branches are characterized by axons of variable diameter that contain a variable number of elementary granules (1000-1600 Å in diameter). Rarely, there are large axon swellings (10-20 µm in diameter) within a nerve or bulging from its periphery. These are densely packed with granules, and are comparable to the Herring bodies of vertebrates. The neurosecretory fibers contain irregularly shaped vacuoles (Fig. 1b). They are accompanied by glial cells of the filamentous type known from the CNS.

Capillaries are distributed near the perineurium of the ganglia, whereas the lacunae lie farther away. The DB region is well supplied with hemolymph entering from the capillaries into the lacunae and from there through ostia at the periphery of the ganglion sheath into the pedal sinus. However, there are no particularly marked accumulations of nerve branches or axons in the

→

Fig. 1. (a) CCN extending from commissure; (b) neurosecretory axons (*A*) within nerve; (c) CCN among dorsal body cells (*DBC*); (d) small granules (*arrows*) in *DBC*s. *G* - glial cell processes, *V* - vacuole. (a) × 5000; (b-d) × 20,000

*I wish to thank Mrs. W. Greven for careful technical help.

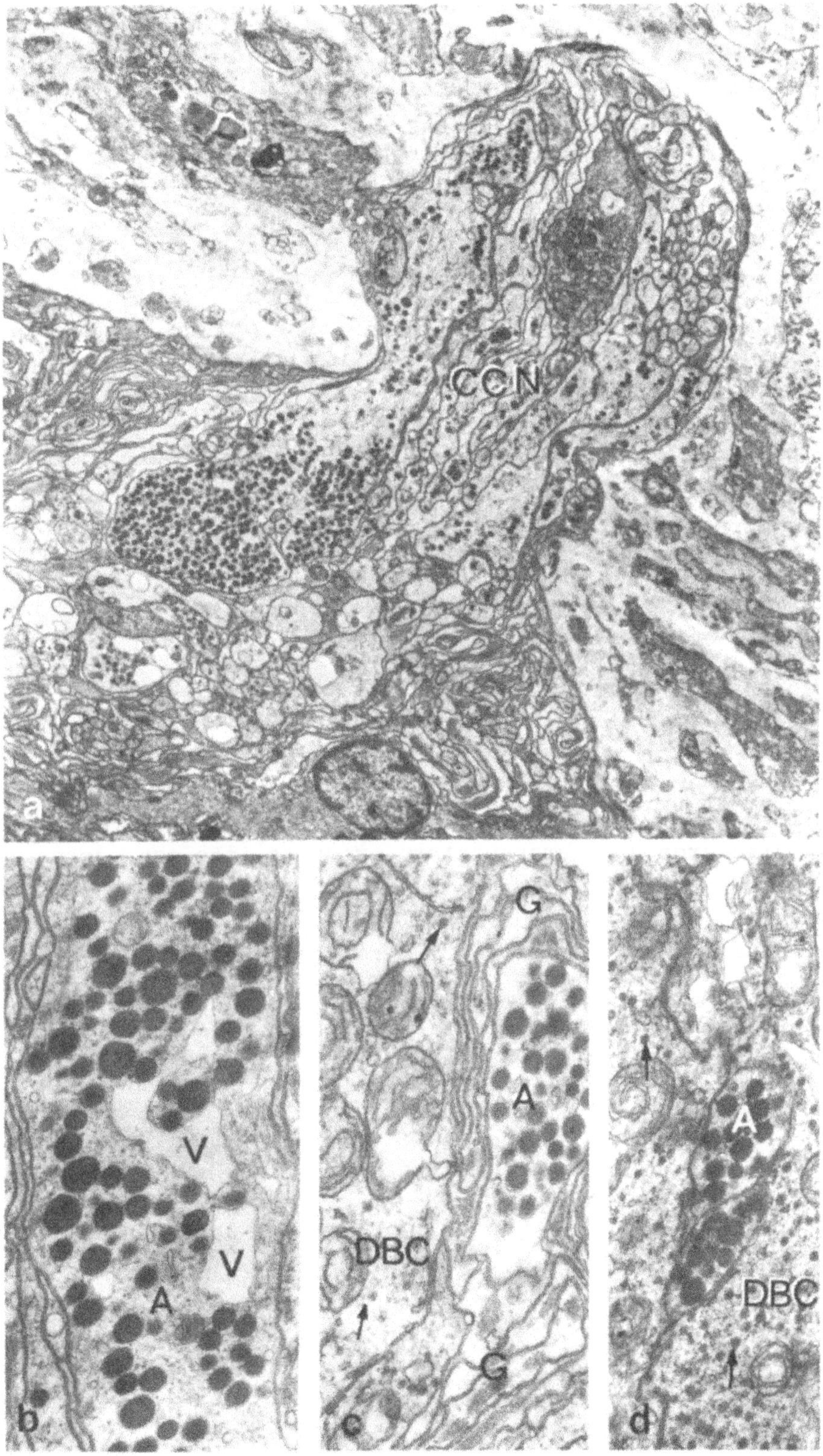
CCN
a
V
V
A
b
G
A
DBC
G
c
A
DBC
d

neighborhood of capillaries or hemolymph lacunae, as would be found in a neurohemal organ.

On the other hand, the morphologic contact between the neurosecretory nerves and the DB cells is far more extensive than we supposed from light-microscopic observations. Small nerves are not only passing by or running through the clusters of DB cells, but are spread between these cells like an irregular network. There is no basal lamina either between adjacent DB cells or between DB cells and axons or glial cell processes. Empty axons can easily be recognized if filamentous glial cells surround them. The DB cells are thought to be endocrine cells. They are rich in mitochondria and lipid droplets and produce small electron-dense granules with a mean diameter of ~ 600 Å. These granules are either spread out in the cytoplasm, lined up at the cell periphery, or clustered within the cell process. These processes may lie in close contact with either the axons or glial-cell fibers. Possibly, the DB granules might be released at the cell periphery by exocytosis into the extracellular fluid. However, the release of the elementary granules, which would characterize the real axon terminals has not yet been observed. No signs of membrane specialization (e.g., thickening) or accumulation of small clear vesicles could be seen. Furthermore, extensive serial sectioning is necessary to decide whether neurosecretory axons discharge their granules at a neuroeffector junction.

It should be mentioned that the CCNs have been developed only in species where the DB is at a certain distance from the cerebral commissure. In the postembryonic stages these nerves grow out only after the DB is visible (SCHLOOT, 1965). In gastropods with DBs lying in more or less direct contact with the commissure, as in Basommatophora, there are no distinct CCNs but only some axons with elementary granules in contact with DB cells. As there is no barrier between tissue fluid and hemolymph within this region, the discharge of neurosecretory products into the extracellular space and the transport from there to the lacunae could occur without difficulties. There seems to be no need for the spreading of the CCNs within the clusters of body cells because the blood passes from the perineurium to the pedal sinus through this endocrine organ. A direct "synaptoid" contact may be an advantage, as is known for insect tissues (see SCHARRER, 1974). In gastropods, too, there are cells other than DB cells that lie in direct contact with neurosecretory fibers such as muscle cells, gliointerstitial cells, and granulated cells (STEINBACH, 1976) of the connective tissue.

References

BOER, H.H., JOOSSE, J.: Endocrinology. In: Pulmonates. FRETTER, V., PEAKE, J. (eds.). London: Academic Press 1975, Vol. I, pp. 245-307

KUHLMANN, D.: Neurosekretion bei Heliciden (Gastropoda). Z. Zellforsch. 60, 909-932 (1963)

KUHLMANN, D.: Der Dorsalkörper der Stylommatophoren (Gastropoda). Z. Wiss. Zool. 173, 218-231 (1966)

MOL, J.J. VAN: Étude morphologique et phylogénétique du ganglion cérébroide des gastéropodes pulmonés (mollusques). Mém. Acad. R. Belg. Cl. Sci. 8°, 37, 1-168 (196)
NOLTE, A.: Neurohämal-"Organe" bei Pulmonaten (Gastropoda). Zool. Jb. Anat. 82, 365-380 (1965)
NOLTE, A.: The mode of release of neurosecretory material in the freshwater pulmonate *Lymnaea stagnalis* L. (Gastropoda). In: Symposium on Neurobiology of Invertebrates. SALANKI, J. (ed.). New York: Plenum Press 1968, pp. 123-133
MARTOJA, M.: Endocrinology of mollusca. In: Chemical Zoology. VII. Mollusca. FLORKIN, M., SCHEER, B.T. (eds.). London: Academic Press 1972, pp. 349-392
SCHARRER, B.: New trends in invertebrate neurosecretion. In: Neurosecretion - The Final Neuroendocrine Pathway. KNOWLES, F., VOLLRATH, L. (eds.). Berlin-Heidelberg-New York: Springer-Verlag 1974, pp. 285-287
SCHLOOT, W.: Postembryogenese des Schlundrings von *Helix pomatia* L. (Gastopoda) unter Berücksichtigung der Sekretion der Nervenzellen. Z. Zellforsch. 67, 406-426 (1965)
STEINBACH, P.: Granular cells in the connective tissue of *Helix pomatia* L. (Gastropoda, Pulmonata). Cell Tissue Res. (1977) (in press)

Perisympathetic Organs of Insects: Their Physiologic Meaning

M. RAABE
Equipe de Neuroendocrinologie des Insectes, Université Pierre et Marie Curie, 12 rue Cuvier, Paris, France

The perisympathetic organs (PO) of insects constitute a segmentally-arranged neurohemal (NH) system involved in the storage and release of neurosecretory (NS) products of the ventral nerve cord (VNC) (RAABE, 1965). It appears from previous experiments that the PO regulate heart rhythm, diuresis, blood protein content, and tanning (RAABE et al., 1973). They are also involved, as seen recently, in the release of an oviposition factor (MESNIER and PROVANSAL, 1975). They thus control numerous processes controlled also by the corpora cardiaca (CC). Their physiologic meaning is not yet known.

One may assume that a widely spread NH system is of value in animals devoid of a good circulatory system. On the other hand, it is advantageous for a control system to be able to perform some local regulation. The ganglia of the VNC, while under the control of the cephalic coordinating centers, also possess some integrative functions. Their NS cells and their NH organs might thus respond to local sensory inputs. If so, the PO are less centralized than the CC, and constitute a link between these, the distal PO of bugs and flies (BAUDRY-PARTIAOGLOU, 1977; MADDRELL, 1974), located far from the VNC in the close vicinity of organs, and the neuroeffector junctions. Some recent findings support this hypothesis. In the coleopteran, *Tenebrio*, the timing of release of Bursicon is not the same throughout the body: it occurs first in the CC, then in the anterior abdominal PO, and last, in the posterior abdominal PO (GRILLOT et al., 1976).

References

BAUDRY-PARTIAOGLOU, N.: Anatomie et histologie des organes neurohémaux de quelques Hémiptères. Int. J. Ins. Morphol. Embryol. (in press)

GRILLOT, J.P., DELACHAMBRE, J., PROVANSAL, A.: Rôle des organes périsympathiques et dynamique de la sécrétion de la bursicon chez *Tenebrio molitor*. J. Insect. Physiol. 22, 763 (1976)

MADDRELL, S.H.P., GEE, J.D.: Potassium-induced release of the diuretic hormones of *Rhodnius prolixus* and *Glossina austeni*: Ca dependence, time course and localization of neurohaemal areas. J. Exp. Biol. 61, 155 (1974)

MESNIER, M., PROVANSAL, A.: Rôle des organes périsympathiques dans l'induction de la ponte chez *Galleria mellonella* (Lépidoptère). C. R. Acad. Sci. (D) (Paris) 281, 905 (1975)

RAABE, M.: Recherches sur la neurosécrétion dans la chaîne nerveuse ventrale du Phasma, *Clitumnus extradentatus:* Les épaississements des nerfs transverses, organes de signification probablement neurohémale. C. R. Acad. Sci. (D) (Paris) 261, 4240 (1965)

RAABE, M., BAUDRY, N., GRILLOT, J.P., PROVANSAL, A.: The perisympathetic Organs of Insects. IV Intern. Symp. Neurosecretion, London. Berlin-Heidelberg-New York: Springer-Verlag 1973

Distribution of Neurosecretory Cells in *Polystoma integerrimum* (Fröhlich, 1791) (Monogenoidea, Polystomatidae)

M. SKOWERSKA
Department of Animal Histology and Embryology, Silesian University, Katowice, Poland

The reason for undertaking this study was the very scarce information concerning neurosecretion in Trematoda, particularly in ectoparasitic species.

The materials studied, specimens of *Polystoma integerrimum*, were taken from the urinary bladder of frogs, fixed in Bouin's fluid, and then paraffin permanent preparations were made. The products of neurosecretion in neurosecretory neurons were identified using the methods of Bargmann (1960), Bock (1966), Gabe (1953), and Steel-Cameron (1959). For the identification of nerve cells and the determination of the nervous-system topography the silver method of Bubenaite was used.

The neurosecretory cells in *P. integerrimum* are located peripherally in cerebral ganglia, in coherent parts of the brain, and along the nerve cord. Vitellarium glands have a dense nerve network in which neurosecretory activity occurs. Neurosecretory elements were also found in the neighborhood of the intestine, reproductive system, and sucker organs.

The neurosecretory cells in the species studied are variform and have different dimensions. There are uni-, bi-, and multipolar cells. The neurosecretory material occurring in these cells is easy to demonstrate by use of Bock's and Steel-Cameron's methods. The amounts of neurosecretory grains and their structure and distribution differ in the perikarya and in axons. In the animals studied, the most intensive neurosecretory activity was found in nerve cells from the neighborhood of the vitellarium glands and the ovary.

Neuroendocrine Control Mechanisms of Gametogenesis in Bivalve Molluscs *Crenomytilus grayanus* (Dunker) and *Patinopecten yessoensis* (Jay)

A. A. VARAKSIN
Institute of Marine Biology, Far East Science Center, Academy of Sciences of the USSR, Vladivostock 690022, USSR

The neuroendocrine system of the molluscs studied is represented by secreting neurons in visceral, cerebropleural, and pedal ganglia. In these cells, Gomori-positive inclusions have been found; the morphologic appearance and tinctorial properties of these inclusions varies throughout the year. Nerve cells containing Gomori-positive material appeared to possess no constant or strict location. The number of cells varies throughout the year. Gomori-positive inclusions have also been found in neuronal branches.

Monthly estimations of the mean volumes of nucleoli, nuclei, and bodies of neurons of visceral, cerebropleural, and pedal ganglia in both male and female mussels and scallops have shown minimum mean volumes to be characteristic of animals in the sexually inert period. This inert period is relatively short in mussels but lasts through the summer season in the scallop. The secretory activity of neurons increases to a considerable extent at active gametogenesis in the prespawning period. The amount of Gomori-positive material in the cytoplasm of nerve cells also increases at that time. The volume of neurons, their nucleoli, and their nuclei are also maximal at that time. The morphologic appearance of Gomori-positive material in the cytoplasm changes significantly when great amounts of Gomori-positive granules appear in axons of almost all the nerve cells shortly before spawning.

Injections of ganglia suspensions from female mussels into immature specimens of the same species result in growth of their gonads and activation of gametogenesis. In the proper environmental conditions, the spawning of these animals seems to be stimulated by the prompt secretion of great amounts of Gomori-positive neurosecretory material into their hematic channels.

Concluding Remarks

Current Trends in the Study of Vertebrate Neurosecretory Systems

K. LEDERIS
Division of Pharmacology and Therapeutics, Faculty of Medicine, University of Calgary, Alberta, Canada

The degree of success of an international gathering of this nature always depends on a number of factors: organization and execution of the program, effectiveness of communication in a multilingual conference, and quality of recent work included in the presentations. On all three counts, this symposium has succeeded admirably: in spite of gaps left in the program by the absence of several important speakers, the day-to-day scientific sessions proceeded with exceptional smoothness. Any linguistic problems, that often detract greatly from the scientific value of presentations in a multilingual gathering, were overcome in this symposium by the professional and accurate simultaneous translations throughout the scientific sessions. I am certain that all participants will also join me in the expression of our appreciation to Professor A. POLENOV and all his colleagues and staff.

As has been the tradition in all previous neurosecretion symposia, many significant new approaches and trends became apparent during this week. The success of this symposium has been greatly enhanced by the presence of the original exponents of the concept of neurosecretion, namely Professors B. SCHARRER and W. BARGMANN. Because of time limitations I can only briefly discuss some of the new trends that were brought to our notice during the lectures and poster presentations. A consideration of the different neurosecretory systems of vertebrates may simplify my task.

A. The Hypothalamo-Neurohypophyseal System

The diversity of cellular components in neurosecretory function (e.g., not only neuronal, but also glial and ependymal), an area of study that has been tackled intensively during recent years, to a great extent in the laboratories of our hosts and symposium organizers, will no doubt lend further impetus to continued studies aimed at the elucidation of the significance of and the role in neurosecretory processes played by "nonneuronal" elements such as the circumventricular, ependymal, and glial components. The review by Professor R. ACHER of the chemical evolution of the neurohypophyseal peptides, together with the evolutionary aspects of the studies by Professor A. POLENOV and his colleagues and Mme J. FLAMENT-DURAND and her co-workers will continue to stimulate further investigations utilizing this admirably suited experimental model (the hypothalamo-neurohypophyseal system).

Significant progress was reported on the hitherto somewhat unexpected extent of distribution, well outside the supraoptic and paraventricular nuclei, and topographic location, of peptidergic neurosecretory neurons. Applications of the relatively novel methodology of immunocytochemistry in the laboratories of Professors G. STERBA, G. WOLF, K. DIERICKX, and G. KOZLOWSKI has not only delineated pathways for the different peptides but has also exposed to further study such structures as choroid plexes and other "extrahypothalamic" areas. Further meaningful studies on nonpeptidergic neurosecretion will result following the important investigations on neurotransmitters or neurotransmitter-like substances, as reported by Drs. M. KONSTANTINOVA, M. PALKOVITS, B. ALESHIN, and D. SCHALYAPINA.

B. Other Hypothalamic Neurosecetory Systems

The sources of production and the loci and control of secretion of other hypothalamic products, the adenohypophyseal hormone-releasing peptides, have long presented a considerable challenge. The significant progress in locating these substances, as presented to this symposium from the laboratories of Professors B. FLERKÓ and colleagues, and A. WEINDL, represent a significant advance, which is likely to improve understanding not only of the sites of production and modes of action of the releasing factors (hormones), but may also represent a milestone in the eventual elucidation of the apparent multiplicity of actions - peripheral as well as central - of this challenging family of peptides, of which few have been identified to date.

The real significance of the occurrence of peptide-protein complexes (A. GALOYAN), apparently originating from Gomori-positive elements, at present included in the hypothalamo-neurohypophyseal system, can not be assessed at this time; the site(s) of origin and possible physiologic roles of these complexes, as well as their pharmacologic importance, may represent another new challenge to those studying neurosecretion.

C. Extrahypothalamic Neurosecretory Relationships

In recent years, diverse actions of neurosecretory products (peptides) have been studied and described. Further progress in this area has come to the fore during the present symposium. The finding of neural links between vasopressin-secreting neurons and, e.g., amygdala (F. STUTINSKY), cochlea-posterior pituitary interaction in stress situations (R. MILIN), the implication of neurosecretory products in processes related to memory (G. STERBA) or to electric activity of the brain (H. UNGER and colleagues), and the interaction between the hypothalamus and the pinael (E. CHAZOV, J. GRACHEVA), all of these examples of neurosecretory-extrahypothalamic interactions give clear indications for expanded areas of interest that will have to be considered in years to come if the full relevance of hypothalamic neurosecretory systems is to be understood.

D. The Caudal Neurosecretory System of Fishes

In the absence of my colleagues Professors H. BERN and H. KOBAYASHI, whose laboratories are actively enganged in the study of caudal neurosecretion and of the active principles of the urophysis, the task falls to me to restate our lack of understanding of the physiologic significance of the neurosecretory system.

Looking at this system optimistically, some satisfaction can be drawn from recent investigations in my laboratory - the elucidation of some chemical and pharmacologic properties of at least two hormonal peptides - and the indication of another system, where the principle of "one neuron-one hormone" may apply (Professor H.A. BERN et al.), and new observations on urophyseal hormone-release phenomena, including the presence and subcellular location of acetylcholine in the urophysis (ICHIKAWA and H. KOBAYASHI). It was even more gratifying to note that a plea by Professor Howard BERN at the previous neurosecretion symposium for other laboratories to accept this challenge has resulted in an active interest in this system by laboratories in Leningrad: the report by Dr. J. SAENKO can be taken as indicating more active studies by Mme. F. BARANNIKOVA and other colleagues. At this time, it may realistically be expected that the elucidation of the physiologic role(s) of this system may be realized in time for the next neurosecretion symposium.

Epilog

B. SCHARRER
Department of Anatomy, Albert Einstein College of Medicine, Bronx, New York 10461, USA

As we come to the close of this the VIIth International Symposium on Neurosecretion, we look back on a memorable week, rich in new information and experience. Many contributions and lively discussions among the participants, who have come to Leningrad from all corners of the world, have brought into focus major current trends in neuroendocrinology. We shall return to our own laboratories not only full of ideas for the continuation of our work, but deeply affected by the warm hospitality we received.

I should like to take this opportunity to express many sincere thanks to the organizers of this symposium, especially to Professor A. POLENOV, and to the Academy of Sciences of the USSR, whose guest I am, for all they have done to make this conference so successful and enjoyable.

It also gives me great pleasure to convey to the local committee, to the participants of this symposium, and particularly to the Academy of Sciences of the USSR, under whose sponsorship it convened, the official greetings and best wishes from its sister organization, the National Academy of Sciences of the USA.

It is not easy to summarize the highlights of this conference. In my own view, one of these is the renewed demonstration of the heuristic value of a broad comparative approach to the interpretation of the phenomenon of neurosecretion. This orientation has proved fruitful ever since the first International Symposium on Neurosecretion at Naples, in 1953, the most pertinent outcome of which was the realization of a remarkable degree of similarity between the neurosecretory systems of vertebrates and higher invertebrates.

The present symposium, the central theme of which was the evolution of neurosecretory activities, has advanced us still further. The extension of ultrastructural and physiological investigations to include the most primitive eumetazoans, the coelenterates, has resulted in the conceptual clarification of the place of neurosecretory neurons within the spectrum of neurochemical communication. The recognition of structural, physiological, and biochemical analogies throughout the animal kingdom has substantiated the concept that neurosecretory neurons are phylogenetically old and pluripotential rather than offshots from the main line that appeared late in the evolutionary history of the neuron.

Another advance in neurobiology, reflected in our present program, is the increasing concern with peptidergic neurons as a distinctive class with multiple and special functional properties. As has become apparent, the products of these neurons engage in modes of information transfer that digress from standard synaptic transmission. Aside from their familiar role in neurohormonal communication, various neuropeptides seem to address themselves to receptor cells via several, more or less shortened extracellular pathways. Some of these arrangements resemble regular neuroeffector sites except for the nonconventional nature of the chemical messengers involved.

Perhaps the most intriguing outcome of these studies, in both vertebrates and invertebrates, is the increase in experimental information concerning neurons as recipients of peptidergic signals. This kind of input seems to modulate neural activities and to result in changes in behavior, learning capacity, and metabolic functions. Another fascinating topic concerns the recently identified endogenous analgesics (endorphins, enkephalins), small peptides that combine with opiate receptors in regions of the brain that are associated with the perceptions of pain. With these newest developments, the time has come for the exploration of potential diagnostic and therapeutic uses of such peptidergic compounds in clinical neuroendocrinology. We have good reason to look forward with anticipation to the next symposium on neurosecretion.

Concluding Remarks

A. L. POLENOV
Laboratory of Neuroendocrinology, Sechenov Institute of Evolutionary Physiology and Biochemistry, Academy of Sciences of the USSR, Leningrad, USSR

In the name of the National Organizing Committee, in the name of all those who took part in the organization of this Symposium and in my own name I wish to thank our dear guests, Prof. Berta SCHARRER, Prof. G. STERBA, and Prof. K. LEDERIS and all delegates from different countries and many cities of the USSR for their warm words of praise and gratitude expressed today in their concluding remarks and earlier at the banquet and in private talks. We organizers of the Symposium see that our efforts were not in vain, and we feel joy and satisfaction. However, we are well aware that some things did not work well, and I have to apologize for all the defects in the organization of the Symposium. It is very regrettable also that our discussions were rather short.

Our symposium has come to an end, and now we have to sum up the results of our work. As Professors B. SCHARRER, STERBA, and LEDERIS have already summarized the scientific results of our meeting, I shall touch only on the formal side of it.

Two hundred and forty-three scientists from 19 countries took part in the symposium, among them 159 Soviet participants. Seventy-five papers were delivered and seventy poster demonstrations were shown.

The problem of neurosecretion is a modern one and its far reaching biologic significance is evident. Many scientists who do not work directly in the field of neurosecretion were very interested in the symposium. In spite of the summer vacation, 64 specialists representing different medical-biologic branches were present in this auditorium.

For us, the Soviet neuroendocrinologists, the Seventh International Symposium was a significant and important event. It was a splendid opportunity for many of us to listen to excellent lectures and to have private talks with outstanding neuroendocrinologists. It was of much value for many of us to have made the personal acquaintance of the pioneers in the study of neurosecretion, Professors B. SCHARRER, W. BARGMANN, and M. GERSCH. Our symposium was a very useful learning experience for young scientists. They could hear skilful examples of reports, see excellent illustrations and preparations, and learn of results achieved by modern techniques of neuroendocrinology, predominantly morphologic analysis. The significance of immunohistochemistry should be especially emphasized. Just as the Gomori technique introduced some years ago by Professor BARGMANN, this new technique will give rise to many new insights in the field of neurosecretion. Of no less importance was that the symposium clearly demonstrated the significance of the widely-used evolutionary and ecologic-histophysiologic approach in elucidating the role of neurosecretory elements in the life of most organisms at different stages of their development. Data concerning relevance to various fields of clinical medicine, agriculture, pisciculture, and air pollution presented in many of the reports delivered are undoubtedly of much value.

It was most pleasant for me, as the chairman of the Organizing Committee, to see smiling and joyful faces of the delegates, and to hear friendly talks and discussions and humorous remarks in the auditorium and during lobby interviews. It gave the impression of a light-hearted and warm atmosphere, of family spirit and comfort throughout our symposium, at the banquet and at our walks and excursions. The weather also favoured us. The sun was shining for us during all these days, and we were warmed by the sun and by the contacts with each other.

Our symposium was a demonstration of a great and warm friendship, a true friendship, which is necessary for real scientists and is a good tradition in the international "neurosecretory family" headed by such sincere and cordial persons as Prof. Berta SCHARRER and Prof. Wolfgang BARGMANN. Let us wish them good health and much energy for many years to come!

Thanks to the friendship among Soviet scientists we managed to hold this important meeting of neuroendocrinologists. I believe that in the name of all delegates present here I may express our gratitude to those who took active part in organizing this symposium. I wish to acknowledge the great and selfless efforts by Dr. O. DANILOVA, Dr. M. KONSTANTINOVA, and Dr. M. BELENKY, and the skilful and accurate work by our simultaneous interpreters, Dr. G. GAUSE and Dr. S. EVMINOV.

Dear Friends! Dear Colleagues! Parting with you today, I wish all of you with all my heart good progress in your further scientific search and good luck. Farewell! I am looking forward to seeing you again at our future meetings, wherever in the world their place may be.

Subject Index

Experimental
Brain Research

Supplement 1

Afferent and Intrinsic Organization of Laminated Structures in the Brain

7th International Neurobiology Meeting

Editor: O. Creutzfeld, Göttingen, Germany

127 figures. XXIII, 579 pages. 1976.
ISBN 3-540-07923-8

This volume contains the proceedings of the 7th International Meeting of Neurobiologists, held in Göttingen in September 1975. Its aim is to give information on the various laminated structures of the brain such as the cerebellar, the allo- and the neocortex as well as some laminated structures in the midbrain. The contributions also include aspects of developmental neurobiology, neurochemistry and theoretical neurobiology as well as classical and modern neuroanatomical and neurophysiological work.
This volume can be regarded as a representative documentation of present day scientific views on the functional organization of various cortical structures in the brain. It is unique in bringing together material for comparison from the different cortical brain structures, in contrast to other monographs concentrating mainly on one aspect such as neo-, allo-, or cerebellar cortex.

Contents: Cerebellum. – Allocortex: Anatomy. Physiology. – Neocortex: Development. Cortical Circuitry. Functional Organization. – Subcortical Laminated Structures: Medial and Lateral Geniculate Body. The Optic Tectum. Electric Lobe.

Springer-Verlag
Berlin
Heidelberg
New York

Monographs on Endocrinology

Editors: F. Gross, M. M. Grumbach, A. Labhart, M. B. Lipsett, T. Mann, L. T. Samuels, J. Zander

Volume 1
S. Ohno
Sex Chromosomes and Sex-linked Genes
33 figures. X, 192 pages. 1967
ISBN 3-540-03934-1

Volume 2
K. B. Eik-Nes, E. C. Horning
Gas Phase Chromotography of Steroids
85 figures. XV, 382 pages. 1968
ISBN 3-540-04277-6

Volume 3
F. G. Sulman
Hypothalamic Control of Lactation
In collaboration with M. Ben-David, A. Danon, S. Dikstein, Y. Givant, K. Khazen, J. Mishkinsky-Shani, I. Nir, C. P. Weller
58 figures. XII, 235 pages. 1970
ISBN 3-540-04973-8

Volume 4
U. Westphal
Steroid-Protein Interactions
144 figures. XIII, 567 pages. 1971
ISBN 3-540-05312-3

Volume 5
J. Müller
Regulation of Aldosterone Biosynthesis
19 figures. VII, 137 pages. 1971
ISBN 3-540-05213-5

Volume 6
K. Federlin
Immunopathology of Insulin
Clinical and Experimental Studies
53 figures. XIII, 185 pages. 1971
ISBN 3-540-05408-1

Volume 7
E. W. Horton
Prostaglandins
97 figures. XI, 197 pages. 1972
ISBN 3-540-05571-1

Volume 8
E. Gurpide
Tracer Methods in Hormone Research
35 figures. XI, 188 pages. 1975
ISBN 3-540-07039-7

Volume 9
R. E. Mancini
Immunologic Aspects of Testicular Function
36 figures, 8 tables. IX, 114 pages. 1976
ISBN 3-540-07496-1

Volume 10
W. I. P. Mainwaring
The Mechanism of Action of Androgens
12 figures, 17 tables. XI, 178 pages. 1977
ISBN 3-540-07941-6

Springer-Verlag
Berlin
Heidelberg
New York

www.ingramcontent.com/pod-product-compliance
Ingram Content Group UK Ltd.
Pitfield, Milton Keynes, MK11 3LW, UK
UKHW051003220926
475831UK00003B/102
* 9 7 8 3 6 4 2 6 6 8 8 7 6 *